Feminist Theology an
Dieting Cu

Feminist Theology and Contemporary Dieting Culture
Sin, Salvation and Women's Weight Loss Narratives

Hannah Bacon

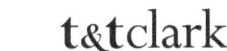

LONDON • NEW YORK • OXFORD • NEW DELHI • SYDNEY

T&T CLARK
Bloomsbury Publishing Plc
50 Bedford Square, London, WC1B 3DP, UK
1385 Broadway, New York, NY 10018, USA

BLOOMSBURY, T&T CLARK and the T&T Clark logo are trademarks of
Bloomsbury Publishing Plc

First published in Great Britain 2019

Copyright © Hannah Bacon, 2019

Hannah Bacon has asserted her right under the Copyright, Designs and
Patents Act, 1988, to be identified as Author of this work.

For legal purposes the Acknowledgements on p. viii constitute an extension of
this copyright page.

Cover design: Terry Woodley
Cover images © The Fall of Man, 1616, Hendrick Goltzius, NGA Images,
Patron's Permanent Fund, and © PhotoAlto sas / Alamy Stock Photo

All rights reserved. No part of this publication may be reproduced or
transmitted in any form or by any means, electronic or mechanical, including
photocopying, recording, or any information storage or retrieval system,
without prior permission in writing from the publishers.

Bloomsbury Publishing Plc does not have any control over, or responsibility
for, any third-party websites referred to or in this book. All internet addresses
given in this book were correct at the time of going to press. The author and
publisher regret any inconvenience caused if addresses have changed or sites
have ceased to exist, but can accept no responsibility for any such changes.

A catalogue record for this book is available from the British Library.

A catalogue record for this book is available from the Library of Congress.
Library of Congress Cataloging-in-Publication Data

ISBN: HB: 978-0-5676-5995-8
PB: 978-0-5676-5997-2
ePDF: 978-0-5676-5996-5
ePUB: 978-0-5676-5994-1

Typeset by Deanta Global Publishing Services, Chennai, India
Printed and bound in Great Britain

To find out more about our authors and books visit www.bloomsbury.com and
sign up for our newsletters.

In memory of Ralph

CONTENTS

Acknowledgements	viii
Introduction THEOLOGY, FOOD AND FAT: A HEALTHY RECIPE?	1
Chapter 1 SYN, DANGER AND DISORDERED DESIRE	49
Chapter 2 SYN, SELF-SURVEILLANCE AND TAKING CARE: TENSIONS AND AMBIGUITIES	99
Chapter 3 SALVATION, 'GETTING RID' AND 'GETTING THERE'	139
Chapter 4 RETHINKING SIN: SIZEISM, THE VICTIMIZATION OF FOOD AND THE DIVIDED SELF	189
Chapter 5 RETHINKING SALVATION: A (RE)TURN TO 'SENSIBLE' EATING	223
Chapter 6 RETHINKING SALVATION: SABBATH AND FAT PRIDE	261
Conclusion FOR THE LOVE OF FOOD, FOR THE LOVE OF FAT	307
Bibliography	311
Index	338

ACKNOWLEDGEMENTS

First and foremost I would like to thank the people in the weight loss group I joined. This book would not have been possible without their willingness to share their experiences with me. I am grateful for their warmth, generosity, trust and honesty. My thanks also to colleagues in the Department of Theology and Religious Studies at the University of Chester who have supported me throughout this project; to Professor Wayne Morris and Dr Dawn Llewellyn especially who kindly read draft chapters at very busy times in the academic year and to Dr Ben Fulford and Professor David Clough whose encouragement always filled me with energy and determination. I would also like to thank Dr Emily Pennington who conducted some preliminary research for me and to Emma Standbrook whose input at the start of this journey was invaluable.

Further afield, my thanks to Professor Lisa Isherwood at The University of Winchester, Dr Lynne Gerber at Harvard University and Dr Rachel Muers at the University of Leeds for reviewing the book proposal for Bloomsbury and for their interest in my work. I also thank my friends and colleagues, Professor Nicola Slee at The Queen's Foundation in Birmingham, Dr Jenny Daggers at Liverpool Hope University, Dr Elizabeth Ursic at Mesa Community College in Phoenix and Dr Susannah Cornwall at the University of Exeter, for their encouragement and for sharing their time with me. A number of academic contexts outside of my own institution have provided creative spaces for the critical engagement and shaping of my ideas. Among them, the BISFT summer school in the UK, the Donner Institute in Turku (Finland), the Faith Lives of Women and Girls' Symposium in Birmingham, UK, and the Body and Religion, and Food and Religion Groups at the American Academy of Religion. I have had many fruitful conversations with numerous individuals, and I extend my thanks to all of them.

The editorial team at Bloomsbury deserve a special mention, not least because it must have felt at times like this book was never going to emerge! Particular thanks to Anna Turton, Miriam Cantwell and Sarah Blake for their patience, consistent enthusiasm and helpful guidance.

Much of this book was written during a sabbatical. By taking temporary leave of my administrative teaching and managerial responsibilities,

I was able to breathe and think – a practice that I suggest in this book to be a crucial method for resisting the hegemony of fat phobia. I therefore want to thank my colleagues and the Head of Department for making this period of leave possible. I spent most of my sabbatical time either working at Gladstone's Library in North Wales or in my study at home. Gladstone's is set in a magnificent Grade-1 listed building in a small village just outside of Chester. Working there was a delight; surrounded by books and plenty of green space filled me with ambition and calm in equal measure. The Gallery Coffee Shop in the village was my regular haven for lunch, and it does the best coronation chicken sandwich on gluten-free bread I have ever tasted! That café was just as important to me, and my time there eating just as significant as the time I spent in the library reading and writing. It gave me time to touch and taste my food and was always utterly rejuvenating. I am truly grateful to the staff in both settings for their role in making this time so special.

At home in my study, the process of writing was aided by my dogs who faithfully sat on the windowsill next to me. Nellie and Jasper have accompanied me in this book in a way nobody else has. I love them dearly, and their presence in this journey lurks behind every page. Ralph also deserves a special mention. He was our first dog but died suddenly at the age of five, a year before we got Nell. He was my companion at the start of this project and sat in the study with Jasper during the early stages. I am only sad that he did not see me complete it. This book is dedicated to him because he gave me so much time and love that I feel I cannot write this work without giving him due credit. *My special boy.*

My friends have been incredibly patient and understanding throughout the writing of this book, especially towards the end as I frequently absented myself from social events and slipped into 'hermit mode'. A special mention must be given again to Wayne who is one of the most reliable and affirming people in my life. I am so lucky to have his friendship and benefit from his love, amazing cooking and fantastic humour.

As ever, my family have been a boundless source of love and encouragement. To my mum, June, my dad, Roger, and my sister, Helen, I offer every ounce of love in my body and my heart-felt appreciation for your consistent support. My twin sister Kate continues to be an ally in all things academic. As a sociologist, she has helped me in more ways than I can say, and her faith and belief in me have been an incredible source of encouragement. She has accompanied me on this journey at every step and without her I would have flagged. Words cannot express how important she is to me. My thanks also to Olivia and Edward, my niece and nephew, and to Keith and G. It is my family that taught me the transforming power of eating with delight and eating together, and it is through food and drink that we continue to reunite from our various locations. I cherish every time we eat together.

As is often the case with things which demand of our time, this book has sometimes pulled me away from my commitments at home. My final thanks and words must, therefore, go to my partner, Berni, who I fear must forgive a multitude of sins for the amount of time I have spent locked away in the study at evenings and weekends. I have often seen our dogs much more than I have seen her, and she has been a rock throughout every stage of writing this book. She has also compiled the index and helped in formatting some aspects of this work; she has helped in more ways than I can name. You are my delight and joy, and I thank God for you. For feeding me with food, reassurance and love; for listening, teaching and contributing; for the love we share – thank you.

INTRODUCTION: THEOLOGY, FOOD AND FAT: A HEALTHY RECIPE?

What would Jesus eat? Perhaps this is a question that might merit historical inquiry, but for Don Colbert, author of the book by the same name, the answer can help ordinary Christians in the twenty-first century eat well, feel great and live longer. Eating what Jesus ate can lead to weight loss and help modern America deal with its obesity epidemic.[1] He is not alone in thinking this. Today countless Americans are committed to fighting fat through faith. Many seek to do this with the help of conservative evangelical weight loss programmes like Carol Showalter's '3D Plan',[2] and through joining Christian weight loss organizations like the 'Weigh Down Workshop' and 'First Place'.

Faith-based dieting is big business. Gwen Shamblin's 'Weigh Down Ministries'[3] is the most successful to date, growing from humble beginnings in 1986 into a multimillion dollar industry with an international market.[4] By the year 2000 it had spread to

---

1. Don Colbert, *What Would Jesus Eat? The Ultimate Program for Eating Well, Feeling Great and Living Longer* (Nashville: Thomas Nelson, 2002).

2. '3D' stands for 'diet', 'discipline' and 'discipleship'. See Carol Showalter, *Your Whole Life: The 3D Plan for Eating Right, Living Well, and Loving God* (Brewster: Paraclete Press, 2007).

3. Shamblin uses the name 'Weigh Down Ministries' interchangeably with 'Weigh Down Workshop'. She notes on her webpage that 'the dream of helping people turn away from the love of food and toward a love of God has turned into a ministry'. Gwen Shamblin, 'The Remnant of the Kingdom of God', http://www.remnantfellowship.org/About-Our-Church/Our-History (accessed 8 May 2018).

4. Rebecca Mead, 'Slim for Him: God Is Watching What You're Eating' (15 January 2001), http://www.spiritwatch.org/rebeccamead.htm (accessed 15 April 2014). Also see 'Gwen Shamblin: The Pioneer of Faith-Based Weight Loss', http://www.gwenshamblin.com/my-biography/ (accessed 2 August 2017). Shamblin notes how she began Weigh Down with 'small classes' taught in a 'retail environment'.

thirty thousand churches, seventy countries and sixty different denominations.[5] Famed in the American tabloid press for suggesting that fat people don't go to heaven because 'grace does not go down into the pigpen',[6] Shamblin boldly contends that fat is a spiritual problem which must be met with a spiritual solution. In her first publication, *The Weigh Down Diet*, she calls her audience away from the 'slavery of overweight' towards becoming 'normal eater[s]',[7] a journey she likens to the Israelites' journey out of slavery into the Promised Land.[8] This is a journey of deliverance since thinness brings freedom from the mastery of food, from yo-yo dieting and from exercise regimens. It is also a journey into righteousness. Eating when hungry rather than to fulfil a spiritual longing prevents the individual from 'going to food for sensual indulgence', replacing their *'desire eating'*[9] with a 'calm, nonmagnetized approach'.[10] Eating is a way of practising obedience to God, giving the heart to God rather than to the '10 o'clock binge', longing after God rather than 'lusting after food'.[11]

When I first came across Shamblin's work I was struck by the way she polarized food and God. She implied that falling in love with God equated to falling out of love with food and that to eat 'well' – to become a 'thin eater'[12] – meant to transcend any desire for food altogether. Desire for food signalled slavery to food, and slavery meant sin. This did not sit well with me as someone who sees food as expressive of God's love, Trinitarian self-sharing and embrace, and as someone who enjoys food and derives considerable pleasure from preparing, sharing and consuming it! She also aligned allegiance to thinness with allegiance to a God she unambiguously imaged in heteronormative and

---

5. R. Marie Griffith, *Born Again Bodies: Flesh and Spirit in American Christianity* (Berkeley, Los Angeles and London: University of California Press, 2004), 176.

6. 'Fat People Don't Go To Heaven', *Globe*, November 2000 cited in Griffith, *Born Again Bodies*, 1.

7. Gwen Shamblin, *The Weigh Down Diet: Inspirational Way to Lose Weight, Stay Slim, and Find a New You* (New York: Galilee Doubleday, 2002), 10.

8. Ibid., 10–11 and 115–25.

9. Ibid., 7. Italics in original.

10. Ibid., 8.

11. Ibid., 149.

12. Ibid., 128.

heteropatriarchal terms.[13] God was charming, good-looking and rich, and she had a 'crush on the Father' and liked to dress for Him.[14]

As troubling as I found Shamblin's position, her faithing of fat shows just how happily Protestant expressions of Christianity in America sit alongside cultural fears about fat and the secular search for the body beautiful. R. Marie Griffith provides an excellent discussion of this in *Born Again Bodies*, arguing that Protestant American desires for the perfect body are nothing new. She notes how derivatives of Protestant Christianity within America, specifically developments within New Thought and evangelicalism, helped establish and sustain dieting and fitness idioms in the United States. Exhorting mind over matter and a steadfast optimism in the self, they promoted the perfectible, eternal, disciplined body and abhorred the deficient, impoverished or languishing body.[15] Such influences, she claims, informed the contemporary Christian weight loss industry in the United States, articulating weight reduction as divine decree and repositioning the thin, white, female body as normative.

For Griffith, what is most alarming about evangelical weight loss culture is its uncritical assent to secular ideals. She accuses weight loss gurus, like Shamblin, of accepting 'ardently and without flinching, the somatic standards of the wider culture'.[16] In a similar tone, Lynne Gerber's ethnographic work inside *First Place* – one of the largest Christian weight loss organizations in the United States – suggests that the 'cultural power' of evangelical weight loss culture is only acquired through the submission of evangelicalism to pervasive cultural ideals to do with appearance, health, morality and cultural legitimacy. Drawing on Pierre Bourdieu, she suggests that the appropriation of secular discourses within Christian diet programmes adds 'cultural capital' to evangelical Christian culture, serving to further the influence of

---

13. In an interview with Shamblin in January 2001, Rebecca Mead notes how her 'depiction of God as the cutest guy on the football team appears to make sense to her audience, which is largely female', with her female followers 'swooning for the Lord'. See Mead, 'Slim for Him'.

14. Gwen Shamblin, *Rise Above: God Can Set You Free from Your Weight Problem Forever* (Nashville: Thomas Nelson Publishers, 2000).

15. Griffith, *Born Again Bodies*, 18.

16. R. Marie Griffith, 'The Promised Land of Weight Loss: Law and Gospel in Christian Dieting', *The Christian Century* 114, no. 15 (7 May 1997), http://www.religion-online.org/showarticle.asp?title=249 (accessed 10 November 2016).

evangelical Christianity in the United States. The Christian weight loss industry perpetuates cultural phobias about fat and the marginalization of fat people through its submission to the forces of 'cultural domination'.[17]

Some may squirm at the way the Christian dieting industry utilizes the tools of faith to sanction the thin ideal, but one of my central claims in this book is that 'secular' forms of weight loss display a similar alliance with Christian devotional practices and schemes of thought. My focus is not on faith-based approaches to slimming or on how Christian diet programmes are resourced by secular ideals. Instead, I suggest that 'secular'[18] forms of dieting can be shown to recycle theological ideas in ways that aid the cultural war on fat. Drawing on qualitative research inside a secular, commercial weight loss group in the northwest of England, I show how one organization implicitly continues and sometimes explicitly adopts Christian theological principles and historic Christian practices. Mapping resonances with the Christian 'tradition',[19] I identify continuities with historical theological propositional thought which has been emitted and established as normative and with the bodily practices of Christianity. Through participant observation and in-depth interviews, I uncover the fascinating and complex ways in which Christian attitudes, beliefs and patterns of action resurface (intendedly or unintendedly) in 'secular' guise. My concerns are distinctly theological. In the first part of the book I show how certain influential theological ideas about sin and salvation generated mainly by early Christian theologians resurface in the group and, in the second, how these Christian categories might be theologically reimagined in light of the fears about food and fat that women narrate in the secular weight loss setting. I suggest that the close analysis of women's

---

17. Lynne Gerber, 'My Body Is a Testimony: Appearance, Health and Sin in an Evangelical Weight-loss Program', *Social Compass* 56, no. 3 (2009): 405–18, esp. 416.

18. By 'secular' I mean those forms of dieting which are not deliberately established upon religious convictions or motivations, or which do not present weight loss as an expression of religious commitment.

19. Following Mary McClintock Fulkerson, I consider tradition to comprise the vision, attitudes and acts of Christians passed on through the generations. Fulkerson, 'Interpreting a Situation: When Is "Empirical" also "Theological"?', in *Perspectives on Ecclesiology and Ethnography*, ed. Pete Ward (Grand Rapids and Cambridge: William B. Eerdmans Publishing Company, 2012), 131.

experiences can provide clues about how we might usefully speak about sin and salvation in relation to dieting culture.

This is not to say that there is a direct relationship between ancient theological perspectives and contemporary weight loss culture as it is expressed by women in this one group but to say that certain theological tropes and idioms inform Western culture (and women's culture specifically) where the legacy of these ideas can still be felt. I suggest that the detail of women's weight loss narratives can be plotted against the particulars of theological systems and ideas concerning sin and salvation, not necessarily because there is an intended or causal link between them but because their happy alliance nevertheless gives us reason for alarm, questioning, scrutiny and review.

My task here is not only to uncover the correlations and intersections between Christian theology and contemporary beliefs about weight but also to engage in an in-depth analysis of the group that will help critique and transform theology and culture. This aligns with what Elizabeth Schüssler Fiorenza sees as the task of a critical feminist theology of liberation, namely, to tender a 'feminist critique of culture'[20] and to remind the church of its 'constant need for renewal'.[21] Indeed, as a feminist theologian informed by the method of liberation theology, I hold that it is not enough to observe with indifference or even interest the symbolic connections between the pursuit of thinness and theological tradition, whether these be positive or negative, intentional or accidental. Christian feminist theology must seek to act and do, and this action must be directed at changing the world rather than just describing it. The feminist theology I develop in this book then presupposes an emancipatory goal. It offers both an analysis of the way this weight loss group recycles certain theological motifs and a constructive response that sets out descriptively and in practical terms how these theological motifs might be recovered and redefined in light of women's experiences of slimming.

Forming a Feminist Theological Response: The Livingness of God

For me, the need for theology to speak constructively is a matter of seeking justice and equality before God. It is caught up with my

---

20. Elisabeth Schüssler Fiorenza, 'Feminist Theology as a Critical Theology of Liberation', *Theological Studies* 36, no. 4 (1975): 607. For Fiorenza, this includes a critique of the 'structures of society that keep women down'.

21. Ibid., 612.

conviction as a feminist Christian that theology must pursue and passionately defend the livingness of all women and of all persons. Born out of Elizabeth Johnson's re-formed Irenaean axiom that '*Gloria Dei vivens mulier*: the glory of God is woman, all women, every woman everywhere, fully alive',[22] what it means to provide a useful theological response to weight loss dieting, I suggest, is to offer a 'lifeful' response – one that brings life to, and cultivates rather than diminishes the aliveness, empowerment and liberation of women and bodies more generally.[23] It is in the first place a theology about, and for, women because slimming continues to be a female-dominated enterprise, as I will outline shortly. It does not claim to be for all women. The theology I offer recognizes the partiality of its starting point, both in terms of the experiences it draws upon – that is, a select group of white, middle-class, heterosexual, mainly able-bodied and not obviously fat people, the majority of whom are women – and in terms of my own privilege and position as a white, middle-class, British, able-bodied Christian. I am starkly aware of the necessarily contextual and limited scope of the constructive proposals I develop in this work. Yet the theology I advance is presented in the hope that it may resonate in different ways and to various degrees with women beyond the confines of the group studied here, in particular, with Christian women who experience their bodies and weight as a site of struggle and contestation and/or with those interested in engaging the tools of faith with contemporary issues around fat.

With Johnson, I hold that prioritizing the aliveness of women is a theological issue because the glory of God and the bodies and lives of women are at stake.[24] If women are indeed fully *imago Dei* and are transformed in the power of the Spirit into the image of Christ,[25] then this theological dignity calls for a critical review of cultural and theological traditions that threaten to deface it.[26] Fat and weight are

---

22. Elizabeth A. Johnson, *She Who Is: The Mystery of God in Feminist Theological Discourse* (New York: The Crossroad Publishing Company, 1992), 15.

23. I am influenced here by the way Nicola Slee speaks about the 'praxis' or 'empowerment' principle evident within feminist research. This depicts research with the explicit goal of furthering the empowerment and liberation of women and which is oriented towards social change. See *Women's Faith Development: Patterns and Processes* (Farnham: Ashgate, 2004), 49.

24. Johnson, *She Who Is*, 13–15.

25. Ibid., 70.

26. Ibid., 71.

inherently theological issues, and they concern much more than shape and size. As Lisa Isherwood argues, they concern 'theological politics and redemptive praxis' because when women are attacked in their bodies, 'it is nothing less than a profound and shocking act of blasphemy'.[27] Valuing women's embodiment reclaims the radical truth of incarnation: the physical is a vehicle for divine presence and embodiment a 'locus of religious meaning'.[28] Specifically, women's bodies are sacred, and the wholeness of women's realities is blessed with the identity of being made fully in God's image.[29] For me, this means taking seriously the ordinary everyday material lives of women who pursue weight loss. Rather than being an apolitical posture, it acknowledges that the personal is always political and that, as Mary Douglas argues, the body as a bounded system is always a symbol of society writ large.[30]

The language of livingness and fullness aptly accompanies a theological work such as this which is inevitably involved in the exploration of food matters and foodways.[31] It is no coincidence that the living God who bids us be full with life (Jn 10.10) is also a God who gives God's self as food for nourishment: as the bread of life (Jn 6.35). Indeed, the theology that this book works towards seeks to be a theology that nourishes: a theology not only *about* food but envisaged *as* food.[32] Unlike some of the ancient theologies lurking behind the vilification of

---

27. Lisa Isherwood, *The Fat Jesus: Feminist Explorations in Boundaries and Transgressions* (London: Darton, Longman and Todd, 2007), 19.

28. Melissa Raphael, *Thealogy and Embodiment: The Post-Patriarchal Reconstruction of Female Sacrality* (Sheffield: Sheffield Academic Press, 1996), 75.

29. Johnson, *She Who Is*, 71.

30. Mary Douglas, *Purity and Danger: An Analysis of Concept of Pollution and Taboo* (London and New York: Routledge, 2002).

31. This book uses the vocabulary of 'foodways' to give expression to members' ways around food: not only how they use food, how they consume it, how they name it and how they measure it but also crucially how they understand it and how they give food meaning. The study of foodways as it appears as a subfield within 'food studies' focuses on how communities and groups behave in relation to food and eating. See Marie W. Dallam, 'Introduction: Religion, Food and Eating', in *Religion, Food, & Eating in North America*, ed. Benjamin Zeller, Marie W. Dallam, Reid L. Neilson and Nora L. Rubel (New York: Columbia University Press, 2014), xxvii-xxxii.

32. Angel F. Méndez Montoya, *The Theology of Food: Eating and the Eucharist* (Chichester: Wiley-Blackwell, 2009).

desire, pleasure, food and fat unearthed within the secular weight loss group, this aims to be a theology which is 'safe' to consume – a theology of bread not stone.[33]

Before moving into the main discussion of this book, however, three questions require further attention: Why write a book on weight loss in the first place, and why from a theological perspective? Why undertake empirical research? And finally, why focus on women given men diet too?

Why Weight Loss?

The Silence of Theology

A project on weight loss dieting is probably not the most predictable for a theologian! When I have introduced my area of research to peers in theology I have often been met by looks of confusion. What has dieting to do with theology? This perceived disconnect is reflected perhaps by the paucity of theological scholarship on dieting, body image and body satisfaction. Mary Bringle's *The God of Thinness* and Lisa Isherwood's more recent *The Fat Jesus* are the only theological works to date that offer lengthy and sustained engagements with the contemporary culture of thinness. Both make valuable contributions, mining the Christian tradition for more body-positive resources: Bringle by drawing on the motifs of creation and incarnation and Isherwood by suggesting that the radicalness of incarnation demands an overhaul of dualistic theology. Isherwood makes a particularly important intervention by confronting cultural obsessions with thinness with the image of a 'Fat Jesus' – a counter-cultural image that calls forth a rebellion against the market-driven, patriarchal thin ideal and that encourages people to live fully in their skin. My study, however, extends such insights by employing empirical methods to analyse the real lives of women who slim and by investigating how slimming is practised within an actual commercial secular weight loss community. Rather than focusing more generally on 'food related problems', on America's obsession with thinness or on

---

33. Elisabeth Schüssler Fiorenza, *Bread Not Stone: The Challenge of Feminist Biblical Interpretation* (Boston: Beacon Press, 1984). Fiorenza draws on Jesus's words in Matthew's gospel (Mt. 7.9) to suggest a transformation of the metaphor of Scripture as 'tablets of stone' to an image of bread that 'nurtures, sustains and energizes women as people of God' (xiii–xiv).

eating disorders, as Bringle does, or on the general question of how Christian theology can speak to cultural obsessions with appearance, body image and thinness, I use qualitative methods to trace and assess the particular ways in which theological meanings resurface in one secular commercial setting. The interpretations I offer provide the basis for a wider discussion of food and fat later in the book.

In my view, Western theology's current silence on food and fat may expose assumptions about what is deemed to constitute 'proper' or 'serious' theology. Towards the start of her book, Bringle ponders theology's reticence around food, sarcastically remarking:

> Theology should, after all, be done in the study, the library, the office – should it not? – and not at the kitchen counter. Theology should be done hunched over a Bible (or a newspaper, or both – thank you, Mr. Barth), and not over a half-gallon of Butter Pecan Fudge ice cream.[34]

She detects a feeling among some constituents that food matters are too fleshy for theologians to concern themselves with, and her assessment of theological opinion may be right. There is perhaps an assumption that theology does not belong in the mundane, traditionally feminine domain of the kitchen. Some may think it is best concerned with the sophisticated, intellectual pursuit of abstract knowledge than with the material and bodily realms of food and eating. This not only suggests that sexism underpins accounts of what constitutes 'proper' theology but may also expose the privilege and plenty most Western theologians enjoy.[35] After all, it is much easier to be quiet about food when we live in contexts where food is plentiful. Theology's even more pronounced

---

34. Mary Louise Bringle, *The God of Thinness: Gluttony and Other Weighty Matters* (Nashville: Abingdon Press, 1992), 12.

35. Theology's silence on food matters has been noted by other theologians, among them Rachel Muers and David Grummet who compare Clement's practical concern with food matters to the 'failure' of modern Christian theologians to attend to the theological importance of 'everyday eating'. They suggest this failure may result from the way theological issues like abortion and war are given preference despite few Christians having to address them in their everyday lives. See *Theology on the Menu: Asceticism, Meat and Christian Diet* (London and New York: Routledge, 2010), vii. This location of theological attention away from the 'everyday' reinforces the point I am forwarding here.

silence on fat and dieting may signal parallel assumptions, indicating that issues to do with weight are deemed too inconsequential for theological attention, caught up with the 'triviality' of female body image and appearance. Losing weight may be assumed to be harmless or of no real concern for theological ethics, given it is obviously good for us – right?

Yet, feminist theology cannot afford to stay silent on food practices and fat politics because women's bodies are often positioned centrally in both, made to bear the burden of guilt, shame and fear attached to them. Food and fat are theological, as well as political, social and cultural issues, and theological systems are among the social and cultural forces that help to malign female appetite and conform women's bodies to a narrow ideal of beauty. Seminal works by Kim Chernin, Naomi Wolf and Shelley Bovey[36] map some aspects of this influence, although religion does not figure prominently in their overall discussions. Wolf, for example, argues that the weight loss industry uses religion to control women's bodies. The 'beauty myth' is 'the gospel of a new religion',[37] and the comparison between religion and an 'obsession' with weight loss dieting is no mere metaphor:

> The rituals of the beauty backlash do not simply echo traditional religions and cults but *functionally supplant them*. They are *literally* reconstituting out of old faiths a new one, *literally* drawing on traditional techniques of mystifications and thought control, to alter women's minds as sweepingly as any past evangelical wave.[38]

The 'Rites of Beauty', she maintains, have taken the place of traditional religion, policing women's appetites and desires even more successfully. In a similar way, Sharlene Nagy Hesse-Biber speaks about the 'Cult of Thinness' in which the 'object of worship' is the '"perfect" body' and the 'primary rituals' dieting and exercise.[39] The most avid in their

---

36. Kim Chernin, *The Obsession: Reflections on the Tyranny of Slenderness* (New York: HarperCollins, 1981); Naomi Wolf, *The Beauty Myth: How Images of Beauty Are Used Against Women* (New York: Doubleday, 1991); Shelley Bovey, *The Forbidden Body: Why Being Fat Is Not a Sin* (London: Pandora, 1989).

37. Wolf, *The Beauty Myth*, 86.

38. Ibid., 88. Italics in original.

39. Sharlene Hesse-Biber, *The Cult of Thinness* (New York and Oxford: Oxford University Press, 2007), 16.

'faith' participate in 'bizarre practices more characteristic of fringe cult movements', she reflects.[40] While I agree with much of this, I suggest that religion does not simply function negatively in weight loss contexts. The discussion I proffer nuances this account by attending to the conflicting ways in which women experience the pursuit of thinness and by highlighting the ambiguous ways in which religious and theological systems intersect with weight loss culture. It also places religion and theology at the centre throughout.

Of course, others have provided more lengthy discussions of the religious and spiritual dimensions of the contemporary pursuit of thinness. In *Starving for Salvation*[41] and *The Religion of Thinness*,[42] Michelle Lelwica argues that 'the religion of thinness' borrows from patriarchal religion's toolkit a number of religious ideas and forms which help control women's bodies. The female body serves as a secular 'icon' and magazines as 'sacred texts'. Both are cultural carriers of ruling ideologies to do with race, class, sexuality and age and help communicate Euro-American norms.[43] The decline of traditional Christianity does not mean that the desire for icons, beliefs, practices and rituals has been replaced but that these desires are met now through other means, including the rituals, beliefs and practices of the religion of thinness. Here, 'the obsessive, imaginary, sacrificial, ritualizing, ascetic, penitential, dogmatic, and devotional aspects of anorexia and bulimia resemble certain features of traditional Christianity'.[44]

Lelwica begins to name some of the theological tropes underlying secular obsessions with thinness, but her emphasis is mainly on secularization which is not my focus here, nor do I wish to attend to the historical, cultural and religious dimensions of eating disorders in America as she does. I am less concerned with how the pursuit of

---

40. She names scientology and Kabbalah as examples of such 'cult-like' movements. Ibid., 17.

41. Michelle Mary Lelwica, *Starving for Salvation: The Spiritual Dimensions of Eating Problems among American Girls and Women* (New York and Oxford: Oxford University Press, 1999).

42. Michelle Mary Lelwica, *The Religion of Thinness: Satisfying the Spiritual Hungers behind Women's Obsession with Food and Weight* (Carlsbad: Gürze Books, 2010).

43. Lelwcia, *Starving for Salvation*, 40.

44. Ibid., 7.

thinness functions 'like religion' or as a form of 'implicit religion'[45] with its own quasi-religious fervour, ritual observances, holy texts and charismatic leaders and more concentrated on uncovering the theological assumptions lurking behind organizational rhetoric and within the weight loss stories that women themselves narrate.

This advances a different approach to those using empirical methods to study secular commercial dieting groups from more sociological perspectives. Kandi Stinson provides this kind of discussion, offering an excellent qualitative sociological study of a secular commercial weight loss group in the United States.[46] Using participant observation, she argues that religious imagery and frameworks of meaning animate the language of members in the group. Themes of temptation, sacrifice and guilt are present, she observes, establishing 'religion' as an important metaphor that works alongside other metaphors of 'self-help' and 'work' to rationalize weight loss. For Stinson, although the metaphor of weight loss as religion has the potential to employ the emotions to a larger extent, members emphasize the (negative) aspects of religion that more easily mesh with notions of discipline and self-control.[47]

Like other feminist researchers, Stinson dedicates only a small portion of her discussion to an analysis of religion and envisages that secular dieting draws on the worst aspects of religion the most. In dedicating the whole of this volume to engaging ethnography with

---

45. Edward Bailey uses the terminology of 'implicit religion' to signal how some community activities have religious dimensions despite not being overtly religious. For him, what appears secular 'might also contain, within itself, the seeds of some other forms of religiosity'. See '"Implicit Religion"? What Might That Be?', *Implicit Religion* 15, no. 2 (2012): 199, and his monograph, *Implicit Religion in Contemporary Society* (Kampen, Netherlands: Kok Pharos, 1997). Implicit religion also has some affinity with the notions of 'invisible religion', 'common religion' and 'diffused religion' discussed by Thomas Luckmann, Robert Towler and Roberto Cipriani, respectively. For more, see Thomas Luckman, *The Invisible Religion: The Problem of Religion in Modern Society* (London: Macmillan, 1967), Robert Towler, *Homo Religiosus: Sociological Problems in the Study of Religion* (London: Constable, 1974), and Roberto Cipriani, '"Diffused Religion" and New Values in Italy', in *The Changing Face of Religion*, ed. J. A. Beckford and T. Luckmann (London: Sage, 1989), 24–48.

46. Kandi Stinson, *Women and Dieting Culture: Inside a Commercial Weight Loss Group* (New Brunswick and London: Rutgers University Press, 2001).

47. Ibid., 121.

critical feminist theological reflection, and by paying close attention to the ambiguous ways in which weight watching operates, I tender a theological response that foregrounds religion and the ordinary lives of women who slim.

Cultural Fears about Fat: Fat as Risk

As well as theology's silence on fat, it also seems to me that at a time when the social and political landscape is saturated with tales of woe about fat, the absence of fat in theological debate appears odd, if not alarming. In Euro-American culture, fat bodies are both visible and invisible, sightly and unsightly, ever present but always nevertheless erased through the commercial, medical, psychological and capitalist discourses which pathologize them.[48] Conjured as diseased or impaired, morally weak and a drain on a nation's economic resources, fat people are represented as freakish and monstrous and take up the position of the spectacle. Whether in fly-on-the-wall documentaries like *Half Ton Son*, TV game shows like *The Biggest Loser* or in TV news reports which routinely show fat people as headless,[49] fat bodies are presented for public entertainment: as objects of the public's fascination and horror.[50]

---

48. Kathleen LeBesco and Janna Evans Braziel, 'Editor's Introduction', in *Bodies out of Bounds: Fatness and Transgression,* ed. J. E. Braziel and K. LeBesco (Berkeley, Los Angeles and London: University of California Press, 2001), 1–15. Also see Le'a Kent, 'Fighting Abjection: Representing Fat Women', in *Bodies out of Bounds*,130–52, and Kathleen LeBesco's, *Revolting Bodies? The Struggle to Redefine Fat Identity* (Amherst and Boston: University of Massachusetts Press, 2004), 1–9.

49. Fat activist Charlotte Cooper discusses the 'headless fatty' in her blog post, 'Headless Fatties', *Obesity Epidemic* (January 2007), available online: http://charlottecooper.net/publishing/digital/headless-fatties-01-07 (accessed 10 February 2016). Also see Chapter 6 of this book.

50. Comparing modern US talk-shows like 'You're Too Fat to Wear That' or 'Mom I Don't Want to be Fat Like You' to the Freak Show, Andrea Stulman Dennett argues that fat bodies are othered in similar ways: 'they' are the freaks and 'we' (the voyeurs) are the normal. Both are about spectacle, and serve to ridicule female fat in particular. See her essay, 'The Dime Museum Freak Show Reconfigured as Talk Show', in *Freakery: Cultural Spectacles of the Extraordinary Body*, ed. Rosemary Garland Thomson (New York and London: New York University Press, 1996), 315–26, esp. 325.

A theological book on dieting and weight is timely, then, not least because fears about fat are growing. It is hard to go a day without being confronted with the apocalyptic vision of a world threatened by fat. Fat, we are told, is the embodiment of risk, to individual health, to economic health and to the health of social values. Obesity is said to be the cause of a number of life-limiting or life-ending conditions, including type-2 diabetes, colon cancer, angina, gall bladder disease, liver disease, ovarian cancer, osteoarthritis, stroke and heart attack.[51] In the United States, the Centers for Disease Control and Prevention (CDC) warns that more than one-third of US adults are obese.[52] In England, the Department of Health cautions that 61.9 per cent of the adult population is overweight or obese.[53] Fat is seen as an unquestionable risk to health even in the midst of growing scepticism about the scientific rigour and defensibility of such conventional wisdom.[54] Health officials warn that the United States and United Kingdom are nations facing an obesity 'epidemic'. The

51. Department of Health, 'Healthy Lives, Healthy People: A Call to Action on Obesity in England' (13 October 2011): 14, https://www.gov.uk/government/uploads/system/uploads/attachment_data/file/213720/dh_130487.pdf (accessed 7 December 2013); Centers for Disease Control and Prevention (CDC), 'Adult Obesity Causes & Consequences', http://www.cdc.gov/obesity/adult/causes.html (accessed 10 November 2016).

52. CDC, 'Adult Overweight and Obesity', https://www.cdc.gov/obesity/adult/index.html (accessed 17 August 2017).

53. Department of Health, 'Policy Paper: 2010 to 2015 Government Policy: Obesity and Healthy Eating' (updated 8 May 2015), https://www.gov.uk/government/publications/2010-to-2015-government-policy-obesity-and-healthy-eating/2010-to-2015-government-policy-obesity-and-healthy-eating (accessed 10 November 2016). The Australian Institute of Health and Welfare states that overweight and obesity are continuing to rise in Australia with two in three adults (63 per cent) overweight or obese. See Australian Institute of Health and Welfare, 'Overweight and Obesity', http://www.aihw.gov.au/risk-factors-overweight-obesity/ (accessed 10 November 2016).

54. For more on this, see Chapter 6. Also see Maria Grazia Franzosi, 'Should We Continue to Use BMI as a Cardiovascular Risk Factor?', *The Lancet* 368 (2006): 624–5, which shows how typical associations between obesity and increased risk of mortality and 'cardiovascular events' are being questioned, and P. Ernsberger, 'Obesity Is an Early Symptom of Diabetes, Not Its Cause', *Health at Every Size Journal* 18 (2004): 67–9; K. R. Fontaine, R. McCubrey, T. Mehta, N. M. Pajewski, S. W. Keith, S. S. Bangalore, C. J. Crespo and D. B. Allison, 'Body Mass Index and Mortality Rate among Hispanic Adults: A Pooled Analysis of

Department of Health in England describes this as 'a health time bomb with the potential to explode over the next three decades'.[55] Adopting an event stronger tone, the US surgeon general appointed by President Bush six months after 9/11 describes obesity as 'the terror within, a threat that is every bit as real to America as the weapons of mass destruction'.[56] Within this political and morally charged rhetoric, fat is indisputably rendered a danger to Western civility, safety and health, and weight loss a moral solution and political virtue.

Of course, the weapons of mass destruction did not turn out to be 'real' after all, but the alignment of fat with the vulnerability of a nation in a post-9/11 and 7/7 context is worth noting. In her discussion of obesity discourse in US life in the wake of the 9/11 attacks, Charlotte Biltekoff argues that anxiety about obesity escalated in conjunction with reactions to these events. Although American phobias of fat were already reaching new levels, news stories about growing waistlines were among the first unrelated stories to be reported after the terror incident. In 2001, shortly after the attacks took place, the US government launched its official anti-obesity campaign.[57] The war on fat, Biltekoff argues, is not unconnected to the war on terror since both coincide in US life to build a sense of threat to the nation and to produce a 'politics of fear'.[58] If US soldiers were getting fatter, as the media reported shortly

Multiple Epidemiologic Data Sets', *International Journal of Obesity* 36 (August 2012): 1121–6.

55. Department of Health, 'Annual Report of the Chief Medical Officer 2002. Health Check: On the State of the Public Health', http://webarchive.nationalarchives.gov.uk/+/www.dh.gov.uk/en/PublicationsAndStatistics/Publications/AnnualReports/DH_4006432 (accessed 16 April 2014).

56. Cable News Network, 'Surgeon General to Cops: Put Down the Donuts', CNN.com/Health (2 March 2003), http://edition.cnn.com/2003/HEALTH/02/28/obesity.police/ (accessed 16 April 2013).

57. Charlotte Biltekoff, 'The Terror Within: Obesity in Post 9/11 U.S. Life', *American Studies* 48, no. 3 (2007): 32.

58. Ibid., 33. Beth Evans has similarly shown that the UK's Department of Health's framing of fat, which is informed by the language of war borrowed from the war on terror, constructs the future of the UK nation as bleak and as demanding drastic action in the present. Just as is the case with the war on terror, the absence of 'evidence' in the war on fat may be equally inconsequential. See 'Anticipating Fatness: Childhood, Affect and the Pre-Emptive "War on Obesity"', *Transactions of the Institute of British Geographers* 35, no. 1 (2010): 21–38.

after 9/11, and the everyday world of the supermarket was the real danger, as the Surgeon General suggested, then fat was a threat to US national security,[59] and one which conveniently justified greater levels of national body surveillance. She argues that by constructing the war on fat in conjunction with the war on terror, the US government was able to direct attention away from its irresponsibility in relation to the Afghanistan–Iraq war – specifically, its poorly defined aims and its defiance to 'fight' an enemy that nevertheless remained elusive – to the irresponsibility of the fat individual, now waging war on an enemy that could be clearly seen. She adds that the war on fat allowed those in minority groups most blamed for fat – specifically blacks, Latinos, the poor and ironically the bulk of the US military fighting the war on terror – an opportunity to become good citizens. It served to control the bodies of those mainly from minority groups, re-securing the priority of the privileged white middle classes.

Biltekoff's argument begins to expose how anti-fat sentiment and the so-called healthy ideal of thinness may operate as a political device which props up the boundaries of white, Western, middle-class normativity, diverting attention away from any signs of social disorder or political dis-ease. Not only is the body symbolic of society and the stage upon which the politics of decency are played out but fat bodies are specifically symbolic of a vulnerable nation and reflective of power which has been denied by the privileged. Thinness is emblematic of a civilized nation and women's bodies in particular tasked with patrolling the borders of civility, and this is a point I discuss at various stages in this book. Christian thought helps construct this body politic, not least through the tropes of sin and salvation that resurface in various ways in the weight loss group I join.

It seems to me, also, that the cultural truth which depicts fat as risk and weight loss as cure may also need challenging. If Britons are 'a nation of dieters', as one news report suggests,[60] but a nation where the obesity 'epidemic' is growing, then the claim that slimming is the solution to the 'problem' of fat is not quite as obvious as it first

59. Biltekoff, 'The Terror Within', 33.
60. Hayley Leaver, 'Companies Growing Fat as You Slim: The Growth of the Weight Loss Market', *Metro* (30 January 2014), http://metro.co.uk/2014/01/30/companies-growing-fat-as-you-slim-the-growth-of-the-weight-loss-market-4282903/ (accessed 3 August 2017). According to this source, over twenty-nine million people tried to lose weight between 2013 and 2014 alone.

appears.[61] This conventional wisdom emerges strongly in the dieting group I attend, and I challenge it in this book. It is also clear that fat is presented in contemporary discourse as an obvious risk to everyone's health, not just those who are obese or overweight according to ideal weight classifications. As Julie Guthman and Melanie DuPuis argue, the focus on prevention rather than cure in anti-obesity policy actually ensures that such discourse is directed at the 'relatively thin' and mostly concerned with 'disciplining the center'.[62] The same message emerges in this slimming group as no-body is considered safe from the threat of fat, and it directs me towards shaping a feminist theological response that attends to the ubiquity of fat phobia.

Accompanying the vilification of fat as risk to physical health are, of course, economic concerns that fatness is draining the nation's purse. In 2008, overall medical care costs related to obesity for US adults were estimated to be $147 billion.[63] In the UK, current costs of excess weight to the NHS are estimated to be over £5 billion[64] and are predicted to rise to £9.7 billion by 2050.[65] The financial impact on public sector services are also believed to be considerable, affecting social care for house-bound people as well as schools which may need to purchase specialized equipment to accommodate larger children.[66] The message that slimming down is good for the nation's financial health is reinforced by talk of 'cuts' resulting from the global economic crisis and the global recession. In Britain, we hear that government spending on public services must be subject to a 'tight squeeze'. Cuts must be deep, bold and severe if the country is to get 'back in shape'. Cutting down, slimming down and eradicating excess, we are led to believe, are crucial

61. See Glenn Gaesser, 'Is "Permanent Weight Loss" and Oxymoron? The Statistics on Weight Loss and the National Weight Control Registry', in *The Fat Studies Reader*, ed. Esther Rothblum and Sondra Solovay (New York and London: New York University Press, 2009), 37.

62. Julie Guthman and Melanie DuPuis, 'Embodying Neoliberalism: Economy, Culture and the Politics of Fat', *Environment and Planning D: Society and Space* 24, no. 3 (2006): 444.

63. CDC, 'Adult Obesity Causes and Consequences'.

64. Department of Health, '2010 to 2015 Government Policy: Obesity and Healthy Eating'.

65. Department of Health, 'Healthy Lives, Healthy People', 16.

66. Ibid., 17.

if public sector organizations are to become leaner, more efficient and more productive.

The worrying thing is that, at the same time as obesity is said to be on the rise and burning a hole in the public purse, weight loss services are profiting from the very 'epidemic' health professionals consider to be such an economic drain. Weight management and weight loss services are commercial services that feed a bourgeoning and highly profitable weight loss market. The value of this market in the United States is thought to be around $59.8 billion[67] with the number of Americans dieting estimated to be 108 million in 2012.[68] Out of a population of c.313 million[69] this puts the estimated percentage of Americans pursuing weight loss in 2012 (35 per cent) on a par with the percentage of Americans considered obese (34.9 per cent).[70] Often, medical practitioners and health professionals can prescribe such commercial services for patients they deem to be in need. Indeed, the slimming organization at the centre of this book offers its weight loss product 'on referral' to the NHS as a means of expanding obesity services. The National Health Service, on its *NHS Choices* website, advises that general practitioners may recommend the use of weight loss programmes which 'may be commercial services that you pay for'.[71]

A theological book on dieting is important, then, because of the suspect ways in which fears of fat and assumptions about health feed the financial markets. Omnipresent discourses about the 'cost' of obesity stigmatize fatness and relegate fat people to the margins of

---

67. Marketdata Enterprises Inc, 'The U.S. Weight Loss Market: 2015 Status Report' (January 2015), http://www.marketresearch.com/Marketdata-Enterprises-Inc-v416/Weight-Loss-Status-8745878/ (accessed 3 November 2016).

68. PRWeb, 'Number of American Dieters Soars to 108 Million', http://www.prweb.com/releases/2012/1/prweb9084688.htm (accessed 23 April 2014).

69. This is the population of the United States on 1 January 2012 according to The United States Census Bureau, US and World Population Clock, http://www.census.gov/popclock/ (accessed 3 November 2016).

70. Statistics are for 2011–2. See Cynthia L. Ogden, Margaret D. Carroll, Brian K. Kit, and Katherine M. Flegal, 'Prevalence of Obesity among Adults: United States, 2011-2012', *NCHS Data Brief* no. 131 (January 2013), http://www.cdc.gov/nchs/data/databriefs/db131.pdf (accessed 3 November 2016).

71. NHS Choices, 'How Your GP Can Help You Lose Weight', http://www.nhs.uk/Livewell/loseweight/Pages/WhataGPcando.aspx (accessed 16 November 2016).

society, while investment into slimming technologies communicate an appetite in government and health care services for correcting fat. Such a concern, however, seems less prevalent when it comes to dealing with eating disorders. A report by the UK eating disorder charity, BEAT, estimates that the total treatment costs of eating disorders to the NHS stand between £3.9 billion and £4.6 billion, with up to a further £1.1 billion estimated for private treatment costs.[72] This is comparable with the economic costs attached to obesity, but far less visible in the public media and considerably removed from the state of emergency declared about fat. BEAT observes that in over 40 per cent of cases, patients are waiting for more than six months to receive appropriate treatment.[73] Long delays for medical help together with reports of women being refused treatment because they are not thin enough indicate not only that the NHS may be unable to cope with an increase in demand but also that some health practitioners may be making patients' lives worse by inferring they need to be thinner to warrant attention.[74] Ultimately, it seems that the economic expense associated with disordered eating matters much less than that incurred in relation to fat, exposing the fat phobic nature of this economic model.

This sketches a rather worrying view of the contemporary landscape, where fears about fat appear to be making a growing number of women and men ill. Fat bodies are also frequently maligned, cast as sloppy, self-indulgent and lazy. The denigrating of fat is fuelled by the commercial media and public health policy presenting excessive weight and excessive thinness as the result of faulty individual choices.[75] However,

---

72. BEAT, 'The Costs of Eating Disorders: Social, Health and Economic Impacts' (February 2015), https://www.b-eat.co.uk/assets/000/000/302/The_ costs_of_eating_disorders_Final_original.pdf (accessed 26 February 2017), 9.

73. Ibid., 29.

74. See, for example, 'Eating Disorder Patients' Lives at Risk Due to Long Waits for NHS Treatment', *The Guardian* (Sunday 14 June 2015), https://www.theguardian.com/society/2015/jun/14/eating-disorders-long-waits-nhs-treatment-lives-risk (accessed 26 February 2017).

75. In health policy, although genetics and economic factors are considered to play a part in the prevalence of obesity, in the end individuals are seen as having ultimate agency to choose 'health', a point evident from the NHS Choices website which carries the strap line, 'your health, your choices' and which aims to 'put you in charge of your health care'. See http://www.nhs.uk/aboutNHSChoices/Pages/NHSChoicesintroduction.aspx (accessed 10 November 2016).

if the aliveness and full dignity of women as *imago Dei* is a theological imperative, then this kind of defamation and commodification of bodies, women's bodies in particular, demands serious theological attention.

Why Empirical Research?

This study begins from the micro-practices of women trying to lose weight rather than providing a purely theoretical discussion. It arises from my conviction that to understand dieting, we must observe and study it in ways that attend to the complexities of women's lives and probe 'the minutiae of its practices, its everyday tropes and demands, its compulsions and liberations'.[76] Feminist research on slimming is at its best when it attends to the ordinary experiences of those directly engaged with the pursuit of weight loss. This avoids dislocating knowledge about fat and dieting from the concrete bodies of women who slim, and foregrounds dieting as a lived, material practice. Accordingly, I select empirical qualitative methods as tools for this investigation – semi-structured interviews and participant observation – and extend the general principle of grounding feminist research in women's experience[77] by 'hearing into speech'[78] the real-life stories of women inside one weight loss group. Such methods

---

76. Cressida J. Heyes, 'Foucault Goes to Weight Watchers', *Hypatia* 21, no. 2 (2006): 127.

77. For excellent studies on the role of women's experience in the doing of feminist theology, see Linda Hogan, *From Women's Experience to Feminist Theology* (Sheffield: Sheffield Academic Press, 1995) and Pamela Dickey Young, *Feminist Theology/Christian Theology: In Search of Method* (Eugene: Wipf and Stock, 1990). For a discussion of some of the difficulties with this as a methodological starting point see Sheila Greeve Davaney, 'The Limits of the Appeal to Women's Experience', in *Shaping New Vision: Gender and Values in American Culture*, ed. Clarissa W. Atkinson, Constance H. Buchanan and Margaret R. Miles (London: UMI Research Press, 1987); Angela Davis, *Women, Race and Class* (New York: Random House, 1981); bell hooks, *Ain't I a Woman? Black Women and Feminism* (Boston: Pluto Press, 1981); Sheila Greeve Davaney, 'Continuing the Story but Departing the Text: A Historicist Interpretations of Feminist Norms in Theology', in *Horizons in Feminist Theology: Identity, Tradition and Norms*, ed. Rebecca S. Chopp and Sheila Greeve Davaney (Minneapolis: Fortress Press, 1997).

78. Nelle Morton, *The Journey Is Home* (Boston: Beacon Press, 1985).

allow me and you, the reader, to understand how women live the pursuit of thinness and to use the experiences of women as a means of testing and exposing the liabilities of theological accounts of sin and salvation as they function to legitimate fears about food and fat. Where Christian theologies emerge as sanctioning or sustaining systems of violence against women's bodies, they are met in this book with challenge and oriented towards more liberating horizons. Where they are shown to be affirming of women's bodies they are employed against the theological traditions which cause harm and are used to help further more just and liberatory accounts of sin and salvation.

I have deliberately selected this organization because it uses the Christian terminology of 'sin' – now spelt 'Syn'[79] – in its weight loss programme. When I first came across the use of this theological trope by the weight loss organization I immediately became interested in how the language of sin functioned. Did the organization and its members recycle normative theological meanings? If so, what purpose did this serve? This line of questioning prompted me to join a regional group as a researcher and fully paying/participating member. I attended the weight loss group weekly for fifteen months, observing the group and following the plan myself. Strictly speaking, there was no need to ask permission from the organization to do the research as anyone can join if they pay the weekly subscription,[80] but I was aware that I would be occasionally pulling out a notebook and speaking to members before, during and after the meetings about their dieting experiences. Conscious that I did not want any of this to arouse undue suspicion or compromise the relationship of trust with the community, I was candid about my role as a researcher and received permission from the consultant[81] to undertake the research.

---

79. 'Sin', or 'Syn' as it is now spelt, is a specialist term employed by the organization to refer to foods like crisps, chocolate, ice cream, cake and alcohol that are high in saturated fats and sugar. For more on this, including the change in spelling, see Chapter 1.

80. This is the reason Kandi Stinson gives for not seeking permission in her ethnographic study inside a secular commercial weight loss group in the United States. See Stinson, *Women and Dieting Culture*, 26.

81. The consultant is the leader of the weight loss group. I use the terms 'consultant' and 'leader' interchangeably throughout this book. According to the organization's website, consultants need no qualifications, just experience of being 'successful' members of the organization who are 'well on the way' to

I conducted thirteen semi-structured interviews with volunteers, twelve women and one man,[82] usually in members' homes. The interviews covered the same general themes – 'you as a dieter', 'motivations for dieting', 'doing the diet', 'feelings about dieting' and 'the group' – and members reflected on each in a conversational exchange.[83] This sometimes involved me sharing my own experiences of being in the group and following the plan; hence, I did not seek to be impartial in the process. Rather, and in keeping with feminist interview research, I approached the interviews as 'encounters' between myself and other members, rejecting the positivist insistence on distance and objectivity.[84] 'Disengagement'[85] in the interview process seemed to be an unreasonable and unethical expectation given I was a fellow dieter and my interviewees knew me as such. To try and occlude this in the interview would be a pretence and would produce an awkwardness and imbalance of power that could detrimentally affect my rapport with participants and their willingness to disclose.

Of course, there is the risk of over-rapport and that by sharing aspects of my own experience, I impacted my participants' responses, but the researcher is always inevitably involved in the shaping of participants' experience. As Marjorie L. De Vault and Glenda Gross argue, the 'telling about experience' in interviews is always-already informed by social, discursive and historical contexts and so is never available in an untarnished form. In this sense, feminist research contributes an awareness that 'telling' always involves a listener, and listening always constitutes an act of interpretation which shapes the account that is heard as well as the telling of it.[86] In the end, sharing something of my

achieving their weight loss goals. For more information on the consultant of my group, see later in this chapter where I introduce the slimming group and weight loss organization.

82. Pseudonyms are used throughout this book to protect the identities of members within this weight loss group. The name of the weight loss organization is also concealed.

83. Anne Oakley, 'Interviewing Women: A Contradiction in Terms', in *Doing Feminist Research*, ed. H. Roberts (London: Routledge, 1982), 55.

84. Ibid.

85. Ibid.

86. Marjorie L. De Vault and Glenda Gross, 'Feminist Qualitative Interviewing: Experience, Talk, and Knowledge', in *The Handbook of Feminist Research: Theory and Praxis*, 2nd edn, ed. Sharlene Nagy Hesse-Biber

own experience felt more equitable and more comfortable. It seemed wrong to ask my interviewees for a form of openness I was not prepared to offer myself, as though my informants were mere vessels of data to be tapped. In reality, however, I shared more of myself with those I came to know the best – with women like Ruth, who joined at the same time as me, and Suzanne, who sat next to me most weeks. My main concern was always to build trust and rapport with my participants and to avoid 'the dilemma of the ethnographer' that R. Marie Griffith outlines, where the researcher does not fully belong to the community they are studying but wants, at the same time, to be trusted by that community.[87]

Participation in the ordinary life of the group enabled me to access the social and cultural worlds of members, to experience in the meetings, through conversations and through my own dieting behaviour, the complex meanings and feelings that losing weight can produce. It allowed me to experience the plan and the environment of the group in my body, for myself, and to fully enter the setting I was studying. It also, however, presented a number of difficulties.

Participant Observation: 'Coming Out' as a Feminist Anxious about Fat

I did not only join the group as a feminist researcher. I also joined the group because I genuinely wanted to lose weight. Starting this project I was acutely aware that I occupied what Cressida Heyes calls a 'fraught standpoint',[88] torn between my feminist convictions which made me suspicious of weight loss dieting and my personal unhappiness with my own size which made me want to lose weight. Other feminists have narrated similar tensions.[89] In the introduction to *Unbearable Weight*,

---

(Los Angeles, London, New Delhi, Singapore and Washington: Sage, 2012), 206–36, esp. 212.

87. R. Marie Griffith, *God's Daughters: Evangelical Women and the Power of Submission* (Berkeley, Los Angeles and London: University of California Press, 2000), 8.

88. Heyes, 'Foucault Goes to Weight Watchers'.

89. See, for example, Robyn Longhurst, 'Becoming Smaller: Autobiographical Spaces of Weight Loss', *Antipode* 44, no. 3 (2012): 871–88. In this article, Longhurst, a geographer, notes how her own experience of weight loss has been 'paradoxical'. 'I have wrestled with critiquing discourses around women and slimness while desiring to be slim,' she says, 'understanding that "fat is a feminist issue"', as well as feeling 'ashamed of my ample body' (877).

Susan Bordo speaks about her own involvement in a national US weight loss programme telling her readers that she lost twenty-four pounds and that some of her colleagues viewed her involvement as hypocritical. She concludes that feminist cultural criticism does not provide a blueprint for the conduct of personal life or political action. 'It does not empower (or require) individuals to "rise above" their culture or to become martyrs to feminist ideals.'[90]

One of the points this book makes is that there is no outside space to which we can retreat, away from our fears and body woes. 'We live in the real world', to quote fat activist Charlotte Cooper, and this is a world where frequently there is much to gain from being or aspiring to be thin.[91] Given these tensions were real for me, I thought there was little point in pretending to rise above my own body, its desires and indeed my own size. To do so would, after all, be to fantasize about somehow leaving my body behind and would, as Throsby and Gimlin argue, restate the body–mind dualism feminists have long since tried to critique.[92] Before joining the group, then, I found myself similarly critical of cultural discourses which push women towards unachievable body ideals while being very aware of my own embeddedness within this discursive culture. I embodied a dilemma, but I could not pretend to be otherwise. I could not take my body and body concerns out of the research. Participating then simply felt more honest.

As a participant, however, I found that my own success as a dieter helped produce the very feelings of celebration in others which sat so

---

She sees her own personal experience of weight gain and weight loss as inseparable from her academic self and suggests that autobiography allows the researcher to narrate such tensions.

90. Susan Bordo, *Unbearable Weight: Feminism, Western Culture, and the Body* (Berkeley, Los Angeles and London: University of California Press, 1993), 30.

91. Charlotte Cooper, *Fat and Proud: The Politics of Size* (London: The Women's Press, 1998), 54.

92. This is a point made by Throsby and Gimlin in their discussion of ethnography inside a commercial weight loss group and with people who are awaiting or who have received weight loss surgery. See their chapter, 'Critiquing Thinness and Wanting to Be Thin', in *Secrecy and Silence in the Research Process: Feminist Reflections*, ed. Róisín Ryan-Flood and Rosalind Gill (London and New York: Routledge, 2013), 106.

uncomfortably with me as a feminist.[93] Other members and the leader herself would assume I was entirely sympathetic with the practice of slimming, would congratulate me on my weight loss and would ask me for advice. I would clap members who had lost weight, engage in the ritual of 'checking' what other women had lost and explain my own loss, gain or maintenance to others, following the conventional practices of the group. I enjoyed receiving affirmation from other women and from the consultant, Louise, but I also felt compelled to say the right thing, bound to use the language of 'good' and 'bad' in the meetings and would sometimes be unsure about how to respond when members celebrated significant weight losses. My compliance meant that the practice of slimming was not questioned and that my feminist and political concerns about slimming were actually rendered unspeakable.[94] This regularly caused me to feel compromised, half wanting to be in the meeting and half wanting to be somewhere else.

Using Women's Experiences

Like other Christian theologians advancing a turn to ethnography in the doing of theology and feminist theology,[95] the use of participant observation and in-depth interviews took me beyond my usual tools of theological investigation – 'beyond the desk and the library'[96] – into

---

93. Gimlin describes a similar situation where her own body impacts the data and research findings. She explains how her dieting 'success' helped to produce in other members of the weight loss group she was interviewing the very sense of failure she was trying to explore. Ibid., 113.

94. Ibid.

95. A number of theologians have turned to qualitative methods as a means of understanding religious practices as they are lived by individuals and communities in concrete settings. Examples include John Swinton and Harriet Mowat, *Practical Theology and Qualitative Research* (London: SCM, 2006); Mary McClintock Fulkerson, *Places of Redemption: Theology for a Worldly Church* (Oxford: Oxford University Press, 2007); Slee, *Women's Faith Development*; Nicola Slee, Fran Porter and Anne Phillips, *The Faith Lives of Women and Girls: Qualitative Research Perspectives* (Farnham: Ashgate, 2013); Ward, *Perspectives on Ecclesiology*; Christian Scharen, *Ethnography in Christian Theology and Ethics* (New York: Continuum, 2011).

96. Elizabeth Phillips, 'Charting the "Ethnographic Turn"', in *Perspectives on Ecclesiology*, 105.

the real lives of women involved in this weight loss organization. Such methods allowed me to listen to women on their own terms. This, however, does not mean that women's experiences and words are used in this book as a neutral foundation upon which to think theologically about weight.[97] Experience is always mediated, located within complex social and discursive contexts,[98] and so it offers no innocent foundation from which to begin theology. As Joan Scott argues, experience can never figure as 'incontestable evidence' because it is historically situated rather than natural or given.[99] As such, this book draws on broader analytical and critical perspectives, including feminist work and the discipline of Fat Studies, to provide a critical reading of informants' narratives and practices.[100] Such perspectives are employed, not to debunk or supersede women's experiences but to subject them to 'a dialectical process'[101] of critical reading and feminist evaluation in keeping with the tradition of feminist liberation theologies.

Insofar as this organization has its own way of speaking about food and weight, replicated to a point by its members, the case study I offer is not generalizable. However, case studies can 'open to view important questions', as feminist theologian Mary McClintock Fulkerson argues, so that the thick description provided nudges the researcher towards 'normative issues'.[102] She describes how her participant observation within the interracial, multi-abled Good Samaritan United Methodist Church 'thickened out' the context of Christian beliefs about inclusive faith for her, making her ask questions about certain notions of tradition. As a result, she determines that theology needs to pay closer attention to bodily forms of communication and interaction and to how communities 'perform' rather than simply read, sing or hear about

---

97. Ibid.

98. See Mary McClintock Fulkerson, *Changing the Subject: Women's Discourses and Feminist Theology* (Minneapolis: Fortress Press, 1994).

99. Joan Scott, 'The Evidence of Experience', *Critical Inquiry* 17, no. 4 (1991): 777. Scott argues that when experience is taken as the self-evident origin of knowledge, 'Questions about the constructed nature of knowledge, about how subjects are constituted as different in the first place, about how one's vision is structured – about language (or discourse) and history – are left aside' (ibid).

100. De Vault and Gross, 'Feminist Qualitative Interviewing', 212.

101. See Fiorenza, *Bread Not Stone*, xiii.

102. Fulkerson, 'Interpreting a Situation', 130.

Jesus.[103] In my case, the close analysis of the slimming group and the theological motifs which surface there compel me towards questions about how food and fat might be re-conceptualized in Christian thought. It causes me to return to the theological classifications of sin and salvation which are salient categories in the weight loss group, to consider how they might speak meaningfully and in more life-affirming ways to women who share similar body concerns to those who attend the group. The descriptions and practical examples of sin and salvation I develop in the last half of the book are theological offerings so they are addressed to communities of Christian women in the first instance, but the principles and practices I promote will have wider application.

My critical review of women's experience is, therefore, expansive in that it pushes me towards the normative task of asking what ought to be going on[104] in a world that is currently obsessed with thin and ideologically opposed to fat. It is also limited in that it draws on a particular set of experiences rendering the theological claims I make partial and rooted in the everyday realities of particular women's lives. Women in the group, however, do not determine to lose weight apart from their wider social relations and communities, in isolation of the social systems and discourses that help to vilify fat or in separation from other women and men who choose to pursue weight loss. Part of my interpretive and constructive task, then, is to understand and respond to the contemporary 'situation'[105] of the group by placing their individual and collective experiences in the context of a wider 'web'[106] of social and

---

103. Ibid., 134.

104. See Richard Osmer's discussion of the normative task of practical theology in his book, *Practical Theology: An Introduction* (Cambridge: Wm. B. Eerdmans Publishing Company, 2008), 129–74.

105. See Richard Osmer's discussion of case studies. Ibid., 51.

106. Bonnie Miller-McLemore presents the notion of a 'living human web' to challenge the individualistic focus of therapeutic care and to stress the need to see individual problems as part of wider social patterns of suffering and injustice. The metaphor of the web, she argues, draws attention to the way individuals are affected and caught up in broader political, social and discursive systems and so identifies the need to attend to social inequalities. See Miller-McLemore, 'Revisiting the living Human Web: Theological Education and the Role of Clinical Pastoral Education', *The Journal of Pastoral Care & Counseling*, 62, nos 1–2 (2008): 10–11, 'The Human Web', and 'The Living Human Web: Pastoral Theology at the Turn of the Century', in *Through the Eyes of Women: Insights for*

political relations. The descriptive and practical meanings of sin and salvation I develop in the final three chapters underline the social and historical dimensions of these theological tropes and the need for such theological ideas to be saturated with the complexities and tensions of the ordinary. Picturing the density of women's experiences as part of a matrix of complex interconnections that extend outwards beyond the individual to include other bodies and social systems, this one situation, I suggest, has the potential to offer 'liberatory lessons'[107] beyond the confines of the group.

Introducing the Weight Loss Organization and Group[108]

The weight loss group at the centre of this book belongs to a very popular and profitable commercial UK organization.[109] Boasting 16,000 groups nationwide, a total of 4,500 trained consultants and 900,000 members weekly, the company estimates a 90 per cent female membership.[110] Statistics suggest that 54 per cent are in full-time employment, that the mean age of members is forty years and that the mean household income of members is £30,000.

My group reflect most of these demographics. The majority who attend seem to be over thirty including the leader, Louise, who appears to be in her mid- to late thirties. Out of the thirteen people interviewed, three are in their twenties, and the remainder aged between thirty-one and sixty-seven. Hevala is the only non-white, non-British woman in the group, identifying herself as 'Middle Eastern'. The socio-economic profile of the group is predominantly middle class, reflecting the affluent social location of the meeting and members' ability to afford

---

Pastoral Care, ed. Jeanne Stevenson Moessner (Philadelphia: Westminster John Knox Press, 1996), 9–26.

107. Fulkerson, *Places of Redemption*, 3.

108. I do not name the organization in this book. This is partly because this was agreed with members and the consultant, but also because identifying the organization is not central to the argument being made. Omitting the name of the organization is not intended to protect its anonymity as the use of 'Syn', along with other distinguishing features, makes it easily identifiable.

109. The company describes itself as 'the most advanced slimming organization in the UK'.

110. According to a presentation by the organization's Food and Nutrition Database Manager in 2004.

the weekly subscription of £4.95. Those interviewed work in various skilled professions, among them, a marketing manager, admin assistant, chartered surveyor, lettings officer, hairstylist, lawyer and play-worker. Three women are retired and one does not work because of a disability. All are UK citizens and identify as heterosexual, with most describing themselves as Christian, although faith is never raised in the interviews as a motivation for weight loss.

Meetings take place in the hall of a local evangelical Anglican church and last for around one and a half hours. Louise leads most of the proceedings, frequently signing members in, weighing members and talking to new recruits about the weight loss plan. The venue is large and set out to facilitate the meeting.[111] Just past the entrance, at the end of a long row of tables, is the registration desk where members sign in. Members queue to pay as soon as they arrive and peruse the various promotional materials displayed on the tables, including corporate recipe books, magazines and flyers. After signing in and purchasing any products, participants walk over to the scale where Louise or a volunteer records their weight. The route to the scale is not always direct. In one meeting, Louise tells me she has deliberately blocked the route in the hope that members will look at the materials she has now placed on the intervening tables and decide to stay for the meeting. These tables sit in the centre of the room and are always replete with food. They house food 'tasters' produced by Louise or other members which are intended to show the kinds of foods which can be eaten on the plan. If Louise brings food items to aid her weekly motivational talk, as is common, these also appear on the tables alongside the 'healthy' food items that members donate for the 'Slimmer of the Week' prize presented at the end of the meeting.[112]

The scale is black, square and plain and displays no numbers. Weight readings appear on a monitor on the weigh-in desk that faces away from the person being weighed and towards the person recording the member's weight. The attendant on the weigh-in desk never audibly communicates an individual's weight. Instead, they write it in the member's weight loss book, pointing to it while verbalizing how much

---

111. 'Image Therapy' is understood by the organization to be a positive peer-group support environment in which members share experiences and achievements and assist one another in making changes to their lifestyles.

112. 'Slimmer of the Week' is an award given to the member who attains the most weight loss in any given week.

weight the member has lost or gained. 'Two on', 'three off', 'maintain', for instance, but all without any reference to 'pounds' as a qualifier. Most members remove their shoes before being weighed, and some remove other items like belts, jumpers and phones. In one meeting, there is talk of a woman who stripped down to her underwear.

After being weighed, those staying for the meeting start to assume their places in the horseshoe formation of chairs that occupy the centre of the room. Some make a drink in the kitchen or help themselves to the tasters while they wait for the meeting to begin. There is always plenty of chatter which sometimes makes it hard to hear the radio Louise plays in the background. Members ask one another how they have got on over the week and rehearse their explanations in advance of Louise's questioning, which is to come. Those who do not stay for the group queue get weighed and then leave abruptly, sometimes running out of the room. Often the number of people being weighed significantly outnumbers the amount of people that stay for the meeting. Once sat in the horseshoe of chairs, members are faced by an array of official and handmade posters that lean up against the legs of the tables in the middle of the room. They display mantras designed to motivate: 'Little pickers wear big knickers', 'You cannot possibly fail until you give up. Never, never give up'.

The meetings are formulaic and predictable. Louise begins by welcoming new members and by handing out awards to those who have reached significant targets: the 'Slimmer of the Week' award, the 'Half Stone' award, the 'Club Ten' award, for instance.[113] Those supplying food tasters are asked to explain what they have cooked and how it coheres with the weight loss plan. Louise then addresses each member in turn about their weight, verbalizing to the group how many pounds they have lost overall and how much weight they have gained or lost that week. Like the person on the weigh-in desk, Louise never verbalizes how much members actually weigh. The group applaud those who have lost weight, and everyone offers their own account of their foodways in explanation of their weight, predictably prompted by Louise's question, 'expected?' At the end of each member's self-reflection, Louise asks the individual to set goals for the following week. She commonly intersperses her profiling of individuals with exercises and talks designed to educate and test members' specialized

113. 'The Club Ten' award is given to members who lose 10 per cent of their body weight. This is usually the first 'target' that members will work towards.

knowledge – a game of 'Higher or Lower'[114] or a talk about how to avoid the excesses of Christmas, for example. The meeting always ends with a raffle and with Louise commissioning the group to 'go forth and shrink!'. Most leave the meeting quickly, and it is not uncommon for members to go direct from the meeting to the takeaway, the time after the meeting depicted by some as an 'eat anything' time or as the 'twilight hours'.

Why Women?

Women's bodies are the primary focus of this book. This is mainly because the majority of people attending the group are women, reflecting the general membership of weight loss organizations. The company does not restrict access to men, but women are the intended market. Mark, a fifty-year-old chartered minerals surveyor, picks up on this in his interview when he suggests that the corporate magazine provides a clue about the organization's assumed audience:

> I can't remember ever seeing a man on the front cover of the [weight loss organization's] magazine. And they had a few case studies, you know, where there were couples doing it. And yeah … I think … there probably isn't a male consultant or if there is there are not many. So it is very female orientated.

Louise also assumes her audience is female, even when Mark is present in the meeting. During one meeting in August, she promotes the organization's 'Woman of the Year Award',[115] apologizing to Mark because he cannot take part. She offers no rationale for the female-centred nature of the award, although none of the women contest it, and Mark even laughs about it. Jane wins the award. She has followed a number of diets in the past but without much success. In the meeting, she proudly tells the group she has lost over five stone (32 kilos) in fourteen months. Louise awards her with a certificate and a silk

---

114. Louise devises this game which mimics the British TV show, 'Play Your Cards Right'. In the game, she shows the group a series of pictures of foods one at a time. After each picture, members are asked to shout out whether they think the Syn value is 'higher' or 'lower' than the previous example.

115. This award is intended to celebrate the 'member' with the best success story.

sash which she wears across her chest. She also presents Jane with a bouquet of pink flowers. Jane is visibly jubilant. In another meeting in September, Louise introduces an exercise she says is designed to help us 'fit into our "frocks" (dresses) for Christmas'. Pieces of paper crackle as they circulate around the room. Each bears a black-and-white drawing of a male and female couple dancing together. The woman is wearing a knee-length ball gown and the man a tuxedo. He holds her close to his body with one arm positioned around her waist. A superimposed grid divides the woman's body into fourteen squares to represent fourteen pounds. Each square is clearly numbered. Louise instructs us to colour in one square for every pound lost. The woman with the most shaded in sections wins the task.

Whether the 'Woman of the Year' award or the picture of the female dancer,[116] it is women who constitute the focus here. It is her body that is divided into pieces and she who must commit to methodically reducing her flesh pound by pound, in the embrace and sight of her male companion, presumably until her entire body has been shaded away and there is nothing left. It is her 'success' that is measured on the scale and through the number of pounds she can eradicate. It is clear too that successful women like flowers, are elegant, wear 'frocks' and reduce their bodies willingly. They also dance with men rather than other women and do not dance alone. Both instances convey to women that they must prepare their bodies in sight of the male gaze. Both confirm that slimming is tied to 'the regime of institutionalized heterosexuality' in which women make themselves '"object and prey"' for men.[117] Such examples convey that it is women who are expected to lose weight and that 'real women are thin, nearly invisible'.[118]

---

116. We might also include here the annual 'Miss Slinky' competition which, according to the organization's website, 'is open to ladies who've slimmed down beautifully and achieved their weight loss dreams. It recognizes and rewards the success of our fantastic slimming superstars.' The use of the term 'ladies' here arguably helps to attach slimness to traditional gender stereotypes, associating the ideal feminine with beauty.

117. Sandra Lee Bartky, *Femininity and Domination: Studies in the Phenomenology of Oppression* (New York and London: Routledge, 1990), 72.

118. Cecilia Hartley, 'Letting Ourselves Go: Making Room for the Fat Body in Feminist Scholarship', in *Bodies out of Bounds*, 61.

The Special Meaning of Weight for Women

These stories suggest that weight carries special meaning for women.[119] It is this feminist position that I forward in this book and which provides an additional justification for my focus on women. Although dieting is now considered to be acceptably masculine with many men feeling increasingly under pressure to reduce their size,[120] levels of body dissatisfaction and fixation upon thinness continue to be higher among women and girls. 'Pro-ana'[121] blogs and online spaces, as well as 'thinspiration' (or 'thinspo') images of thin and predominantly female bodies, expose just how important avoiding fat and maintaining a low body weight is, especially for women. In the United States, it is estimated that twenty million women have an eating disorder.[122] One in 200 women are affected by anorexia, and two to three in 100 by

---

119. S. Bear Bergman argues that as a trans person who is taken for a man most of the time, whether they are seen as fat depends on the way their body is gendered by onlookers. Bergman reflects that 'as a man, I'm a big dude, but not outside the norm for such things. ... As a woman, I am revolting. I am not only unattractively mannish but also grossly fat' (141). This further supports the view that what constitutes fat is determined by the gendered coding of bodies. See S. Bear Bergman, 'Part-Time Fatso', in *The Fat Studies Reader*, 139–42.

120. Lee F. Monaghan argues that masculinity does not provide a shield for deflecting anti-fat prejudice. He notes that men contacted during his research reported feeling increasingly under pressure to attend to their appearance. *Men and the War on Obesity: A Sociological Study* (London and New York: Routledge, 2008), 73–6.

121. Pro-ana and pro-mia websites tend to promote positive and non-medicalized views of anorexia and bulimia and are usually formed and used by people with anorexic and bulimia who do not wish to recover. First emerging in the late 1990s, these online platforms tended to present anorexia and bulimia as lifestyle choices rather than as illnesses that required cure. In more recent years, pro-ana sites have sought to advocate how to live 'safely' as anorectic. For more, see Ashley C. Rondini, 'The Internet and Medicalization: Reshaping the Global Body and Illness', in *Bodies and the Sociology of Health*, ed. Elizabeth Ettorre (London and New York: Routledge, 2010), 107–20.

122. NEDA, 'Research on Males and Eating Disorders', https://www.nationaleatingdisorders.org/research-males-and-eating-disorders (accessed 6 August 2017).

bulimia.[123] American women and girls aged between fifteen and twenty-four are twelve times more likely to die from anorexia nervosa than any other illness.[124] In the UK, more than 725,000 people are reported to have an eating disorder, the majority of whom are women.[125] Dieting, weight loss and purging behaviours are said to be even more common and sometimes just as fatal.[126] The vast numbers of women intentionally pursuing weight loss through dieting also show no sign of abating. In the United States alone, 91 per cent of college-aged women are reportedly trying to lose weight,[127] 80 per cent of thirteen-year-old girls have attempted to lose weight and 50 per cent of girls aged between eleven and thirteen see themselves as overweight.[128]

Faced with such evidence of diminished physical and mental health, and alarmingly high mortality rates associated with eating disorders and dieting behaviour among women in particular, the need for feminist theologies to pay attention is self-evident. These statistics and trends also suggest that fat may not be the real enemy but fear of fat and the

123. South Carolina Department of Mental Health, 'Eating Disorder Statistics', http://www.state.sc.us/dmh/anorexia/statistics.htm (accessed 3 November 2016).

124. Ibid. A study of 14,686 Australian women between the ages of eighteen and twenty-three shows that one in five underweight women reported dieting to lose weight, that dieting was associated with higher levels of depression, decreased physical health and greater body dissatisfaction (Justin Kenardy, Wendy J. Brown and Emma Yogt, 'Dieting and Health in Young Australian Women', *European Eating Disorders Review* 9 (2001): 247–8 and 250).

125. BEAT, 'The Costs of Eating Disorders: Social, Health and Economic Impacts' (February 2015), https://www.beateatingdisorders.org.uk/uploads/documents/2017/10/the-costs-of-eating-disorders-final-original.pdf (accessed 18 February 2019). The report notes that underreporting among men may contribute to this (23).

126. National Collaborating Centre for Mental Health, 'Eating Disorders: Core Interventions in the Treatment and Management of Anorexia Nervosa, Bulimia Nervosa and Related Eating Disorders' (2004): 7, https://www.nice.org.uk/guidance/cg9/evidence/full-guideline-243824221 (accessed 3 November 2016).

127. Marketdata Enterprises Inc., 'The U.S. Weight Loss Market: 2014 Status Report & Forecast' (1 February 2014), available online: http://www.marketresearch.com/Marketdata-Enterprises-Inc-v416/Weight-Loss-Status-Forecast-8016030/ (accessed 23 April 2014).

128. South Carolina Department of Mental Health, 'Eating Disorder Statistics'.

quest for an ideal (thin) body.[129] According to one source, 54 per cent of American women aged eighteen to twenty-five would rather be run over by a truck than be extremely fat.[130] This not only reveals 'thin' as the 'invisible, unmarked counterpart' to the category of obesity[131] but also suggests that any feminist theological discussion of weight loss dieting must engage critically with the politics of fat phobia as well as with the cultural appetite for thinness. This book offers such a response.

But Men Diet Too!

Feminist engagements with weight loss and the compulsion for thinness need, however, to acknowledge that women are not the only people concerned about their weight. Although statistics confirms the prevalence of dieting and eating disorders among women, it also shows that men are being increasingly affected. In the United States, it is estimated that ten million men will have an eating disorder at some point in their lives.[132] Body dis-ease among men may also be more common what statistics suggest. According to the National Eating Disorders Association (NEDA), men may face a 'double stigma' for having an eating disorder typically branded as 'feminine or gay' and for seeking psychological help.[133] Lower recorded levels of eating disorders among boys and men then may reflect a reluctance to disclose struggle because of stigma. Statistics that expose the prevalence of disordered eating and dieting behaviour among women and girls may, therefore, need closer inspection.

---

129. Michelle Lelwica warns that 'the real epidemic is among those with seemingly "normal" eating habits, who regularly police their appetites with the aim of getting or staying noticeably slim'. See M. Lelwica, E. Hoglund and J. McNallie, 'Spreading the Religion of Thinness from California to Calcutta', *Journal of Feminist Studies in Religion* 25, no. 1 (2009): 20.

130. Rina Rossignol, 'Fat Liberation (?) Assumptions of a Thin World', *Journal of Progressive Human Services* 14, no. 1 (2003): 6.

131. Elena Levy-Navarro, 'Fattening Queer History', in *The Fat Studies Reader*, 16.

132. NEDA, 'Research on Males and Eating Disorders'. One study also suggests that exposure to muscular male figures in the commercial media produces a measurable effect on levels of body dissatisfaction among men. Richard A. Leit, James J. Gray and Harrison G. Pope, 'The Media Representation of the Ideal Male', *International Journal of Eating Disorders* 31, no. 3 (March 2002): 337.

133. NEDA, 'Research on Males and Eating Disorders'.

Bell and McNaughton criticize feminist narratives on weight loss dieting for playing down men's involvement and for seeing this as either a recent development or relatively insignificant in comparison to women's weight loss practices. They suggest that statistics relating to patterns of dieting among men may not be an accurate indicator of levels of body anxiety among men. Men may feel uncomfortable attending organized weight loss groups or feel unable to voice their concerns about weight, but this does not mean that men are not engaging in weight loss activities.[134] Drawing on the work of Hillel Schwartz, Peter Streams and Sander Gilman, they argue that evidence shows men actively participating in weight loss dieting, even if they are silent about it. Such historical analyses, they claim, reveal a particular emphasis for men on muscle development and also signal that men have been just as readily confronted with images of slender male models. Bell and McNaughton, therefore, conclude that although men are encouraged to get big by gaining muscle, this does not equate to a relaxation of the fat-free norm. Fat is maligned in men because it is symbolic of the feminine and viewed as a threat to masculinity, but fat carries multiple meanings for men and for women that cannot simply be understood from the perspective of gender analysis.[135] They thus warn against one-dimensional studies that do not take account of how weight intersects with ethnicity, gender and sexuality.

I am sympathetic to much of this. It is true that cultural fears about fatness and obsessions about thinness intersect with cultural and theological constructs of gender, race, sexuality, disability and other sites of difference. However, if fat is feared in men as a symbol of a feminized body which undermines masculinity, then this only supports the feminist critique which would locate fear of fat with an entrenched fear of the female body. Fear of the feminized male body exposes the same disdain for the female body, and I suggest this is rightly theorized as an outworking of patriarchy and appropriately met by feminist challenge.[136] It may be that the male pressure to bulk up does not erase the pressure to be slim, however this is possibly

---

134. Kristen Bell and Darlene McNaughton, 'Feminism and the Invisible Fat Man', *Body & Society* 13, no. 1 (2007): 116.

135. They argue that in black rap culture, fat is often seen as hyper-masculine and as an assertion of, rather than a threat to, masculinity. Ibid., 195 ff.

136. Also see Jana Evans Braziel, 'Deterritorializing the Fat Female Body', in *Bodies Out of Bounds*. 'Even today fatness in men marks them as "effeminate", "emasculated", and "soft"' (238).

because leanness is subsumed into the muscular-masculine ideal. While thinness is an integral feature of this, muscle often matters more.[137] While muscle is intended to lower the body's fat percentage and so remains connected with reducing fat, this association is arguably more indirect than the pressure placed on women, which is a more unilateral pressure to be thin.

In the case of the group at the centre of this book, its majority female demographic is actually experienced by Mark as an environment in which he feels more at ease to name his body concerns without fear of embarrassment. He tells me in his interview: 'It's easier to be a bloke that's overweight and 50 [because] you just sort of look like every other 50 year old bloke, you know, apart from one or two.' Women, on the other hand, are 'more self-conscious about their image', and this makes him feel happier in their company. 'I actually prefer the company of women in a situation like that,' he remarks. He finds the group to be a positive space where he can meet with like-minded people to voice concerns about weight: concerns he believes men are not expected to have, especially in their fifties. Unlike Bell and McNaughton who argue that low levels of dieting reported among men may suggest they are uncomfortable attending organized weight loss groups or feel awkward speaking about their weight concerns,[138] Mark's comments suggest that majority-women weight loss groups may, in some cases, provide important contexts for men to voice body anxieties. They may offer important settings in which men can break with cultural taboos and silence surrounding masculinity, fat and age.

---

137. In their study, Leit, Gray, and Pope found that exposure to adverts featuring muscular men increased the discrepancy between men's actual muscularity and their body ideals. Such images produced increased levels of body dissatisfaction in some men, however 'this dissatisfaction was primarily with respect to musculature, rather than body fat' (Leit, Gray and Pope, 'The Media Representation of the Ideal Male'). For more, see Harrison G. Pope, Jr, Amanda J. Gruber, Barbara Mangweth, Benjamin Bureau, Christine deCol, Roland Jouvent and James I. Hudson, 'Body Image Perception Among Men in Three Countries', *American Journal of Psychiatry* 157, no. 8 (2000): 1297-301.

138. Bell and McNaughton, 'Feminism and the Invisible Fat Man', 116.

Fat, Feminism and Intersectionality: Limitations and Opportunities

This book suggests that the construction of female embodiment under patriarchy means that women's bodies are seen as especially dangerous and in need of discipline. Within this system, fatness takes on special meaning because it signifies a body that refuses to be bound, a body 'out of bounds', to cite the title of Braziel and LeBesco's edited collection.[139] Unlike LeBesco and other feminist voices within the field of Fat Studies, I pay particular attention to how religion assists with this coding of fat. It is striking how religion is absent from interdisciplinary debate on fat.[140] Although intersectionality figures strongly as authors probe the complex ways in which fatness is configured in relation to other matrices of power relating to gender, sexuality, nationality and class, for example, such debate often overlooks the way religion intersects with discourses about fat or with fat identity.[141] By providing a distinctly theological contribution to feminist studies and fat studies, I probe the intersections between Christian systems of belief and fat and between religion and thin, while engaging a feminist analysis that addresses

139. LeBesco and Braziel (eds), *Bodies out of Bounds*.

140. This point is raised by Lynne Gerber, Susan Hill and LeRhonda Manigault-Bryant in their special issue of the international journal *Fat Studies* that deliberately engages with the intersection between religion and fat in light of this deficit. See Lynne Gerber, Susan Hill and LeRhonda Manigault-Bryant, 'Religion and Fat = Protestant Christianity and Weight Loss? On the Intersections of Fat Studies and Religious Studies', *Fat Studies* 4, no. 2 (2015): 82–91.

141. The under-representation of religion in critical discussion of fat is also evidenced by the way *The Fat Studies Reader* edited by Esther Rothblum and Sondra Solovay addresses subjects like the history of fat, the queerness of fat, class and fatness, race and fatness, gender and fatness, public policy and fat, age and fat, education and fat, but without any consideration of the intersection between religion and fat. This may be evidence of a more general tendency among intersectional approaches to overlook the place of religion in their analysis and theorizing. Dawn Llewellyn and Sonya Sharma note that it is only recently that religion has undergone intersectional analysis. This may reflect how religion and theology are sometimes side-lined outside of theology and religious studies academic departments and a tendency within feminist theory and gender studies to neglect religion. See their 'Introduction', in *Religion, Equalities, and Inequalities*, ed. Dawn Llewellyn and Sonya Sharma (London and New York: Routledge, 2016), xix.

the way the gendering of fat is tied to other structures of domination, including philosophical, classist, racist, heterosexist, ableist and colonial systems. I show how one slimming organization appropriates the Christian moral rhetoric of sin (Syn) and related ideas about salvation to feed cultural fears about fat. As such, I extend Bell and McNaughton's claim that fatness and thinness are cultural carriers of multiple forms of privilege and discrimination surrounding gender, class, ethnicity, age, sexuality and dis/ability, to argue that religion assists with moralizing and polarizing these constructs. Religion and theology, I argue, provide an important explanatory tool for making sense of women's weight loss practices and beliefs.

Of course, early feminist studies on dieting and fat can seem quite limited today due to their failure to attend sufficiently to the complex intersections between fat and other aspects of identity. Yet these works have helped establish fat and thin as weighty issues in need of feminist critique. Susie Orbach, for example, has been incredibly important for emphasizing the ways in which women are often judged on the basis of their looks. For her, the pressure on women to comply with the slim ideal means that the thought of rebellion against such pressures leads to feelings of 'uneasiness' and 'freakishness' among women,[142] and similar feelings are expressed by women in the group. So normal is the expectation that women's bodies should be slim and fat maligned that questioning these norms becomes practically impossible, Orbach argues. This enables the problem underlying the 'thinness campaign' to go untapped – namely, the construction of femininity under patriarchy.

As examples of second wave feminism, such accounts frame the pursuit of thinness as a response to the shift in gender roles at the end of the twentieth century and resultant advances made by women in terms of status and social influence. Orbach, Naomi Wolf, Kim Chernin and others explain the quest for thinness as a backlash against women's power,[143] what Orbach terms a 'skewed reaction to women's desires to be regarded seriously'.[144] It functions to remind women that they 'must

---

142. Susie Orbach, *Fat Is a Feminist Issue* (London: Arrow Books, 1978), 203.

143. See, for example, also Susan Faludi, *Backlash: The Undeclared War against Women* (London: Vintage, 1993), who links the rise of women's sexual liberation with an increased emphasis on women's appearance and the thin ideal.

144. Orbach, *Fat Is a Feminist Issue*, 203. Also see Wolf, *The Beauty Myth*.

not occupy more than a little space'[145] and to 'checkmate power at every level in individual women's lives'.[146] For Wolf, it replaces the 'Feminine Mystique' described by Betty Friedan, by relocating women's fulfilment from 'housework' to 'beauty work'.[147] In committing to weight loss, women exchange the frustrations of daily life and of living in a world of gender and other inequalities for control over their appetites. In so doing, they are robbed of their bodies, spending time and energy on perfecting their appearance rather than on changing the social circumstances that cause them to pursue weight loss as a 'solution' in the first place.[148]

Although this book is in broad agreement with this position, it troubles the assumption that women are co-opted into the 'Beauty Myth'. Such a critique, I suggest, fails to sufficiently take account of women as social agents. In addition to this, it is important to recognize that women do not experience embodiment in the same way nor do they experience fat or the pressures of thin in identical ways. For Hevala in this weight loss group, for example, the pursuit of thinness is not simply about weight; it provides a way of Westernizing her non-Western body. She moved to the UK from Kurdistan when she was three and tells me about a humiliating experience when she was weighed in her school class:

> I was eight years old and we were having some kind of project, and everybody was doing something. And they were talking about weight and the teacher's going 'right everybody, these are scales and they weigh you'. And she said, 'I want somebody to volunteer to come and stand on them' and I didn't obviously, I sort of like didn't volunteer. Then the teacher goes, 'Hevala, you can do it.' An' I remember going, walking up to it and just, it's like the longest walk in my life, and my whole body was shaking. I stood on it and it was, I was 8 years old and 8 stone and all my friends were like 5 ½ [stone] or something – you know, what the average weight is – and I was quite big, obviously, compared to them all. I was mortified, cos she went 'oh, oh, right'. I don't think she expected it to be that much and she just sort of like, quite embarrassed, carried on talking.

145. Orbach, *Fat Is a Feminist Issue*, 204.
146. Wolf, *The Beauty Myth*, 19.
147. Ibid., 16–17.
148. Orbach, *Fat Is a Feminist Issue*, 202–3.

Hevala explains that it is from this point that she comes to see her body as too big. In the interview she blames her mother's excessive feeding for her size, defining this as a 'Middle Eastern thing' that her mother failed to curb after moving to the UK. In making these connections, Hevala depicts weight loss as an opportunity to reverse the harm done by her mother's (over)feeding and to assimilate into normative (white, Eurocentric) culture. It is arguably because she employs the Eurocentric lens adopted by her teacher in this story that Hevala comes to understand her Kurdish body as 'obviously' big and distinct from the 'average' bodies of her (white?) classmates. Weight loss becomes a means by which her Middle Eastern female body can gain validation as 'normal' (read: white). Moreover, attending the group grants her access to a 'white' social network.

This brings to the fore the importance of feminist work on the colonial dimensions of the thin ideal. Michelle Lelwica claims that the rise of eating disorders among non-white women in Westernized, postcolonial societies shows how women across the globe are embracing this 'homogenizing export'.[149] Such an ideal, she suggests, testifies to the 'missionizing' reach of the elite white-Western vision of womanhood which is produced and disseminated by the popular media.[150] It not only reinforces women's subordination in comparison with men but also establishes 'the hierarchical position of a select few women (those who are tall, white, wealthy and thin) above a diversity of "others"'.[151] The white-Western-thin feminine ideal thus becomes the lens through which all women's bodies are judged across the globe, and this is arguably why Hevala judges her own body to be inadequate.

It is this colonial, Eurocentric, middle-class, able-bodied, heteropatriarchal account of femininity which surfaces in the weight loss group depicted in this book. Yet it is important to appreciate that such an identification of thinness with economic and cultural privilege has not always been the case. In the Middle Ages and at the start of the Renaissance in Europe, for example, the fuller female figure was valued. At this time, Europe was plagued by disease and so the larger woman came to be a sign of life, fertility and health.[152] In eighteenth-century

---

149. Lelwica, Hoglund and McNallie, 'Spreading the Religion of Thinness.', 32.
150. Ibid., 25 and 30.
151. Ibid., 26.
152. Catrina Brown and Karin Jasper, 'Why Weight? Why Women? Why Now?', in *Consuming Passions: Feminist Approaches to Weight Preoccupation and Eating Disorders,* ed. Catrina Brown and Karin Jasper (Toronto: Second

Europe, when food supply started to be more reliable, resistance to food started to be a symbol of refinement. With the rise of the middle class towards the end of the nineteenth century, eating and appearance came to operate as markers to separate the middle class from the working class.[153] Thinness among women thus came to be a sign of distinction, and women learnt the etiquette of 'the cult of the lady'. It was only at this point that women who could eat well deliberately chose not to with the regulation of food and eating seen as a sign of wealth.[154]

Today, however, reports show that non-Western cultures which have experienced economic growth and growing levels of industrialization and Westernization are seeing similar patterns of obesity and body dissatisfaction as the West.[155] Cross-cultural studies suggest that disturbed eating among girls is also evident in non-industrialized societies which have been heavily influenced by Western norms and institutions.[156] As such, it seems that poor socio-economic status and

---

Story Press, 1993), 20-1. Brown and Jasper note that the fuller female figure tends to be valued more in times of economic hardship, when food production is unreliable or in shortage, and the thinner female body valued more in times of economic affluence (Ibid., 20).

153. See Mervant Nasser, *Culture and Weight Consciousness* (London and New York: Routledge, 1997), 3.

154. Brown and Jasper, 'Why Weight? Why Women? Why Now?', 22.

155. Maho Isono, Patti Lou Watkins and Lee Ee Lian, 'Bon Bon Fatty Girl: A Qualitative Exploration of Weight Bias in Singapore', in *The Fat Studies Reader*, 127-38. This study shows women in modern Singapore impacted by weight-related remarks and weight bias. It suggests that Singapore emulates Western culture's rise in 'obesity' and eating disorders partly because of its transition from a relatively poor nation (where fat was previously desirable) to a richer power. With industrialization comes an increase in body weight and an increase in fat stigma; hence, Singapore is now seeing fat bodies regulated through slimming centres and weight loss products much like other Western nations. Also see Sing Lee, Y. Y. Lydia Chan and L. K. George Hsu, 'The Intermediate-Term Outcome of Chinese Patients with Anorexia Nervosa in Hong Kong', *The American Journal of Psychiatry* 160 (May 2003): 967-72. This study observes similar rising trends in anorexia among women in societies such as Hong Kong, Japan, Singapore and Taiwan. Even in China, rising trends in anorexia echo Western patterns of body dissatisfaction and a growing propensity towards fat phobia.

156. Lelwica, *Starving for Salvation*, 20.

non-whiteness do not protect women from the thin ideal. According to NEDA, the view that eating disorders only affect white wealthy women is a 'myth'. 'We do know', it remarks, 'that the prevalence of eating disorders is similar among Non-Hispanic Whites, Hispanics, African-Americans, and Asians in the United States, with the exception that anorexia nervosa is more common among Non-Hispanic Whites'.[157] Even where many do not have enough to eat, women struggle to resist the hegemonic white-Western-thin feminine ideal. Once again, this substantiates the 'missionizing' reach of the elite white-Western vision of womanhood.

My focus on women in this book then does not dismiss the way gender intersects with race, class, age, nation, sexuality and other signifiers in order to locate women's bodies as cultural carriers of various expressions of civility and decency. It focuses on the particular pressures women feel to reduce their size but without assuming all women are similarly positioned in the hegemony of thinness (as victims) and without reducing the 'tyranny of slenderness'[158] to a matter of gender alone.[159]

157. The National Eating Disorders Association, 'Race, Ethnicity and Culture', http://www.nationaleatingdisorders.org/race-ethnicity-and-culture (accessed 11 November 2016). Soh, Tonuyz and Surgenor similarly observe that 'the treasured ideal of slimness has percolated through all levels of society via the media' lending increasing support to the view that eating pathology is no longer restricted to the wealthy. 'Eating and Body Image Disturbances across Cultures: A Review', *European Eating Disorders Review* 14, no. 1 (2006): 54–65, esp. 59.

158. This phrase is used by Kim Chernin in her classic work, *The Obsession: Reflections on the Tyranny of Slenderness*.

159. Thinness may, for instance, be a way for non-heterosexual women to gain recognition, acceptance and achievement in a heteronormative society. Hesse-Biber suggests that even though thinness is tied up with a heterosexual view of femininity, lesbian women may still feel compelled to submit to its stringent demands, not to attract a man but to succeed in a heterosexist world, especially when it comes to employment (*The Cult of Thinness*, 208). Also see M. Feldman and I. Meyer, 'Eating Disorders in Diverse, Lesbian, Gay, and Bisexual Populations', *International Journal of Eating Disorders* 40, no. 3 (2007): 218–26. Race and class are also important markers. According to Public Health England, women from black African groups have the highest prevalence of obesity and people with disabilities more likely to be obese (Public Health England,

Go Forth and Shrink!

Before I outline the shape this book will take, I want to draw the reader's attention to certain terminology. First, as far as possible, from this point on I avoid the term 'dieting'. Members of the weight loss group mainly do not use it, and the organization advocates a strong anti-diet message that places deliberate emphasis on what members can eat rather than focusing on deprivation. I thus refer to 'slimming' and 'weight loss' rather than 'dieting', employing both terms interchangeably to mean the process of pursuing a thinner body. I refer to the weight loss programme as the 'plan' because this is the terminology employed by members and the consultant.

I also avoid terms like 'obese' or 'overweight', except where members choose to use them. These are medical terms which employ scientific measures of ideal body weight, such as the body mass index (BMI), to categorize bodies according to their perceived level of risk. What constitutes 'overweight' or 'obese' depends on the measures used and the borderlines of these categories have changed and shifted over time and in tandem with social attitudes and prejudices about body size. As such, I see them as ideologically loaded (premised on certain ideas about normality and health), politically driven and as culturally positioned rather than as providing objective, dispassionate measures

---

'Health Inequalities', http://www.noo.org.uk/NOO_about_obesity/inequalities (accessed 11 November 2016). In the United States, obesity is reported to be more prevalent among black and Latina communities, linked in the latter case with food insecurity (Trust for America's Health and Robert Wood Johnson Foundation, 'Race and Ethnic Disparities in Obesity', http://stateofobesity.org/disparities/ [accessed 11 November 2016]). Some studies also confirm that in the West there is a correlation between economic status and weight. Women of higher socio-economic status are more likely to diet and have a lower body weight (see Sog, Touyz and Surgenor, 'Eating and Body Image Disturbances Across Cultures: A Review', 58). Also, obesity (which is more prevalent among women) tends to increase with greater levels of deprivation (Public Health England, Health Inequalities). Fat is a negative marker of distinction and class difference, as Lynne Gerber argues, 'Few seeking cultural participation or authority can afford to be tainted with its stain.' Gerber, *Seeking the Straight and Narrow: Weight Loss and Sexual Reorientation in Evangelical America* (Chicago and London: University of Chicago Press, 2011), 230.

of health.[160] I prefer to use the term 'fat' as this more accurately locates notions of the ideal body within social, historical, cultural and political discourses, rather than in relation to seemingly pre-determined, neutral categories. It is a subjective term with undecided meaning. Many members see or think of themselves as fat despite their average and sometimes even small size. Helen, for example, tells me, 'I know that I'm overweight again, but I'm not like *overweight*. But to me that's how I think of myself.' She, like others, implies that 'overweight' reflects her own perception of her body, rather than being an objective category. This follows Colls in suggesting it is possible to 'feel' as well as 'look' fat, and that fat cannot be reduced to a simple visual descriptor.[161] It also reflects wider cultural trends with Anglo-American society where women see their bodies as 'too fat' regardless of their size.[162]

The Shape of This Book

This book begins by exploring the categories of Syn and salvation narrated and embodied by women in the weight loss group. Chapter 1 uncovers the negative meanings attributed to Syn by members and Louise, drawing out prominent associations with defilement, danger, death, guilt and shame and how these continue normative theological

---

160. I will say more about this in Chapter 6.

161. See R. Colls, 'Review of Bodies Out of Bounds: Fatness and Transgression', *Gender, Place and Culture: A Journal of Feminist Geography* 9, no. 2 (2002): 219.

162. Kim Chernin in *The Obsession* recognizes that fat is not necessarily an indication of weight. 'I am concerned ... with the large numbers of us who think we are overweight when we are not and spend the better part of every waking moment pursued by a nagging worry about the pseudo-obesity we suffer from,' she comments (35). Ellen Granberg, in highlighting that it is not uncommon for 'normal-sized' people to see themselves as overweight, argues that 'these perceptions can influence behaviour as strongly as weight itself, or more so'. See her article, '"Is That All There Is?" Possible Selves, Self-Change, and Weight Loss', *Social Psychology Quarterly* 69, no. 2 (2006): 110. April Herndon argues that 'culturally "fat" can mark any woman, referencing body size in general, a jiggle of a thigh, or the slight swell of a tummy'. Such a lack of clarity, she suggests, exposes all women to the danger of discrimination. See 'Disparate but Disabled: Fat Embodiment and Disability Studies', *NWSA Journal* 14, no. 3 (2002): 132.

meanings in helping to locate women's bodies and appetites as especial sites of suspicion and danger. Chapter 2 complexifies this landscape by exposing the way traditional theological discourse is adapted through a positive association of Syn with permission. It explores how various methods of self-surveillance help participants to skilfully negotiate the ambiguities of Syn. I argue that tensions between self-care and self-harm and between agency and domination continue historic, theological ambivalences in approaching embodiment. Chapter 3 considers the relationship between weight loss and salvation, identifying the ways in which the organization and its members frame weight loss in redemptive terms. Given the appropriation of the Christian lexicon of Syn, these connections are once again plotted against a specifically Christian theological background. Through the course of these initial chapters, Christian theologies emerge alongside other social systems as disciplinary frameworks which help restrain women's bodies and temper their desire, and as systems which might encourage practices of self-care, facilitate women's freedom and cultivate concern for the body's wholeness, aliveness and fullness.

Chapters 4–6 use the insights from my ethnography to think again about the categories of sin and salvation asking how they might be usefully employed in response to a culture where fears about fat are reaching epic proportions and the quest for thinness among women shows no sign of abating. Emphasis here is on amplifying the aspects of women's Syn and salvation narratives together with related theological traditions which have been shown in Chapters 1–3 to be worthwhile and liberating, while modifying, limiting or rejecting those aspects which have been shown to engender harm.[163] Chapter 4 focuses on the theme of sin suggesting that this Christian moral terminology expresses the complex material realities that diminish bodies and which prevent bodies from thriving alongside other bodies. Sin, I suggest, is an historical material reality that disrupts people's God-intended, original createdness for relation, aliveness and flourishing and can be appropriately named as 'sizeism', the 'victimization of food' and the 'divided self'. Extending the feminist hamartiology of Rosemary Radford Ruether and her account of sin as sexism and as distorted

---

163. I am influenced here by Stephen Pattison's proposal of how to theologically deal with shame. See *Shame: Theory, Therapy, Theology* (Cambridge: Cambridge University Press, 2000), 298.

relationality, I propose that sin describes distorted ways of relating to food, fat and the 'bodyself'.[164]

The final two chapters return to the notion of 'salvation' arguing that this takes on meaning in relation to the daily lived experience of ordinary women. Salvation, I argue, is a form of reconciliatory action, a praxis that emerges from a refusal to let the sins of sizeism, the victimization of food and the divided self have the last word. In Chapter 5, I present salvation as the alimentary and erotic practice of 'sensible eating' – a mode of eating that reconnects food with feeling, pleasure, sensuality, desire and passion and which orients women towards the alimentary and relational practices of touch and taste. In Chapter 6, I identify salvation with the observance of Sabbath arguing that rest and repose from fat hatred and from the frenetic sacrificial work of burning fat have the potential to open up a redemptive space for faith-based expressions of fat pride and for practices intent on making peace with fat rather than waging war against it. Both chapters call for a theological reinterpretation of cultural and Christian attitudes towards food and fat. They return to many of the themes uncovered in women's weight loss narratives, sometimes using overlooked theologies to turn harmful renditions of sin and salvation towards more liberating, lifeful ends and sometimes using the worthwhile features of women's Syn and salvation narratives to challenge harmful theological traditions and practices, and help redirect theological perspectives. In both cases, I offer practical theologies of sin and salvation in the hope that they may be sources of nourishment for women with whom the issues in this book resonate.

164. Carter Heyward presents the notion of the 'bodyself' to depict the body and self as one integrated unit. See, for example, *Touching Our Strength: The Erotic as Power and the Love of God* (New York: Harper San Francisco, 1989), 8.

Chapter 1

SYN, DANGER AND DISORDERED DESIRE

This chapter begins to uncover the ways in which Christian attitudes, beliefs and patterns of action resurface in secular guise in the slimming group.[1] It describes and discusses the notion of 'Syn' at the centre of the weight loss plan, charting its meaning for the organization and its members.

Alliances between sin, food and fat are ubiquitous in contemporary Western capitalist culture. According to Lynne Gerber, most Americans experience feelings of goodness and badness, 'even sinfulness and redemption' in relation to their eating.[2] She argues that Protestant religion has helped to imbue the secular quest for thinness with quasi-religious meaning. Up to the close of the nineteenth century, Protestant Christianity in the United States played an important role in offsetting fears about excessive consumption and indulgence generated by capitalism, but its increasingly permissive approach to consumption saw a need to employ other mechanisms to contain modern excess.[3] Dieting and food regulation emerged as important restraints at the turn of the twentieth century, she suggests, infusing the secular pursuit of weight loss with the moral and the sacred, and framing fat as a 'secular sin'.[4]

The salience of this constructive alignment between fat and sin can be glimpsed by the way it surfaces in medical research and public

---

1. Some parts of this chapter are taken or adapted from the following articles: Hannah Bacon, 'Fat, Syn, and Disordered Eating: The Dangers and Powers of Excess', *Fat Studies* 4 (2015): 92–111; Hannah Bacon, 'Sin or Slim? Christian Morality and the Politics of Personal Choice in a Secular Commercial Weight Loss Setting', *Fieldwork in Religion* 8, no. 1 (2013): 92–109, © Equinox Publishing Ltd 2013. They are used with kind permission of the publishers.
2. Gerber, *Seeking the Straight and Narrow*, 21.
3. Ibid., 24.
4. Peter Stearns cited by Gerber, ibid., 25. Also see Griffith, *Born Again Bodies*.

health policy. In 1995, the *British Medical Journal* published an article titled 'Obesity in Britain: Gluttony or Sloth?' causally relating obesity to excess consumption and sedentary lifestyles. According to the authors, Andrew Prentice and Susan Jebb, increased levels of fat in the British diet and increased levels of inactivity among the British public are both to blame for obesity. However, although both are causal factors, it is sloth that plays a more dominant role because energy needs have decreased at a faster rate than the increase in energy/calorie consumption.[5] A later report by the House of Commons borrows this moral language from Prentice and Jebb to construct fat in a similar way. Here, the heading 'Gluttony or Sloth?' is employed to frame discussion of the 'root causes' of obesity. Quoting directly from this earlier article, it dismisses genetics as an aetiological factor and claims that 'instead, the key question remains that articulated by Susan Jebb and Andrew Prentice in 1995: … "Should obesity be blamed on **gluttony**, **sloth**, or both?"'.[6] By placing the terms gluttony and sloth in bold type, the report ensures that even greater emphasis is placed on the language of sin.[7]

Neither document acknowledges how 'gluttony' and 'sloth' tie obesity discourse to the Christian language of sin.[8] Indeed, the terms appear to be used without much critical consideration, but gluttony and sloth have both been labelled as 'deadly sins' by the Church.[9] Rendered

---

5. Andrew M. Prentice and Susan A. Jebb, 'Obesity in Britain: Gluttony or Sloth?', *British Medical Journal* 311 (1995): 437–9.

6. House of Commons, *Obesity: Third Report of Session 2003-04*, vol. 1 (London: The Stationery Office Limited), 23. Emphasis in original.

7. William James Hoverd also makes this point in his discussion of the House of Commons report. See his essay, 'Deadly Sin: Gluttony, Obesity and Health Policy', in *Medicine, Religion and the Body*, ed. Elizabeth Burns Coleman and Kevin White (Leiden and Boston: Brill, 2010), 208.

8. For social historian Roberta Seid, the ancient sins of gluttony and sloth have become inculcated in a 'new faith' of slimming such that Americans believe that controlling what they eat will lead to virtue. She maintains that politics, fashion, medicine, the food industry and the rise of feminism have all contributed to 'the new American creed of slenderness and fitness' (20) in which 'eating for pleasure is sin' (25) and 'eating right' means not to eat at all (30). Roberta P. Seid, *Never Too Thin: Why Women Are at War with Their Bodies* (New York: Prentice Hall Press, 1989).

9. Susan Hill, *Eating to Excess: The Meaning of Gluttony and the Fat Body in the Ancient World* (Santa Barbara: Praeger, 2011), 121. Also see Chapter 6.

thus, they have been constructed as inappropriate behaviours and as personal faults which stand to drag the righteous away from spiritual purity and love for others.[10] For human geographer Bethan Evans, the deliberate use of the terms in the House of Commons report implicates the notion of 'sin' and provides an instance of how medical and moral discourses on fat combine to legitimize the stigmatization, medicalization and othering of fat bodies. She suggests that the language of gluttony and sloth 'draws on and reproduces particular moralities regarding (fat) bodies',[11] framing fat in terms of remorseless weight gain and complacency.[12] Yet Evans also fails to probe the theologies of sin operating in the background of such policy documentation.

In the weight loss group I attend, the concept and terminology of 'Syn' is foregrounded. The word 'Syn' is seen, spoken and heard, albeit without any acknowledgement of its religious roots. This overt use of Syn-talk departs from other weight loss programmes where concepts of sin may be more hidden and unspoken. Sociologist Kandi Stinson, for example, finds that in the group she studies, 'though rarely mentioned explicitly, notions of sin lie close to the surface as food and eating are dichotomized into good and bad'.[13] Like Evans, she is not inclined to probe the theological meanings at work, but she does detect that notions of sin are camouflaged in 'red light foods' that are difficult to eat in small amounts.[14]

In this chapter, I scrutinize the weight loss narratives and micro-practices of members in the group to plot the complex ways in which the association between fat and sin develops. Syn forms part of the specialized language and knowledge that members are expected to learn and accurately reproduce. As such, food and weight are not simply talked about through the moralizing categories of 'good' and 'bad', as Stinson observes, but are explicitly tied to the notion of 'Syn'. This goes beyond identifying fat and thin with an abstract or vicarious concept of the sacred and instead weds members' Syn-talk to a Christian moral symbolic and to a number of nuanced theological meanings. Although some commentators have seen the association between fat and sin

10. Hoverd, 'Deadly Sin: Gluttony, Obesity and Health Policy', 215.
11. Bethan Evans, '"Gluttony or Sloth": Critical Geographies of Bodies in (Anti)Obesity Policy', *Area* 38, no. 3 (2006): 260.
12. Ibid., 264.
13. Stinson, *Women and Dieting Culture*, 121.
14. Ibid., 120.

in popular discourse as a trivial connection that lacks any serious grounding in religion,[15] I claim that the identification of fat with Syn draws upon a rich theological history that supplies the slimming organization with a powerful discursive mechanism for disciplining women's bodies and appetites. As well as joining with other feminists to argue that early Christian approaches to the female body are the 'taproot [of a] two thousand year old hatred and fear of flesh'[16] helping fuel Christianity's restrictive attitude to food,[17] I draw on the real, ordinary lives of women to show how religion continues to inform everyday speech about weight.

Syn: Tensions and Ambiguities

The terminology of 'Syn' is fundamental to the organization's approach to weight loss and has been claimed as its own intellectual property and trademark. In fact, so important is the term to the company's brand, that it has threatened legal action against various commercial businesses for aligning their products too closely to its weight loss service and characteristic feature of Syn. In 2005, the organization opposed a trademark application by *Sin and Slim* (another UK slimming company), contesting the use of 'sin' in its weight loss plan.[18] In 2016, the 'No! Sins Cafe' in Linthorpe, North East England, was forced to change its name or risk legal proceedings, as the company claimed it alone had

---

15. See, for example, Robert Soloman (ed.), *Wicked Pleasures: Meditations on the Seven Deadly Sins* (Lanham: Rowman and Littlefield Publishers, 1999).

16. Bovey, *The Forbidden Body*, 27.

17. Isherwood, *The Fat Jesus*, 63.

18. *Sin and Slim* have since ceased trading. For full details of legal proceedings, see M. Reynolds, 'In the Matter of Application No. 2389949 in the Name of a Different Limited and in the Matter of Opposition Thereto under No. 93939 by Miles-Bramwell Executive Services Limited' (17 December 2007), http://www.ipo.gov.uk/t-challenge-decision-results/o36607.pdf (accessed 4 December 2014). For media coverage see Rosie Murray-West, 'Slimming Clubs Weigh into Trademark War over Who Has the Right to "Sin"', *The Telegraph* (14 February 2006), http://www.telegraph.co.uk/news/uknews/1510451/Slimming-clubs-weigh-into-trademark-war-over-whohas-the-right-to-sin.html (accessed 4 December 2014).

ownership of the words 'Sin', 'Sins', 'Sin Free', and 'Syn'.[19] In 2017, the British supermarket, Asda, was made to remove its 'Slimzone' meals from its shelves which it advertised as 'Syn-Free' and as compatible with one of the slimming plans marketed by the organization.[20]

Syn, though, is not the only category employed by the company to speak about food. 'Free Foods' and 'Healthy Extras' accompany 'Syn' to make up the three classifications used in the weight loss plan to organize members' eating. Free Foods include lean meats, fish, pasta, fruit and vegetables and are presented as the way members satisfy their hunger. Members can eat as much Free Food as they choose. Healthy Extras typically refer to foods like bread, cereal, milk and cheese which are either rich in calcium or high in fibre, and these must be carefully quantified. Syn, however, is arguably the most controversial of the three categories because it depicts foods that members often see as 'bad' and is commonly saturated with angst and panic. That the term has been at the centre of so much legal wrangling testifies to its centrality not only in relation to the weight loss programme but also in relation to the company's profits.

'Syn' is a specialist term that typically depicts foods like crisps, chocolate, ice cream, cake and alcohol that are high in saturated fats and sugar. Independent of which plan members decide to follow, foods are allocated different Syn 'values' and members are advised to consume between five and fifteen Syns a day. This forms what is commonly known as the 'Syn allowance', and Louise frequently reminds those attending the meeting that they should keep a log of their daily intake. Syn values are calculated by 'Head Office' and appear as a seventeen-page list in the middle of the weight loss guide that members receive when they join. Louise never informs the group about how these are determined, and it is common for values to change as 'experts' test and tweak established calculations. Members can ascertain the most up-to-date values by consulting the

19. Bethany Lodge, 'No Sins Cafe Forced to Change Its Name after Slimming World Threatens Legal Action' (7 July 2016), https://www.gazettelive.co.uk/news/teesside-news/no-sins-cafe-forced-change-11580726 (accessed 10 May 2018).

20. Fiona Parker, 'Asda Pulls Diet Ready Meals from Shelves after Slimming World Dispute', *The Telegraph* (19 March 2017), https://www.telegraph.co.uk/news/2017/03/19/asda-pulls-diet-ready-meals-shelves-slimming-world-dispute/ (accessed 10 May 2018).

company's website, by using the online 'Syn calculator' or by calling the 'Syns Hotline.'[21]

The fine detail of what actually counts as Syn, Free Foods or Healthy Extras depends on which of the plans members follow.[22] In my group, participants mainly combine the 'Original' and 'Green' plans, oscillating between them. On the Original plan members observe what are colloquially termed as 'red' or 'meat' days, where meat, fish, fruit and vegetables are Free and items like pasta, rice, potatoes, bread, cheese, milk and cereal are classified as Healthy Extras. Whereas those foods identified as Free are unrestricted, those categorized as Healthy Extras must adhere to the portion sizes stipulated in the weight loss guide. On the Green plan members observe what are informally known as 'green days', where fruit and vegetables are Free along with rice, pasta and grains (which, it is important to note, are *not*-Free on red days). Meat and fish (which are unrestricted on red days) now accompany cheese, milk, cereals or bread in being categorized as Healthy Extras. In both plans, exceeding the permitted allocation of Healthy Extras results in Syn and negatively impacts a member's Syn allowance. The undecidability of these categories means that Syn is a slippery and indeterminate concept that evades fixed meaning. Whereas on a red day, 28 grams of lean beef is Free, on a green day it counts as two Syns; a 300-gram vegetable lasagne is eleven Syns on a red day but six Syns on a green day.[23]

Interestingly, the official definition of Syn forwarded by the organization avoids a negative overlay. The guide members receive when they join states that 'Syn' stands for 'Synergy' and portrays the way the three food groups of Healthy Extras, Free Foods and Syns work together

---

21. The company has also developed its own app that allows members to search for foods and track Syn.

22. Although members in my group tend to follow the Green and Original plans, there are other options available. The 'Extra Easy' plan has members choose Free Foods, Healthy Extras and Syns but names fish, meat, fruit, vegetables, pasta, grains, pulses and rice all as Free. This effectively means that those following this programme can combine protein and carbohydrate without weighing or measuring either. 'Mix2Max' is designed for 'days when you want to fit in with eating out or a busy schedule', according to the guide, and allows members to switch between 'Original' and 'Green' through the course of one day.

23. According to the weight loss guide published in March 2009.

to 'optimize'[24] weight loss. Members are encouraged to select Synful foods so that they do not deprive themselves of the things they enjoy, and I will say more about this positive rendering of Syn in the next chapter. It is important to acknowledge, however, at this stage, that Syn is allied with a strong anti-diet stance which places the term at a distance from normative Christian interpretation. According to the guide, Syn is to be embraced because it allows members to eat what they want without regret.

The spelling of 'Syn' though has undergone careful modification. From its inception in the late 1960s until 2004, the organization adopted the conventional Christian spelling of the term ('sin'), albeit without making any reference to its religious foundations. The 'Sin-a-Day' eating plan was promoted as a slimming tool that allowed more choice than other competitors, yet disgruntlement from members around the term's guilt-inducing capacity appears to have provoked the company to change tack.[25] In the early 2000s, the organization modified the spelling of sin to 'Syn' and marketed Synergy as a more scientific concept. Synergy spoke about nutritional balance and required members to limit consumption of saturated fats, alcohol and sugar while eating at least five portions of fruit and vegetables a day and a mix of carbohydrates and lean protein foods. By re-spelling the word, the company managed to retain the distinctive feature of their brand while attempting to adjust its meaning.

What will become apparent in this chapter is that while Syn is framed positively by the organization on its website, in other corporate materials and sometimes by Louise in the weekly meetings, members and Louise also continue to hold to well-established religious understandings and to notions of sin that connect the term to naughtiness, guilt and wilful disobedience. This exposes the system of Syn as divided within itself as it both permits and prohibits members to eat.[26] What this chapter shows is that women learn to fear Syn and to align it with personal failure, shame and moral disorder. In this respect, members restate

---

24. The general approach to weight loss promoted by this organization is called 'Food Optimising'.

25. In one online forum, 'fleur' notes that 'way back when, Syns were indeed Sins (as in naughty things, LOL). The change in spelling is a relatively new thing.' 'Jaylou' also comments, 'Over the years the word "Sins" has been much loved but greatly debated. We wanted a new word unique to [the organization].' MiniMins.com, 'Syns' (4 March 2010), https://www.minimins.com/threads/syns.139980/ (accessed 8 December 2016).

26. I will say more about this tension in Chapter 2.

the normative theological position that sin is a state from which those in danger need rescuing, and this exposes the group's Syn-talk as more closely located to traditional theological discourse than the organization's positive stance suggests.

Missing the Mark: Sin within Christian Thought

In Christianity, the notion of 'sin' has been, and continues to be, an important device for naming and shaming certain groups, individuals and behaviours. Traditional associations with dirt, pollution, impairment, disease, death, guilt and offence present the self as out of sorts, rebellious, disordered, deformed and defiled. The Greek verb translated as sin, ἁμαρτάνω (transliterated as *hamartánō*), means 'to miss the mark', to err or go wrong.[27] Sin signals a predicament of alienation, loss of potential and rebellion.[28] In Western Christianity, it has been defined most prominently as a self turned inwards upon itself (*incurvatus in se*) and as closely aligned with hubris or pride.[29] This has served to locate sin as an individual offence against God. As we will see, the notion of 'Syn' employed in the group retains this feature of individualism and continues to foreground the voluntary will. If traditional Christian theology teaches that human beings have become estranged from God, their own authentic good selves and created capacity, then women in the group reflect a similar position, albeit without reference to God, believing that Syn causes their bodies to become out of sorts and 'bad' (i.e. fat), placing them in need of repair.

Syn, Danger and Disobedience

Louise plays a vital role in establishing Syn as dangerous. She tells the group repeatedly that all foods that are not Free carry a Syn value

---

27. Regularly used in ancient times, in works by Homer and Plato, for example, the Greek verb depicts an archer missing the target. See Bible Hub, *Strong's Exhaustive Concordance of the Bible*, http://biblehub.com/greek/264.htm (accessed 18 August 2017).

28. For a discussion of these, see Paul Fiddes, *Past Event and Present Salvation: The Christian Idea of Atonement* (London: Darton Longman and Todd, 1989), 6–7.

29. For more on this, see Chapter 6.

and this serves to construct Syn and Free Food in opposition to one another. Free Foods are 'safe', she advises, because they do not need regulating; Syn, on the other hand, is unsafe and in need of tight control. Comparing a pastry sausage roll to one she has made which substitutes the pastry for wholemeal bread, she remarks that it is 'scary' how many Syns are in the proper sausage roll: eleven to be precise. In one September meeting I explain to her that I am surprised by my one pound weight loss. My family had been over, and this had meant eating food which was not strictly 'on plan' so I had anticipated a gain. Louise responds by cautioning me: thinking I can have a 'day off' places me in a 'danger zone'. I must remember to count my Syns, and not simply think I can let my hair down. I feel suitably chastised. In another meeting she recounts the instance of a woman who, on Christmas day, ate seventy Syns[30] just by not watching the food she polished off between courses. It is the Syns we don't see which stand to get us into the most trouble, she warns – the Syns lurking in salad dressings and in the bits of cereal at the bottom of the cereal box.

Louise's recurring message is that our eating must be watched and watched carefully. One evening she recounts the time when she handed out fake eye balls to the group to place in their lunch boxes as a reminder that she was watching them, and it is this eye for detail that she encourages us to develop. We must cut the rind off of our bacon she instructs, even those fiddly bits between the meat, otherwise what we think is 'Free' (on a red day) becomes Syn and unsafe. Part of the alarm surrounding Syn, then, is that Free Food might suddenly mutate and tip the member over into the kind of Syn which is irrecoverable. Vigilance is, therefore, crucial.

Members share Louise's anxiety about the dangers of Syn. Sarah, who is twenty-three and a play worker, tells me that it is the taste of crisps that threatens to stall her weight loss potential:

> The only thing I find hard is [the] Syns. When I have a sandwich – so that's like the bread's Syns – I just have this thing where I want to eat crisps. But we get like these velvet crisps. I don't know what they're called, what the name is, but they're like four Syns. But they're *so* tasty. Or we'll get *Quavers* and um. I just like find a sandwich with a few crisps on the side. And I have done that quite a lot and it's still worked but I know if I *didn't* have them.

---

30. This is presented as excessive given the weekly recommendation is between thirty-five and one hundred and five Syns.

Here Sarah implies that although she is losing weight, abstaining from crisps would accelerate her success, but she finds them too difficult to resist. Mark similarly defines savoury foods like sausage rolls and meatballs as his 'downfall'. Although feeling good about his weight loss, he wonders why this is not enough motivation to prevent him from 'slipping'.

It is customary for members to associate weight gain with Syn and moral downfall. Common parlance is that Syn causes a person to fall 'off the wagon', 'slip' or 'slide', go 'backwards' and/or 'downwards'. Ruth is sixty-seven and joins because she realizes she is putting on a stone every ten years and has decided to try and stop this. She perceives a danger with her own foodways which makes it 'very easy to just slide back into your wicked ways ... and eat all these things which are responsible for how you got where you are in the first place'. Joy tells me that in the last four years she has 'probably gone down a slippery slide', consuming more wine and causing her to put on weight. She talks too about 'not doing enough' to avoid tempting Synful foods and admits that she is 'still slipping'.

Syn also 'creeps' and surprises. Joy is a hairstylist who has attended the group for ten months at the point of her interview. She tells me,

> [It is the] wine at night and just silly things that creep on without you knowing at the time, until you look in the mirror! You go to put something on and you think, oh, what have you done? Get the wine back out and drown your sorrows!

Like Louise, she suggests that Syn is dangerous because it hides in unsuspecting places and can have serious unforeseen implications. A poster in the meeting room reiterates the point, warning that 'little pickers wear big knickers!' Syn, it would seem, can have weighty consequences.

Reconceiving the Fall: Sliding into Syn

Sausage rolls, crisps and alcohol are all defined as Syn by the organization. By identifying their consumption and taste with a slip or slide downwards, members reproduce the ancient theological principle of the Fall that aligns eating with individual moral decline and a lapse into an unintended state of moral disorder. Indeed, it is this theological trope that resurfaces most strongly in members' Syn-talk.

1. Syn, Danger and Disordered Desire 59

According to the *J* (Yahwist) creation narrative in Genesis (2.4b-24 and 3), sin enters the world through food. God commands the first human being[31] not to eat from the tree of the knowledge of good and evil, warning that 'in the day that you eat of it you shall die' (2.17). Intent that this creature should not be alone, God creates 'every animal of the field and every bird of the air' (2.19-20), but no partner is found. Taking the rib from the creature's side, God then fashions a woman, finally producing a suitable companion. After speaking with the serpent the woman concludes that the tree is 'good for food', 'a delight to the eyes' and 'to be desired to make one wise' (3.6). She eats and gives some to the man, and their eyes are subsequently opened (3.7). They see that they are naked and hide from God who is walking in the Garden. When they are questioned by God, the man blames the woman (3.12) and the woman blames the serpent (3.13), but both name eating as their sin and, together with the serpent, are punished by God (3.14-19).[32] God declares that the man has become 'like one of us knowing good and evil' and to prevent the pair from eating the fruit from the tree of life which would cause them to live forever, banishes them from the Garden (3.24).

According to Ken Stone, many early Christian thinkers reading this story considered it to speak of the dangers of food and appetite. The significant role of food in the creation narrative was something that ancient thinkers took seriously, he argues, because they believed it spoke about the realities of temptation which they experienced in their own lives and served as a warning about the temptation of food.[33]

---

31. I am influenced here by Phyllis Trible. She draws attention to the similarity between the Hebrew terms *hā-'ādām* and *hā-ᵃdāmâ* to suggest that the first human creature God creates is a sexually undifferentiated 'earth creature'. According to Trible, when God uses the rib from *hā-'ādām* to fashion the woman, the original earth creature disappears and two new beings emerge. It is at this point that sexual division is introduced hence human sexuality is introduced simultaneously. According to Trible, this renders inaccurate the common theological assumption that God creates man first. For more, see *God and the Rhetoric of Sexuality* (Philadelphia: Fortress, 1978), 78.

32. Ken Stone observes how this punishment also concerns food and eating: the serpent will eat dust (3.14) and the man will toil to produce food from the ground to eat (3.17-19). See his book, *Practicing Safer Texts: Food, Sex and Bible in Queer Perspective* (London and New York: T & T Clark, 2005).

33. Ibid., 27.

This is not difficult to detect. In *The Confessions*, Augustine laments his desire for food and drink: 'Beset by these temptations I struggle every day against gluttony for eating and drinking.'[34] Aggrieved that he cannot give up eating like he can fornication, he expresses frustration at his inability to move from hunger to satiation without passing through the 'snare of concupiscence'.[35] While he maintains that eating and drinking repair the body until such a time when both 'food and belly' will be destroyed by God,[36] the fact that he cannot avoid eating and that eating for necessity is pleasurable is deeply troubling for him. 'I fight against the pleasure in order not to be captivated by it,' he admits. 'By fasting I wage a daily warfare, and habitually force my body to obey me.'[37]

Many ancient readers held similar views considering gluttony to be the first sin. For Tertullian, for example, Adam 'yielded more readily to his belly than to God' and 'sold salvation for his gullet!' Fasting was a way to expiate the 'primordial sin' of Eden, a way to 'make God satisfaction through the self-same causative material through which he had offended, that is, through interdiction of food'.[38] Basil of Caesarea similarly considered that 'it was gluttony that betrayed Adam to death and brought wickedness upon the world, thanks to the lust of the belly'.[39] God's command not to eat from the tree of knowledge was actually 'the law of fasting and abstinence'.[40] Because Eve did not fast then, fasting was a means of making amends for the sin of Eden.[41] Fasting offered a way of returning to paradise, specifically to the diet of Eden which he

---

34. Augustine, *The Confessions*, introduction, trans. and notes Maria Boulding, ed. John E. Rotelle (New York: New City Press, 1997), X.31.47.

35. Ibid., X.31.44. According to Augustine, concupiscence signals disordered desire or 'lust', not simply sexual lust but the longing for other earthly pleasures, including enjoyment from eating. For more on this see Anthony N. S. Lane, 'Lust: The Human Person as Affected by Disordered Desires', *Evangelical Quarterly* 78, no. 1 (2006): 21–35.

36. Augustine, *The Confessions*, X.31.43.

37. Ibid.

38. Tertullian, 'On Fasting', in *Ante-Nicene Fathers*, vol. 4, ed. Alexander Roberts and James Donaldson (Peabody: Hendrickson Publishers Inc., 1995), VIII.3.

39. Stone, *Practicing Safer Texts*, 27.

40. Basil the Great, *On Fasting*, I.3, https://www.crkvenikalendar.com/post/post-svetivasilije_en.php (accessed 10 July 2018).

41. Ibid.

believed did not contain any wine or meat.[42] Aquinas, writing much later, thought that the deadly sin of gluttony was responsible for the Fall, and that it was rightly named 'sin' because it denoted 'inordinate concupiscence', that is, 'lust' for food which was 'unregulated by reason'.[43]

Traditional accounts of the Adam and Eve story have thus been firm in naming the carnal desire to feed one's appetite as the original source of sin. The notion of the 'Fall', as a theological interpretation of Genesis, has situated Adam and Eve's transgressive eating at the heart of a monumental slip or lapse into a state of estrangement from God. However, the association between gluttony and lust, seen already in the comments by Basil, was common among early Christians informed by the ancient world. Food and sex were considered to be intimately connected. Clement of Alexandria, for example, believed we should discipline the belly and the organs beneath it; Jerome claimed that eating turned Adam and Eve into sexual creatures; Augustine was suspicious of chillies because he believed they would inflame the passions.[44] Associations between food and sexual passion also figure in the writings of the desert fathers as lust and gluttony are named as two *logismoi* ('passionate thoughts')[45] that stand to distract the monk and hinder prayer. According to the fourth-century monk Evagrius Ponticus, 'Whenever the demons attempt to dislodge one's thinking with shameful pleasures, they introduce the warfare of gluttony, so that once they have fired the stomach beforehand they can the more effortlessly cast the soul into the pit of lust.'[46] This assumed connection

42. Ibid., 1.5.
43. See Thomas Aquinas, *Summa Theologiæ*, 43 (2a2æ. 141–54), Temperance, trans. Thomas Gilby (Cambridge and New York: Cambridge University Press, 2006), Q148.1. According to Aquinas, 'Gluttony is the term for an immoderate appetite in eating and drinking, not for any appetite. And we regard an appetite as immoderate when it departs from the reasonable order of life in which moral good is found' (148.1). The sin of gluttony is not inherent to food itself, it is a 'disorder' in the sensory appetite that drives a person to 'exceed his measure from desire for pleasure'.
44. Isherwood, *The Fat Jesus*, 38.
45. Hill, *Eating to Excess*, 126.
46. Evagrius Ponticus, 'To Eulogios: On the Confession of Thoughts and Counsel in Their Regard', in *Evagrius of Pontus: The Greek Ascetic Corpus*, ed. and trans., introduction and commentary by Robert E. Sinkewicz (Oxford: Oxford University Press, 2003), 39.

between the belly and lust is continued with the development of the 'seven deadly sins' that presents gluttony and lust as two related vices.[47]

Of course, it is Augustine who stands out in Christianity as being especially suspicious of sexual passion. His impact on the church and its theologies of sin and grace is hard to overstate. Described by Tatha Wiley as 'incalculable',[48] such influence has been formative not only in shaping the Western theological tradition and its views about sin but also in cementing fears about sexuality. His classical account of original sin has food, lust and sin combine in the primordial act of disobedience. Augustine's thought, though, is intricately informed by his own sexual phobias. Tormented by his sexual desires and sexual behaviour, he sees in his personal experience evidence of an acute tension between reason and the emotions, rationality and the appetites/passions. His struggle to control his 'member' and his loathing for the 'animal movement'[49] of the erect penis informs his distrust of sexuality which then infiltrates his theology of sin. It also forms the context for his conversion to Christianity in 386 CE, which is a conversion into continence and celibacy as he renounces marriage and sexual activity.

Augustine certainly conceives that the Eden story speaks about sexual passion because he depicts the use of fig leaves in the story as an attempt by Adam to shield his shameful penis.[50] But his fears about food emerge in tandem with his sexual phobias. For Augustine, sin signals a profound disharmony within the soul and one that originates with Adam and Eve, but mainly with Eve's lustful appetite. Eden displays the power of food to sabotage the divine order and enslave the soul within the body. When Eve eats and seduces Adam to do the same, God's holy order is turned upside down because irrational, sensible, covetous desire is placed in control of the rational soul.[51] As a result,

---

47. For more on this, see Chapter 6. Also see Hill, *Eating to Excess*, 121–43.

48. Tatha Wiley, *Original Sin: Origins, Developments, Contemporary Meanings* (New York and Mahwah: Paulist Press, 2002), 56.

49. Augustine, *Answer to the Pelagians*, introduction, trans. and notes Roland J. Teske, ed. John E. Rotelle (New York: New City Press, 1997), II.43.38.

50. Ibid., II.39.34.

51. Augustine, *Answer to the Pelagians*, 36.22. Here Augustine argues that after the disobedience in Eden, the rational soul is no longer able to control the body's sexual impulses. The genitals are aroused against their will, 'as if they are in their own power'. The weaknesses that we inherit, which sees the flesh no longer obedient to the will, is a 'sin dwelling in our members'.

humanity becomes enslaved to sin. The inner struggle Paul confesses in Rom. 7.15,[52] where he finds himself unable to do the good he wills, is a predicament Augustine relates to and that he identifies with the post-lapsarian human condition.[53] Humanity is now marked by the 'morbid lust'[54] and disease of concupiscence, he argues – an anxious grasping that more often than not seeks fulfilment in material and sensible things (like food and sex), rather than in God. Concupiscence depicts 'the capacity of desire to overwhelm the rational determination of our willing',[55] and in Eden it is Adam and Eve's lust that topples their rational knowledge of the good God has disclosed. As a consequence, human nature becomes weakened ('wounded') because of the Fall and in its weakened state is not always strong enough to resist the temptation to act in ways uncoordinated by reason:[56] it is now prone to sin, not able not to sin (*non posse non peccare*). Despite conscious efforts to orientate the will towards the good, humans constantly find themselves

---

52. Paul laments that as flesh, he does not understand his own actions since he does the very things he hates and does not want: 'So I find it to be a law that when I want to do what is good, evil lies close at hand. For I delight in the law of God in my inmost self, but I see in my members another law at war with the law of the mind, making me captive to the law of sin that dwells in my members. Wretched man that I am! Who will rescue me from this body of death? (Rom. 7.21-24). Paul frames this tension as an inner conflict between the spirit and flesh, maintaining that 'these are opposed to each other, to prevent you from doing what you want' (Gal. 5.17). In *Religion and the Body* (Cambridge: Cambridge University Press, 2000), Sarah Coakley reminds us that this battle is not between body (*soma*) and soul (*psyche*) but between the flesh (*sarx*) – understood as the whole human person in its rebellion against God – and spirit (*pneuma*) – understood as the whole human person in obedience to God (93). Also see Jane Barter Moulaison, '"Our Bodies, Our Selves?" The Body as Source in Feminist Theology', *Scottish Journal of Theology* 60, no. 3 (2007): 341–59 (352, n. 19).

53. Augustine, *Answer to the Pelagians II*, introduction, trans. and notes Roland J. Teske, ed. John E. Rotelle (New York: New City Press, 1998), I.18-22.

54. Augustine, *The Confessions*, VIII.7.17.

55. Alistair McFadyen, *Bound to Sin: Abuse, Holocaust and the Christian Doctrine of Sin* (Cambridge: Cambridge University Press, 2000), 190. The sins of concupiscence are irrational because they signal a failure to coordinate knowledge of the good with action (192).

56. Ibid., 190.

willing against themselves. The human will has become divided, says Augustine, and the single soul 'torn apart in its distress'.[57]

This notion of 'original sin', developed in the fourth and fifth centuries by Augustine and his teacher Ambrose,[58] retains Paul's insistence in the New Testament on the fleshiness of human beings as a result of the Fall.[59] It is a doctrine Augustine develops as a polemic against Pelagius who teaches that the will is in no sense prone towards choosing certain options. For all its problems and unpalatable implications, not least the highly controversial claim that human beings are born guilty of the sin of others and are rightly punished for it, the idea of original sin has continued to exert its influence. Developed subsequently by thinkers like Anselm, Aquinas, Calvin and Luther, it communicates that sin somehow perverts the whole of humankind and is inescapable. Prominent reformers promote the total depravity of human being and even though the Renaissance and Enlightenment herald a counter-belief in progress imploring that human beings are actually getting better, the sense that human beings are in some sense 'born bad' has continued to stick.

Syn, Inner Conflict and the Battle for Self-control

According to James Boyce, the Christian story of creation provides the spiritual foundation of the Western world, shaping Western people's understanding of themselves and moulding a sense of inherent badness. For him, even if we want to dismiss original sin as illegitimate and tied to a past we don't even remember, 'no religious inheritance can be banished by such feeble weapons as amnesia or scorn'.[60] He notes that the legacy of original sin lives on in the Western cultural imaginary to

---

57. Augustine, *The Confessions*, VIII.10.24.

58. Although it should be noted that similar theologies were circulating beforehand by thinkers such as Anthony the Great, Athanasius, Tertullian and Cyprian of Carthage.

59. Deborah Sawyer, 'Hidden Subjects: Rereading Eve and Mary', *Theology and Sexuality* 14, no. 3 (2008): 315.

60. James Boyce, *Born Bad: Original Sin and the Making of the Western Mind* (London: SPCK, 2014), 5.

this day, seen in 'trendy diets' and a culture of self-help concerned not so much with 'doing wrong, but with being wrong'.[61]

Certainly the notion of 'original sin' conceives of sin more as an ontological disorder or as what Aquinas images as a distortion of our God-created telos and God-given (natural) inclination towards virtue.[62] Women in the group, on the other hand, tend to see Syn as something they do. In this sense, Syn is more axiological and moral than ontological. However, the distinction between being and doing wrong is blurred because of the way Syn is embodied. Participants assume that the result of (wilful) disobedience is weight gain (fat) and a body that becomes other than what it should be. Jane, for example, experiences her larger body as 'alien', and this fuels her need to hide: 'And I got that I didn't want to go out, because I was so big. I really was in a state with the size that I was because it was alien to me.' For Jane, as with other women, Syn is tied to identity – it not only disfigures the body by making it fat but causes the person to feel out of character and out of sorts in their own skin. Syn is thus certainly not only an action but also a state of alienation where women are separated from their perceived true selves.

The classical association of sin with a disintegrated or disharmonious self that acts against its best interests shows up quite obviously in women's weight loss narratives. Participants mimic the sentiments of Paul and Augustine communicating the frustration of Syn and speaking of an inability to prevent themselves from doing the good they know by reason. Joy, for example, tells me that she feels 'fed up' with herself when she attends the meeting and gains weight because 'I know in my heart of hearts that I could do it, but I'm just getting a bit too relaxed some weeks'. Wendy is similarly frustrated because she keeps repeating the same pattern of getting comfortable when losing weight and then eating a bag of chips (i.e. fries) to celebrate.

---

61. James Boyce, 'How Original Sin Led to a Western Obsession with Self-Help', *The Guardian* (23 July 2015), https://www.theguardian.com/culture/australia-culture-blog/2014/jul/23/how-original-sin-led-to-a-western-obsession-with-self-help (accessed 7 March 2017).

62. Note that, for Aquinas, the rational capacities of the soul are 'in a sense lacking the order proper to them, their natural order to virtue, and the deprivation is called the "wounding of nature"'. Thomas Aquinas, *Summa Theologiæ*, 26 (Ia2æ. 81-85), Original Sin, trans. T. C. O'Brien (Cambridge and New York: Cambridge University Press, 2006), Q.85.3.

Drawing on her own observations inside a commercial weight loss group, Kandi Stinson finds that women are encouraged to see their selves as a duality characterized by internal conflict. She describes one occasion when her group are made to watch a video in which the central protagonist, Gail, is depicted as two selves – one good and one bad. In the video, Gail sits down to eat but is interrupted by a phone call from a colleague. As she speaks to him, she begins to nibble on a cake. By the end of the conversation, Gail realizes that she has practically eaten the entire cake. Another Gail then appears – the bad self – telling Gail that she might as well finish off the whole thing. Then the positive Gail makes an entrance, reassuring Gail that she doesn't have to eat it and can throw the rest away. Gail is torn but in the end heeds to the voice of the good self realizing this is her true self. For Stinson, the video clearly communicates that whereas the bad self gives into temptation and loses control, the good self maintains self-control and feels the required guilt when this is lost.[63] Such a message, she claims, is compatible with the religious metaphor of a battle between good and evil.

She is certainly right but it is important to observe that the particular battle being waged in Gail's case and in the case of women like Joy and Wendy above is an inward struggle more commensurate with Augustine's inner turmoil than with a cosmic battle between supernatural forces. As with Augustine, this battle is materialized and played out in and through the body. It is a battle specifically between the inferior carnal desire for pleasure and the superior rational will, and so one that aligns well with the particular tradition of original sin. In my group, participants similarly experience their wills as deficient, but unlike Augustine, they conceive of themselves as being utterly able to follow their own rational inclinations. Women believe that they should be able to transcend their passions and control their bodies, and this is ultimately demonstrated by the way losing weight is reduced to a simple matter of will power: 'What do I want more?' asks Suzanne. 'Do I want to lose a pound or have a glass of wine? Do I want to feel good when I'm in the class?' The implication is that if she *really* wanted to lose weight, she would forfeit the wine. A poster in the meeting room unequivocally confirms the need to engage the will against any emotional attachment to food:

We all have it. If you have the true 'WILL' to lose weight and believe you can, you have the 'POWER' to achieve it.

63. Stinson, *Women and Dieting Culture*, 127.

Augustine is more pessimistic about our human ability to choose the good for ourselves, but he nevertheless emphasizes the need for the rational will to subdue the passions and exert its influence.

It is not simply Christianity, however, that has helped secure the prominence of the will and erect a combative relationship between the mind and body. The European Enlightenment played a major role in establishing reason as sovereign. Offering a vision of the (male) rational, self-actualizing subject, Enlightenment philosophies venerated the critical power of reason and, in so doing, dethroned superstition, nature, religion and emotion that were considered opposite. Descartes's rationalism provided one of the most important foundations for Enlightenment thought, imagining the mind and body as two distinct substances. Indeed, it is with Cartesian thought that 'an unbridgeable gulf'[64] is established between the body and mind, and the body presented as an autonomous machine and vessel for the non-spatial mind.[65]

According to Bethan Evans, such Cartesian logic directs obesity politics to this day, helping divide body and mind and present fat as a disorder of the body that can be diagnosed mechanically through BMI and other measuring devices.[66] Cartesianism, she argues, establishes bodies as unruly and dangerous and constructs obese bodies as flawed. It also considers rationality as acting through science and technology,[67] allowing the rationalizing enterprises of science and medicine to be presented as compelling solutions to fat. In identifying fat with the body, Cartesian logic overlooks the emotional and social aspects of eating and body size.[68]

In my group, this logic is clearly operative. The notion of 'Syn' assists members with the inner struggle they narrate between their rational wills and appetites by reducing food items to a number (i.e. to a Syn value) and eating to a mathematical equation and mechanical act. Syn helps to rationalize members' appetites and distract from any emotional

---

64. Elizabeth Grosz, *Volatile Bodies: Toward a Corporeal Feminism* (Bloomington and Indianapolis: Indiana University Press, 1994), 7.

65. Lisa Isherwood and Elizabeth Stuart similarly stress that Rene Descartes ushered in the era of 'profound body/soul dualism' – see *Introducing Body Theology* (Cleveland: The Pilgrim Press, 1998), 71–2.

66. Evans, "'Gluttony or Sloth?'", 261.

67. Ibid., 261–2.

68. Ibid., 263.

connection with food. It also constructs eating as a solitary affair that can be managed entirely by the individual and so minimizes the social significance of food. This leads some members to resent social occasions where they cannot easily predict or control the dishes being served.

Yet the antagonism between body and mind also mimics earlier theologies which have informed Christian dualism. Indeed, the emphasis on willpower and on the success in controlling the body channelled by weight loss culture would have delighted the Church Fathers.[69] Asserting the dominance of the rational will reflects the patriarchal theological schema that places 'the passions' in opposition to reason and in alignment with women, bodiliness and corruption. In early Christianity, writers as distinct as Tertullian, Irenaeus, Clement of Alexandria and Ignatius of Antioch echoed Paul in affirming the body as good and were united in opposing the Gnostics who tended to view the body as a creation of an evil power and drag on the soul.[70] This however did not prevent such thinkers, and others besides, from viewing the body as a foil and hindrance for the soul. In one of his earlier works, Augustine dialogues with the (male) figure of Reason who advises him accordingly:

> You must entirely flee from things of sense. So long as we bear this body we must beware lest our wings are hindered by their birdlime. We need sound and perfect wings if we are to fly from this darkness to yonder light, which does not deign to manifest itself to men shut up in a cave unless they can escape, leaving sensible things broken and dissolved.[71]

For Origen, the body is a 'shadow' of the soul. Marred by corruption, it is firmly planted at the bottom of the hierarchy of human being and the mind firmly established at the top. It is the mind that is in the image of God, and the corrupt body will be transformed in the resurrection so that it shares the incorruptibility of the soul.[72] I will return to similar theological positions in subsequent chapters, but this theologically

---

69. Isherwood, *The Fat Jesus*, 4.

70. Margaret Miles, *Fullness of Life: Historical Foundations for a New Asceticism* (Eugene: Wipf & Stock, 1981), 19.

71. Augustine, 'The Soliloquies', in *Augustine: Earlier Writings*, vol. VI, trans. John H. S. Burleigh (London: SCM, 1953), I.xiv.24.

72. Miles, *Fullness of Life*, 50.

informed need to master the unruliness of the flesh by imposing the force of the will onto the sensible passions of the body has been worked out through various projects that seek to control women's bodies, and it takes renewed form in the weight loss group. Here, the theological alignment of virtue with transcendence of the appetitive and sensible self resurfaces as women attempt to assert the dominance of their rational wills over their bodies. In this dualistic system, it is the desire for pleasure that emerges as especially hazardous.

Syn and Eating What We Do Not Need: The Snare of Pleasure versus 'Sensible' Eating

Indeed, women in the group consider the pleasure of eating to be dangerous and unsafe, whether the tastiness of crisps or other Synful items. For Ruth, taste is associated with the consumption of foods that are not 'sensible' to eat. Speaking about the plan she comments: 'You have to say well, if that's a sensible way of eating, what was going wrong before? And what was going wrong before was all the stuff that you ate as well as the stuff that you needed.' She continues to explain the problem as 'eating too much of the kind of food which is very tasty' – food like pastas loaded with cheese. Such items are 'addictive' and 'garbage', so the only answer is to locate such 'wrong' foods and avoid them altogether: 'If you don't have them at all, you're all right.' Eating the wrong foods is not sensible because these are not foods we need, but are foods we eat for pleasure in excess of what we need, and they are foods that hook us with their taste.

Other members make similar judgements about the dangers of taste. Tracy explains in her interview that she tries to select 'something quite plainish' when eating out in order to stick to the plan. The food 'tasters' supplied by Louise and other members also often appear to forfeit taste for the sake of creating 'sensible' dishes that are low in Syn: a chocolate brownie made from Scan Bran;[73] a quiche made from corned beef and cottage cheese; a curry made with baked beans, mushy peas and Indian spices. None of these seemed especially appetising to me, yet many in the group partake of them. In this economy, good sense may dictate what makes for good taste, but what certainly dominates is the need to

---

73. Scan Bran is a Scandinavian high-fibre crisp bread (similar to Ryveta) which is available for purchase at the weight loss meetings.

rationalize one's appetite and curb the desire for pleasure. For Ruth, this kind of sensible consumption that replaces impulse with control and eating for necessity is an 'obvious' and intelligent way to eat; it is 'one of these things that's in the general domain of what we know about how we ought to behave'.[74]

Such a schema echoes ancient Christian concerns about the pleasure of eating, not unlike the fears expressed by Augustine earlier in this chapter. Following the Greek philosophers that informed them, early Christian thinkers were suspicious of modes of eating that were not governed by moderation and necessity. Clement of Alexandria, in his *Paidagogos*, cites Phil. 3.19 where Paul speaks against those whose 'god is their belly' to claim that Christ 'the Instructor' calls humans to eat to live rather than live to eat.[75] 'For neither is food our business, nor is pleasure our aim,' he advises. Humans should eat to sustain the body so that it can receive and obey the Word.[76] It should be plain, intended towards health and 'conducive both to digestion and lightness of body'.[77]

---

74. In her qualitative study of 'overweight' and 'obese' women, Carof Solenn finds that eating forbidden food engenders greater degrees of guilt when appreciated for its taste, a point she likens to Eve's eating of the forbidden fruit where her enjoyment makes her even guiltier. See Carof Solenn, 'Eating with the Fear of Weight Gain: The Relationship with Food for Overweight Women in France', *Menu: Journal of Food and Hospitality Research* 1, no. 1 (2012): 72. Prata Gaspar and Maria Clara de Moraes also observe in their qualitative study of eating behaviour among French female college students that pleasure is dichotomized with necessity. In the end, food associated with enjoyment is viewed as unessential and as that which stands to make the individual fat. See their article, 'Control of Eating Behaviour and Eating Pleasure among French Female College Students', *Menu: Journal of Food and Hospitality Research* 1, no. 1 (2012), 94. We can see in this preference for necessity over taste, another assertion of the dualism between affect and reason as food is once more stripped of its emotional components. If foods are 'good' because they are low in Syn or because we eat them for health rather than pleasure, then the staple binary of modernity between mind and matter is repeated once more.

75. Clement of Alexandria, 'The Instructor', in *Ante-Nicene Fathers: Translations of the Writings of the Fathers Down to AD 325*, ed. Rev. Alexander Roberts and James Donaldson, vol. II (Grand Rapids: WM. B. Eerdmans Publishing Company, 1977), II.2.

76. Ibid., II.1.

77. Ibid., II.1.

Convinced that the best way to improve spiritual health was by working on the body, he insists that the 'good' Christian should not be ruled by their belly since lack of self-control over food produces 'insanity in reference to the belly'.[78] The body occupies a female submissive role in his view, and following the Stoics of his day, he places great value on moderation and calm.[79]

Over a century later and in his ninth sermon of the *Hexæmeron*, Basil warns that a person who degrades themselves by indulging the 'passions of the flesh' becomes a 'slave of thy belly' and 'approachest animals without reason and becomest like one of them'.[80] Food ought to function like clothes, meeting the practical needs of the body and nothing more: 'For a man in good health bread will suffice, and water will quench thirst.'[81] Eating for health is not the same as eating for pleasure, and 'savage gluttony' should be confronted by 'moderation, quiet, and self-control'.[82] He warns about the dangers of 'nibbling in secret'.[83]

The concept of 'weight' fits squarely into this system of fear, taking on symbolic meaning as the corruptible, sensible and appetitive self that drags the soul away from God. Augustine, for example, laments that he is 'dragged back by my own weight'[84] – the weight of his own sexual habits and his lust for other pleasures, including food. He speaks about the weight and drag of concupiscence that pulls us 'headlong into the deep',[85] and the lightness of body that fattens the soul making it more like the resurrected body which will rise 'without blemish, without deformity, without mortality, without being a burden or a weight'.[86] The

---

78. Ibid., II.1. Also see Michel Desjardins, 'Clement's Bound Body', in *Mapping Gender in Ancient Religious Discourses*, ed. Todd Penner and Caroline Vander Stichele (Leiden and Boston: Brill, 2007), 417.

79. Desjardins, 'Clement's Bound Body', 424.

80. Basil the Great, 'The Hexaemeron', in *The Nicene and Post-Nicene Fathers*, vol. VIII, trans. with notes Rev. Blomfield Jackson, ed. Philip Schaff and Henry Wace (Grand Rapids: WM. B. Eerdmans Publishing, 1978), IX.2.

81. Basil the Great, 'The Letters', in *The Nicene and Post-Nicene Fathers*, II.6.

82. Ibid.

83. Bringle, *The God of Thinness*, 65.

84. Augustine, *The Confessions*, X.4.5.

85. Ibid., XIII.7.8.

86. Augustine, *Sermons*, III/7 (230-272B) 'On the Liturgical Seasons', trans. and notes E. Hill, ed. J. Rotelle (New York: New City Press, 1993), 240.3.

mind, in 'tending upward', is 'held back by a weight',[87] and the body literally dragged down to earth/mortality by its hefty flesh. Those who indulge the flesh by lavishing in earthly delights like eating for pleasure are 'bent down to the ground' and become like beasts.[88] 'When you achieve the condition of finding no delight at all in earthly things, in that moment, believe me, at that point of time, you will see what you desire', he writes in *The Soliloquies*.[89] Augustine conceives that in exacerbating appetite through fasting, the soul's hunger grows and the person becomes 'capacious'.[90] In this view, sin is a weight produced by an inordinate desire for food and other earthly pleasures that must be escaped in pursuit of union with God.

The alliance between weight and sin, however, is not only symbolic. For some early Christian theologians, fatness itself manifests irrationality and an indulgence in pleasure characteristic of inordinate desire. Slimness or 'lightness of body' is thus a sign of moral purity and self-control. The fourth-century thinker John Chrysostom speaks about those who become fat through 'luxurious living'. Such people are like animals, he claims, for 'it is only for brute beasts to be feeding from morning to night'.[91] He speaks of the 'disgusting spectacle' of 'a man cultivating obesity', who is seen 'dragging himself along like a seal'.[92] Writing in the second century, Clement of Alexandria similarly encourages his readers to 'let not food weigh us down, but lighten us'.[93] Fasting empties the soul of matter, making the body clear and light for the receipt of divine truth.[94] Jerome after him instructs that 'the slenderness, the deliverance of the body from the encumbrance of much

---

87. Augustine, *Sermons* III/10 (341-400) 'On Various Subjects', trans. Edmund Hill, ed. John E. Rotelle (New York: New City Press, 1995), 400.2.

88. Ibid.

89. Augustine, 'The Soliloquies', I.xiv.24.

90. Augustine, *Sermons*, III/7, 240.3.

91. John Chrysostom, 'Homily XXXV on the Acts of the Apostles', in *Nicene and Post-Nicene Fathers:* First Series, vol. XI, ed. Philip Schaff (Edinburgh: T & T Clark, 1889), XXXV, https://www.ccel.org/ccel/schaff/npnf111.vi.xxxv.html (accessed 5 February 2018).

92. Ibid.

93. Clement of Alexandria, 'The Instructor', II.9.

94. Caroline Walker Bynum, *Holy Feast and Holy Fast: The Religious Significance of Food to Medieval Women* (London: University of California Press, 1987), 36.

flesh gives us some conformity to God and His angels'.[95] Weightlessness is next to Godli(ke)ness, and this, for John Donne writing much later in the 1600s, provides a theological mandate for staying trim. Citing this passage from Jerome in his sermon on Easter Day in 1626, Donne recommends slimness to his congregation instructing that 'the flesh that we have built up by curious diet, by meats of provocation, and witty sauces [is] artificial flesh of our own making'.[96] All flesh is sinful, so the more we have the deeper we bury the soul. The soul, he instructs, does not require 'so vast a house of sinful flesh, to dwell in'.[97]

Women in the weight loss group similarly consider Syn to be both a symbolic and an actual weight; it not only causes them to slip and slide, dragging them away from their sensible/rational projects of weight loss, but also manifests on their bodies as excess pounds that need to be removed. Members thus reach similar conclusions about fat as these ancient thinkers. Lucy sees that her bad behaviour is the reason for her anticipated weight gain. Samantha says that if she has eaten out then she will expect a gain to follow: 'In the back of my head it's "that's gonna catch up with me at some point"'. Women assume that Syn is worn on the body as fat and that virtue takes on material form as thinness. Fat also makes the body beastly. In a manner reflective of Chrysostom, Ruth depicts fat as base and monstrous: 'You don't want to be lurching through the town knocking people out of the way with your vast size!'

Taking the Wrap for Fat

That members are individually culpable for Syn is further communicated through the categories of 'good' and 'bad' that members employ to speak about themselves and their food choices. Women talk about having 'good' and 'bad' weeks, 'good' and 'bad' days, but these seldom refer to successes or problems encountered at work, in family, personal or social life. To have a bad week generally means to have failed to follow the plan effectively and to have exceeded the Syn allowance. Syn, as an expression of bad foodways, is thus closely aligned with rebellion: 'Sometimes if you've had a really bad week or you've been out for say

---

95. Jerome cited by John Donne, *The Works of John Donne*, vol. I, ed. Henry Alford (London: John W. Parker, 1839), 314.
96. Ibid.
97. Ibid.

a lot of meals, I'll think, oh God, what is it [i.e. the scale] gonna say?' says Samantha, reflecting on how she can dread the weigh-in when her eating strays from the plan. Being bad is also conjured by members as a transgression against Louise or themselves. Kerry is retired and has been off and on diets all her life. She has joined a number of slimming clubs over the years to prevent herself from having to confront familiar faces when she inevitably gains weight and has to return. 'It's easy to have a bad week and feel that you've blown it and feel that, you know, you've let yourself down, you've let her [Louise] down,' she explains.

Interestingly, however, members are not always very comfortable with this type of morally loaded speech. Ruth, also retired, comments that she does not like it when people speak about being 'naughty'. Although 'the group *does* encourage people', she remarks, 'there's just a slight element of um, this word "naughty" creeps in every now and then, not very often, but often enough to jar.' Leanne, too, has her reservations. She tells me before one meeting that she has 'tried everything' when it comes to dieting, including a cardio diet usually intended for people preparing for heart surgery. Unlike other members, she refers to herself as 'fat' in our conversation and explains that she is in the group for the 'long haul' because she loathes her size. Although she feels uncomfortable with the judgemental nature of Louise's language of 'good' and 'bad', she admits that she nevertheless finds herself using it because it is hard to avoid.

In employing this moral terminology, members come to locate the blame for Syn and fat squarely with themselves, absorbing the burden of guilt. Lucy, a hairdresser who joins the group with her friend and colleague, Joy, comments:

> If I know I've been bad, well that's my own fault isn't it. I kind of go [to the meeting] expecting to have put weight on. ... Don't blame your age, don't blame ... things like that, which you do don't you? You know. Don't blame your periods! It's you! So that's it, do something about it!

The only appropriate response to fat is the acknowledgement of guilt and acceptance of the need for personal reform: do something about it! As with the Augustinian–Lutheran tradition, Syn is here localizable in the distorted will of the individual, presented primarily as a personal offence that results from a misuse of freedom. The notion of 'sin' as a private and insular affair thus resurfaces in members' Syn-talk in ways that mesh with cultural assumptions about personal culpability for fat, helping to blame the individual for their weight and compel weight loss as a moral obligation.

Corporeal Freedom and Syn as the Great Equalizer: Choosing and Losing the Body

It is not simply the power to impose the rational will against the body that members see themselves as possessing. They also come to think that they can choose what kind of bodies they have, being active in their own material construction. 'You *are* in control of how you look ... , you can look the way you want to,' says Hevala during her interview. Suzanne, in planning for a forthcoming trip to New York, tells me that she can lose seven pounds in five weeks because 'other people do it, so why can't I?' Suzanne's belief that her mind and will can be employed to fashion a body that is transformed according to the time-bound targets she sets herself shows just how much weight loss is rationalized, universalized and abstracted from the material limits of the body.

Feminists have seen in this kind of practice a worrying tendency towards material transcendence and disembodiment. For Susan Bordo, this emphasis on choosing our own bodies is a manifestation of the 'ideology of limitless improvement and change' that defies the very materiality of the body.[98] It conceives of the body as 'cultural plastic' and establishes ourselves as 'master sculptors of that plastic'.[99] According to Bordo, the Cartesian vision of a disembodied mind and fantasy about transcendence here resurfaces as a new 'postmodern configuration of detachment, a new imagination of disembodiment'.[100] Now, the vision is of a body unaffected by material limits, a body that can choose its shape and size at will and be any-body and go anywhere. Such an enactment of the postmodern body in cultural practice, Bordo claims, gives expression to the postmodern discourse of 'life as plastic possibility and weightless choice, undetermined by history, social location, or even individual biography'.[101] 'What sort of body is it that is free to change its shape and location at will, that can become anyone and travel anywhere?' she asks. 'No body at all', she replies.[102]

---

98. Bordo, *Unbearable Weight*, 245.
99. Ibid., 246.
100. Ibid., 227.
101. Ibid., 251.
102. Ibid., 229.

This stress on limitless choice and self-determination clearly aligns with capitalist ideology, positioning weight loss as a consumer/market choice. More specifically, it is expressive of neoliberal rationality,[103] where choices about the body are framed as market choices, and citizens fashioned as rational economic actors and entrepreneurs who have the ability to service their own ambitions.[104] In the group, such entrepreneurial freedom exacerbates the unease and guilt experienced by women about their bodies because the promise of freedom materializes as a new form of restriction. As Eva Chen argues, neoliberalism's insistence that women must actively choose and enjoy their bodies actually results in a new type of pressure – the pressure to 'follow and not deviate, and to constantly live up to its promise by actively choosing and enjoying'.[105] In this system, women have no choice *but* to choose thinness, and in the context of the slimming group, the compulsion to choose and to design their own thinner bodies makes women even more anxious about making the right choices – weight loss or wine, which do I want more?

The assumption that all have Synned and are capable of achieving thinness and restructuring their bodies is an outworking of neoliberalism that conveniently masks economic, racial, cultural and other differences between members so that thinness can be established as a universal norm. This, though, shares with the doctrine of original sin the understanding that all bodies are positioned identically in sin. According to Augustine, all are equally culpable, and although the will is disordered rather than entirely free to determine its own destiny, all are equally afflicted. So too, members conceive that they are equally positioned in Syn. In the group, this causes women to believe they each have a level of capacity to shape and remake their bodies. Herein features of the theological logic of original sin align with the market rationality of neoliberalism to confirm that no-body is innocent.

---

103. Rosalind Gill and Jane Arthurs, 'Editors' Introduction: New Femininities?', *Feminist Media Studies* 6, no. 4 (2006): 445.

104. This is integral to Wendy Brown's account of neoliberalism in 'American Nightmare: Neoliberalism, Neoconservatism, and De-Democratization', *Political Theory* 34, no. 6 (2006): 694.

105. Eva Chen, 'Neoliberalism and Popular Women's Culture: Rethinking Choice, Freedom and Agency', *European Journal of Cultural Studies* 16, no. 4 (2013): 448.

1. Syn, Danger and Disordered Desire 77

This concealing of difference is especially obvious in Helen's interview. Helen is twenty-four and has been attending the group for two years. She joins the group with her friend Sarah, determined to lose weight in time for her wedding. She identifies as disabled and tells me that she has a condition that impairs her mobility, preventing her from being able to work. Recalling the period immediately after her diagnosis when she was in hospital, she explains that the doctor had prescribed total bed rest. For four months she did not move, although she did attend the weight loss meetings:

> I was going to [the group], still losing weight, cos obviously I was losing muscle and thinking like, wow at least I'm losing weight while I'm doing this. But then obviously, through the physio and gradually having to do it myself, I started to put on weight because I was building back my muscle. That was a bit of a weird time cos it was like, well, I need to build the muscle up, but I want to lose weight. I was on morphine during that time, so I wasn't really on the planet. And then I kind of got myself off the morphine onto other medications and it was like, okay, I don't know what's been going on but I need to get back in. It's like only six months till the wedding and I was like, I've just got to lose as much as I can now, really go for it.

In this passage, Helen's personal circumstances and disability offer no defence against the universal compulsion to slim. Although she loses weight because of muscle wastage and gains weight because she is getting better, her weight gain leaves her feeling conflicted – pleased that she is building up her strength but concerned that her improved muscle is making her heavier. Adamant that she must redouble her efforts and commit once more to her weight loss goals, her disability appears as a controllable outcome she may be able to alter or influence through hard work. Later in her interview, she expresses frustration that her current medication makes her gain weight, throwing her off target. When I ask how she feels sitting among other women who do not have the same health challenges, she suggests that this just confirms the need for her to persevere and apply more effort: 'It is a bit difficult, but you know, you've just got to kind of keep going and keep trying.' If her weight continues to rise, she says, she will probably ask her doctor to take her off the medication.

Striking here is the way Helen's desire for thinness seems to trump her willingness to give her body what she needs for her own well-being. To be sure, the emphasis she places on hard work is a further expression of the Protestant work ethic discussed by Max Weber and observed by others as an important feature of body improvement culture in Euro-America.[106] Her adamance that fat can be controlled through hard work fuels a more determined effort to master her body's size,[107] hence she inhabits the space of the good Protestant, approaching life with 'constant thought',[108] 'restless effort'[109] and a 'purposeful will'.[110] Yet, the compulsion to choose self-improvement manifests here also as a compulsion to shape a thin *able* body. As such, it is not only fat which is framed as a controllable outcome but disability as well. Similarly for Hevala who chooses to lose weight to reverse the effects of her mother's 'Middle Eastern' feeding and in response to a public weighing in her primary school,[111] the compulsion to fashion a thinner self is a compulsion to curate a body that adheres to a white Eurocentric feminine ideal.

These instances expose the way a conservative individualistic ethic constructs other sites of difference – such as race and dis/ability – as cultural plastic. Belief in the plasticity of the body shores up what Michelle Lelwica calls the 'imperial paradigm',[112] not only concealing differences between women but also compelling all women to choose for themselves the white, able-bodied, middle-class, Eurocentric image of femininity.

---

106. Quinn and Crocker, for example, find that the Protestant ethic emerges as a risk factor for women who feel overweight, making them especially vulnerable to psychological distress. Given the Protestant ethic holds that self-discipline and hard work lead to positive results, it makes women who view their weight as a salient factor more likely to judge themselves negatively. For more, see Diane M. Quinn and Jennifer Crocker, 'When Ideology Hurts: Effects of Belief in the Protestant Ethic and Feeling Overweight on the Psychological Well-Being of Women', *Journal of Personality and Social Psychology* 77, no. 2 (1999): 409.

107. It also produces psychological distress for Helen as we will see in Chapter 3.

108. Max Weber, *The Protestant Ethic and the Spirit of Capitalism* (London and New York: Routledge, 1992), 118.

109. Ibid., 170.

110. Ibid., 119.

111. For more, see the introduction of this book.

112. Lelwica, Hoglund and McNallie, 'Spreading the Religion of Thinness', 22.

Syn, Death and Disease

In the group, Syn is also considered to carry deadly consequences. Not only does it produce the fat that uncovers a person's guilt but the Syn that is worn on the body as fat is also presumed to cause ill health and even death. Mark tells me about a heart scare which although probably unrelated to his weight, nevertheless makes him have a 'mortality moment', prompting him to lose weight. Ruth attends a consultation with her doctor and subsequently identifies her high blood pressure with her weight, and her weight with excessive foodways, despite her doctor not making the connection. In all of these cases, members assume ill health and death are causally related to fat and fat causally related to 'bad' foodways (Syn), even when such connections are not made by medical professionals.

It has been a common feature of Christian teaching to associate Adam and Eve's consumption of the forbidden fruit with the arrival of human death.[113] This view has been heavily influenced by Paul's claim in the New Testament that 'sin came into the world through one man, and death came through sin, and so death spread to all because all have sinned' (Rom. 5.12). For Paul, human beings have lost their original righteousness but have gained restoration in Christ, for while 'the wages of sin is death' (Rom. 6.22-23), Christ makes possible eternal life.

In the Hebrew Bible, fat more specifically is identified with depravity and death. In the book of Judges, the story is told of the Moabite king, Eglon, who defeats Israel with the help of the Ammonites and Amalekites. Eglon is described as 'a very fat man' (Judg. 3.17). In hearing the cries of the Israelites who have lived under Eglon's rule for eighteen years, God sends Ehud son of Gera, the Benjaminite, to deliver them. Thrusting a sword into Eglon's (fat) belly, Ehud kills the Moabite king, and Moab is subdued by Israel. According to Susan Hill, Eglon is not killed because he is fat, but because of what his fat represents, namely, 'greed, decadence, and wilful disregard of God',[114] behaviours directly opposed to Israelite values. For Hill, Eglon's death marks a triumph over fat, that is, over the behaviours his fat represents. Death is not only a symbolic end of what his fat signifies but also the literal eradication of this girth.

---

113. The assumption that humankind were created immortal has been challenged by numerous thinkers, for example, Stone, *Practicing Safer Texts*, 23–45.

114. See Hill, *Eating to Excess*, 32–3.

Once again fat emerges as both a symbolic and an actual weight. For women in my group, death is also assumed to be the outcome and likely end for the wayward greed and disobedience their physical fatness represents. This is particularly apparent in the 'Let's Beat It Together' campaign which Louise launches during one meeting in February. There are red balloons in the room which bear the imprint of this motto. Louise describes the campaign as a twelve-week weight loss challenge intended to educate the local community about the dangers of obesity. It rewards new members and those who recruit them with free weigh-ins. The new set of posters displayed in the meeting room clearly communicates the campaign's message: 'Ours is the first generation ever where parents might outlive their children because of obesity.' Another warns that 'every year 40,000 people die from weight-related illnesses'. The source of these claims is not cited, but this does not seem to matter. The sentiments of Paul resurface as members learn that the wages of Syn is indeed death. Conflating the medical with the moral, these statements present fat as a deadly disease and also relate fatness in children to parental neglect.

The association between sin, death and disease is an obvious one in Christianity. According to the New Testament, the sickness from which humans suffer is sin, and Christ comes as a physician to heal and restore sinners to 'health' (e.g. Mt. 9.12; Lk. 5.31). As already noted, it is with Augustine that this is worked into an understanding of sin as a congenital disease that infects the whole of humanity. Reflecting on Lk. 5.31-32,[115] he maintains that even infants require healing by *Christus medicus* (Christ the Physician) because they share in the guilt of original sin.[116] Calvin, although critical of Augustine's understanding of original sin as a biological defect, nevertheless considers that the sin which is 'imputed' and 'inborn' is akin to a type of disease: 'All of us ... are born infected with the contagion of sin. In fact, before we saw the light of this life, we were soiled and spotted in God's sight.'[117]

---

115. 'Those who are well have no need of a physician, but those who are sick; I have come to call not the righteous but sinners to repentance' (Lk. 5.31-32).

116. See, for example, Augustine, *Answer to the Pelagians*, III.8.

117. Calvin cited in Serene Jones, *Feminist Theory and Christian Theology: Cartographies of Grace* (Minneapolis: Fortress, 2000), 104. Jones explains that for Calvin, the 'imputation' of sin means that humans wear a judgement that is not theirs by nature but which they impose on themselves and on other generations. Sin is not a genetic condition as with Augustine but a judgement

Of course, we might agree with critics of Augustine that such a view defies common sense[118] and is morally repugnant, but this organization seems to share Augustine's conviction that the disease of sin is passed on through the generations. The weight loss company assumes that Syn is displayed on the body as fat and that fat is linked to disease and death, standing to have a catastrophic effect both now and in the years to come. 'One million of our children are obese storing up health problems for the future,' declares a poster in the room. The power of this discourse to generate fear and fuel arguments about the cost of fat to the nation's health and economy cannot be overstated. Indeed, it reiterates a feature of anti-obesity discourse captured by the 2014 annual report of the Chief Medical Officer in England where obesity is advocated as a 'national risk' alongside threats such as terrorism and climate change. In this report, Sally Davis suggests that rising levels of obesity among pregnant women threaten their own well-being as well as the health of future generations.[119] The implication is that women are to blame for generations of sick people and so are responsible for rescuing themselves and their children from the devastating effects of fat. The 'Let's Beat It Together' campaign which addresses a majority female audience similarly holds women responsible for the future: not just their own future, but the futures of their children and their children's children. Mirroring traditional beliefs about the Fall and original sin, fat is identified with women's faulty choices and is viewed as a disease that stands to impede the lives of generations.

that we willingly put on, like clothes, and which is contrasted by the garment of 'alien righteousness' supplied by God.

118. William Harmless, 'Christ the Paediatrician: Augustine on the Diagnosis and Treatment of the Injured Vocation of the Child', in *The Vocation of the Child*, ed. Patrick McKinley Brennan (Cambridge and Grand Rapids: William B. Eerdmans Publishing Company, 2008), 128.

119. Sally Davis, *Annual Report of the Chief Medical Officer, 2014. The Health of the 51%: Women* (London: Department of Health, 2015). Davis outlines her case in the introduction to this report: 'In women obesity can affect the outcomes of any pregnancies they have and impacts on the health of any future children they may have. In pregnant women, the developmental environment can affect the fetus and its germline cells, e.g. their eggs (primary oocytes) and so a woman's health whilst she is pregnant also impacts on the health of her children and grandchildren' (10).

Syn, Guilt and Shame

From the discussions so far, it should be clear that guilt and shame constitute an important feature of women's Syn-talk. In her interview, Suzanne describes how the shame she experiences as a result of gaining weight can make her anxious about Tuesday's weigh-in:

> I feel ashamed or like I've let myself down in a way cos I think I'm like, Wednesday, Thursday ... Friday and then it just like goes downhill from there and I think, oh God, it's Tuesday! I'm going tonight and there's nothing I can do about it now.

While some fear the consequences of missing the meeting, others are afraid of what will happen if they stay:

> If I've been quite naughty and I think I am going to put weight on, then sometimes I do think, uh [*sighs*] I really don't want to sit there and have the 'oh, a little gain this week' [*imitates Louise*], you know, or whatever. And I just think I really don't want to do this. So there are times when I'll just go and get weighed and then just go, and I won't stay for group. (Helen)

Louise's predictable refrain, mimicked here by Helen, means Helen can be sure that Louise will compel a confession from her in front of the group. The only way she can refuse to confess is by missing the meeting. This presents shame as closely tied to experiences of hiding and exposure.

According to Stephen Pattison, the incentive to '*hide, disappear or flee*'[120] is central to the experience of shame. It is related to the fear of 'losing face' and of being judged to be inferior and defective.[121] Shame, for Pattison, is also linked with feelings of powerlessness and passivity: 'The person experiencing shame has no power of herself to help her self – or anyone else.'[122] This self feels helpless and out of control, 'lacking in power and agency in the face of the hostile "other"'.[123] In the group, women fear losing face/respect and envisage their fat as moving them

---

120. Pattison, *Shame: Theory, Therapy, Theology*, 75. Emphasis in original.
121. Ibid., 75–6.
122. Ibid., 75.
123. Ibid.

into a position of feeling judged in the company of others,[124] whether by Louise or other members. Those who suspect weight gain often worry that the meeting will expose their weakness and cause them to feel ridiculed in public. The sense of powerlessness this produces is clearly communicated in an earlier extract by Suzanne who explains her hopelessness when Tuesday arrives and the week has not gone well. Understandably, meetings can be fraught with anxiety. Samantha speaks about the 'fear factor' of having to sit there knowing that you have put weight on. The problem with gaining weight is that 'you let yourself down in front of a load of other people', she tells me. For Sarah, it is the 'guilt' that compels her towards obedience. She explains that having a bad week and knowing she will have to talk about it makes her more inclined to stick to the programme. The prospect of being exposed in public compels women's obedience helping establish an economy of fear in which the only acceptable response to fat is shame and hiding.

Shame and fear are powerful components of Christian confession. In *The Confessions*, Augustine admits that his disclosures before God are 'tinged with fear and secret sorrow'.[125] His natural inclination is to take cover from God who sees all and knows all, but God thrusts him into his own sight so that Augustine can 'perceive [his own] sin and hate it'.[126] As a result Augustine is filled with 'self-abhorrence' and finds himself 'loathsome'.[127] Louise occupies a similar space as God or the community in this confessionary paradigm. Fearing her all-seeing eye and the embarrassment of being exposed in front of others, many dread the meeting because they can predict how they will feel when they are thrust in front of their own faces and made to confront their Syn. It is not only members' verbal confessions which produce shame and guilt, however. As we have already seen, participants consider that Syn is worn on the body as fat, and this means bodies can be shamed before they even voice their confessions in the meeting. Fat is a 'virtual confession'[128] of Syn and a discursive construction that produces a particular kind of truth-telling.

---

124. Pattison identifies this as a feature of shame. Ibid., 72.
125. Augustine, *The Confessions*, X.4.6.
126. Ibid., VIII.7.16.
127. Ibid., VIII.7.17.
128. I borrow this language from Samantha Murray, *The 'Fat' Female Body* (New York: Palgrave, 2008), 74.

According to feminist philosopher Elizabeth Grosz, bodies often speak without talking because they become coded with signs, laws, norms and ideals. In Western capitalism, the body is considered to be expressive of an interior subjectivity,[129] she argues, seen to confess truths about the inner self. The body thus 'becomes a text, a system of signs to be deciphered, read, and read into'.[130] Social laws, norms and ideals are incarnated and 'corporealized' in bodies, and bodies are also 'textualized', '"read" by others as expressive of a subject's psychic interior'.[131] Drawing on Grosz's insights, Samantha Murray states that fat bodies are routinely read as immoral and as expressive of unhealthiness and unethical living, exposing the fat person as 'a moral and aesthetic failure'.[132] 'The confession', she says, 'is one of necessary pathology, indulgence and excess, and before the "fat" subject even speaks, this confession is produced as truth.'[133]

In my group, fat similarly speaks for itself. Guilt and shame are worn on the body as excess weight without members having to say a word, but this virtual confession does not negate the need to audibly disclose Syn. In their weekly confessions, women usually reproduce the truths their bodies already display, taking the wrap for fat and blaming their gains on their 'bad' foodways. If women do not accept responsibility for their gains, Louise often compels their guilt by reminding them of the need for remorse. We see this in the exchange below, where Lisa describes to me what aspects of the meeting she does not like:

> **Lisa** Maybe when she [Louise] says, you've put on weight you're like, oh, I dunno. I don't feel embarrassed, I just feel ashamed. But then I remember actually, it was after Christmas. I put on half a pound and then the next week I put on half a pound and then Louise was like, 'are you ok with that?' And I just went, 'oh

---

129. Elizabeth Grosz, *Space, Time and Perversion* (New York, Abingdon and Oxon: Routledge, 1995), 34.

130. Ibid., 34–5.

131. Ibid.

132. Murray, *The 'Fat' Female Body*, 69–70. Also see Kimberly Dark, 'Coming Out Fat', in *Fat Sex: New Directions in Theory and Activism*, ed. Helen Hester and Caroline Walters (Farnham and Burlington: Ashgate, 2015), 215–22. Dark argues that 'for many onlookers, fat is actually proof of failure and poor moral character' (216–17).

133. Murray, *The 'Fat' Female Body*, 75.

yeah, I'm fine, it's only half a pound'. And then she said, 'oh, well you've put on half a pound in two weeks so you need to lose this week, don't you?' like this, and I was like, 'oh yeah, okay'.
Hannah It was a bit of a telling off?
Lisa Yeah it was a little bit but actually, I'm glad she said it cos I thought, actually yeah, why am I saying I'm happy with putting on weight two weeks on the run? I know it's only half a pound each week but I shouldn't be like, oh yeah, I'm happy 'cos I hadn't gone oh I'm definitely gonna lose *so* much next week. I didn't like her saying that; made me think oh, actually, yeah.

What is striking here is that although Lisa is originally quite happy to accommodate her small weight gain, Louise's 'telling off' makes her adjust her confessing narrative so that it adheres to the normative pattern of guilt–shame. In this way, confession provides a mechanism not only for 'managing' shame but also for evoking it.

Such an observation departs from the findings of Daniel Martin who draws on interviews and participant observation inside *Weight Watchers* to argue that the company emphasizes shame control rather than shame avowal.[134] He charts the way *Weight Watchers* changed tack from a system of 'card calling' to a new system where consultants step back and allow the group to resolve fraught situations for themselves. Instead of evoking shame by announcing the names and weight losses/gains of each individual (as happens in my group), this shift in *Weight Watchers*, Martin reflects, suggests a move towards shame management rather than production.

In my group, shame management strategies are evident as Louise invites members to counsel and encourage one another. She frequently supplies participants with excuses that they can use to explain unexpected gains (of which 'water retention' is the most popular) and invites those who are deflated and demotivated to focus on what they

---

134. Daniel D. Martin, 'Organizational Approaches to Shame: Avowal, Management, and Contestation', *The Sociological Quarterly* 41, no. 1 (2000): 137–40. According to Martin, until the 1970s *Weight Watchers* relied on a system of 'card-calling' but the loss of revenue resulting from members terminating their subscriptions, prompted a change in approach, as did concerns about corporate liability. This is not unlike the shift in spelling from 'Sin' to 'Syn' implemented by the organization at the centre of this book which similarly occurs as a means of deflecting shame and securing revenue.

have achieved. Confession functions as one of the most important mechanisms for managing shame as many consider it to expose Syn thereby enabling them to move on.[135] As well as repeating the Christian pattern of repentance and absolution, this ensures members do not feel so ashamed that they entirely disengage from the weight loss process (which would be financially hazardous), while guaranteeing that they feel enough shame to be motivated to carry on directing their finances towards the amelioration of their fat. Yet the way Louise compels Lisa's confession (above) suggests that she does more than simply 'contain' women's shame experiences. By adjusting members' confessing narratives, Louise actually evokes shame and reveals the cultural truth about fat that women are already compelled to know as 'obvious' and 'common sense' – that, as Levy-Navarro puts it, fat must be beaten, blamed and changed; that the fat self is 'all that we must hate, avoid, and finally control'.[136]

In her discussion of confession in weight loss discourse, Levy-Navarro contends that confession narratives '[tell] us what we already know';[137] they are coercive because even though they may be experienced as liberating, they also 'have the effect of compelling us to acknowledge their truth'.[138] Confession, in her view, corroborates cultural knowledges about fat[139] rather than revealing something hidden within the self. This applies a Foucauldian lens to the activity of confession. Observing confession as one of the West's most valuable techniques for producing truth, Foucault acknowledges that when confession is not offered freely, it is forced out of the body, 'driven from its hiding place in the soul, or

---

135. Hevala tells me, 'I think just being there [in the meeting] makes you kind of think like you've reset everything so you've reset the balance and you kind of feel like, right that's it. Back in control a bit now. You don't feel like you're hiding from it; you're kind of ... you've faced what happened and you've openly said this is what's happened to me this week and that's it, and I'm drawing a line under it. And you can start a new week. But if you don't do that I think you can still sort of hide away from it a little bit.'

136. Elena Levy-Navarro, 'I'm the New Me: Compelled Confession Diet Discourse', *The Journal of Popular Culture* 45, no. 2 (2012): 250.

137. Ibid., 348.

138. Ibid., 349.

139. Samantha Murray talks about this in terms of a '*tacit* investment in dominant aesthetics'. Murray, *The 'Fat' Female Body*, 92 (emphasis in original).

extracted from the body'.[140] We misunderstand confession, he claims, if we consider it to be extracting a truth 'lodged in our most secret nature'.[141] Instead, it is a product of power that works to validate certain knowledges.

In my group, although women conceive that confession allows them to face up to hidden truths (like Augustine suggests), the acknowledgement of guilt is driven out of their bodies by Louise in the way Foucault describes. Louise is 'not simply the interlocutor but the authority who requires the confession, prescribes and appreciates it, and intervenes in order to judge, punish, forgive, console, and reconcile'.[142] She is positioned as already knowing the truth that members' bodies disclose, even before they speak. Confession then is a device through which members are made to corroborate her truth and forced to know it for themselves. It is an 'obligatory act of speech'[143] that helps validate implicit knowledges about fat which structure the power relations between Louise as judge and members as confessors.[144] Bodily shame, then, is dispelled through confession, as Martin suggests, but it is also manufactured and harnessed to realign women's thoughts and actions with prominent social values.[145]

The assumption that fat virtually confesses Syn repeats the feature of Western capitalism that presents the outer body as expressive of the inner self. In this setting, curating and controlling the outer stands to represent the inner more favourably and to align the body with the will. In 'appearance organizations'[146] like this one, such an enterprise is a marketable commodity. It is also an important feature of Christian asceticism where food restraint and sexual abstinence figure as important methods of practising the relationship between the body and soul. R. Marie Griffith observes that although diverse in type

---

140. Michel Foucault, *The History of Sexuality, Vol. 1, The Will to Knowledge*, trans. Robert Hurley (London: Penguin, 1978), 59.

141. Ibid., 60.

142. Ibid., 61–2.

143. Ibid., 62.

144. Murray, *The 'Fat' Female Body*, 74–5.

145. Also see Carole Spitzack, *Confessing Excess: Women and the Politics of Body Reduction* (Albany: State University of New York Press, 1990), 60.

146. Daniel Martin describes appearance organizations as 'organizations for whom the physical appearance of members is a primary concern'. Martin, 'Organizational Approaches to Shame', 126.

and meaning, Christian practices of discipline designed to control the appetite and desire for food and sex are all rooted in the assumption that the visible body is expressive of the invisible soul. That is why Christian thinkers hold that the body can be 'scoured for indications of damnation and salvation'.[147] Participants in my group are not fasting in pursuit of a spiritual quest like the spiritual athletes of the past, but they do anticipate that their bodies and the number on the scale can be read as visible evidence of their moral character, and thus of Syn. In this way, women continue in the ascetic tradition by foregrounding the outer body as a gateway to the inner self.

Fat, however, is not always visible. Fat is not just a visible stigma that shames individuals – what Erving Goffman names as a 'discredited identity'[148] – because what counts as fat is often so miniscule that assistance is needed to bring it out into the open so it can be shamed. Much like Syn, fat hides in unsuspecting places. Frequently, it is the scale, members' coerced confessions and Louise's public announcement of their weight gain that make fat visible and Syn apparent. In this way, the scale, confession and Louise actually produce members' fat rather than it being self-evident.

The meeting then allows women's bodies to be shamed and stigmatized, sometimes quite apart from what they look like. It also confirms that fat is a stigma with which almost any woman can be identified, challenging assumptions about who qualifies as fat in the first place. Nita McKinley suggests that 'the hostility that is directed toward fat women who do not "confess excess" is evidence of the challenge that the fat woman presents to dominant cultural discourse, especially those of the ideal woman'.[149] The fact that Lisa (in the dialogue with me above) is not large heightens and nuances this critique, showing that refusing to confess excess, even when a woman is not fat, protests against normative cultural scripts about gender and fatness. Women are expected to admit guilt and confess excess, independent of their size.

---

147. Griffith, *Born Again Bodies*, 23.

148. Erving Goffman, *Stigma: Notes on the Management of a Spoiled Identity* (New York: Prentice Hall, 1963). For a discussion of this in relation to fat, see Abigail C. Saguy and Anna Ward, 'Coming Out as Fat: Rethinking Stigma', *Social Psychology Quarterly* 74, no. 1 (2011): 53–75.

149. Nita Mary McKinley, 'Ideal Weight/Ideal Women: Society Constructs the Female', in *Weighty Issues: Fatness and Thinness as Social Problems*, ed. Jeffrey Sobal and Donna Maurer (New York: Aldine de Gruyter, 1999), 110.

The Gendered Nature of Syn

So far, I have argued that by identifying Syn with danger, irrationality, disobedience, death, disease, shame, pleasure and excessive eating, the slimming group reproduce dominant theological discourses about sin. Such meanings help vilify fat and bolster cultural and organizational assumptions about thinness and corpulence. Any amount of 'excess' is established as a virtual confession of Syn, confirming all women's bodies as deviant and in need of repair. Repeating the individualism and assumed 'badness' promulgated by Western understandings of sin, the meanings that members attribute to Syn also mesh with the capitalist and neoliberal enterprises of freedom and consumer choice. Stress on the individuated will, on choosing the good, on shaming bodies and foodways that move out of their appropriate places fulfils the agenda of constructing members as autonomous, active consumer agents who are always already free to make rational choices. This ideology is driven by an incessant consumerism that compels women to practise their entrepreneurial freedom through the purchase of a slimmer self. The marking of food and fat through association with Syn confirms that women must choose to lose their fat if they are to become 'good'. The extent to which women are free to choose slimming for themselves in these circumstances will be the subject of the next chapter, but I want to end this section by drawing out more explicitly the gendered theological nature of these discursive constructions.

Syn as Feminine

The gendering of Syn is exposed most obviously by the way the organization targets a female audience and by the way it attracts a predominantly female membership. This follows normative theological tradition in locating women in closer proximity to sin and food-related failure. Syn is also exposed as being gender-coded by the way the organization reproduces symbolic linkages integral to classical theologies of sin which are already gendered. Associations with corporeality, death, defilement, desire, irrationality, pleasure and the realm of the non-human animal are integral components of the discursive system of sin that have been historically and consistently affiliated with women and used against them. By aligning Syn-talk with these dominant theological components, the organization and its members vicariously repeat the misogynist assumptions of these ancient systems.

The Christian gendering of sin and the related spheres of corporeality and affect has its roots in the 'samatophobia' of Greek metaphysics and philosophical dualism.[150] For Plato and Aristotle, for example, corporeality is not simply base and corrupt but gendered female. The body is a prison for the soul, according to Plato, and escaping the dungeon of the body akin to escaping the excesses of the female that lacks form and reason. Aristotle continues this tradition assuming that in reproduction, the mother is the passive incubator that supplies the formless matter that the father then shapes.[151] He identifies corporeality with softness and softness with incontinence, the female and corpulence.[152] In this philosophical model, fat occupies the symbolic space of the female, aligned with excessiveness and with a lack of restraint.

Such meanings not only continue to hold sway in Western cultural constructs of fatness but also inform early Christian writers who tend to classify the female principle as corporeal and the male as incorporeal. Many classical Judeo-Christian texts use the masculine and feminine as symbols which represent the superior and inferior capacity for rationality, morality and strength,[153] reflecting the influence of the philosophies of the ancient Greco-Roman world. Augustine, for example, distinguishes between the masculine dimension of the mind which he terms 'wisdom' or *sapientia* that was that part of the mind concerned with 'intellectual cognition of eternal things',[154] and

---

150. See Grosz, *Volatile Bodies*. She argues that Western philosophy has 'established itself on the foundations of a profound somatophobia', in which the body is regarded as 'a source of interference in, and a danger to, the operations of reason' (5).

151. Ibid.

152. Jana Evans Braziel, 'Sex and Fat Chics: Deterritorializing the Fat Female Body', in *Bodies out of Bounds*, 239-40.

153. Kim Power, *Veiled Desire: Augustine's Writings on Women* (London: Darman, Longman and Todd, 1995), 113.

154. Augustine, *On the Trinity*, Books 8-15, ed. Gareth B. Matthews, trans. Stephen McKenna (Cambridge and New York: Cambridge University Press, 2002), 12.15.25. *Scientia* was helpmeet to *sapientia* in the same way that Eve was a helpmeet to Adam, according to Augustine: 'For just as among all the beasts, a help like unto himself was not found for man, unless one were taken from himself and formed into his consort, so for our mind, by which we consult the superior and inner things, for such employment of corporeal things as the

the feminine dimension of 'knowledge' or *scientia* concerned with 'reasonable cognition of temporal things'.[155] Despite insisting that *scientia* and *sapientia* are features of both male and female minds, his association of the masculine with the person of Adam and the feminine with the person of Eve aligns women with the temporal realm and men with the superior realm of the eternal.

Participants recreate associations between corporeality, irrationality, death and disordered desire that are already symbolically aligned with the feminine. In so doing, they repeat the Western problematic construction of consumption and bodies Christian thought helps to cement. If corporeality is feminine, then fatness is a hyperbolic expression of corporeality and an exaggerated manifestation of the feminine.[156] Fat is expressive of *too much* corporeality and *too much* femininity. This places fatness in the feminine discursive position of the 'residue', described by Luce Irigaray as that (excess) which the male symbolic expels as 'scraps' and 'uncollected debris'.[157] For Irigaray, the residue is homeless in the realm of discourse and meaning, rendered as waste or as a discarded fragment. Women occupy the place of the residue, she argues, having been expelled from the realm of discourse so that the male can establish himself as subject. According to Irigaray, women exist in a state of *déréliction* or abandonment,[158] serving as 'sacrificial objects' to protect men from 'the violence of their death drives'.[159]

---

nature of man requires, no help like unto itself was found in the parts of the soul which we have in common with the beasts' (12.3.3). When the mind was dragged away from contemplation of eternal things towards lust and desire for sensual pleasure, this was akin to the serpent once again tempting Eve (12.12.17). In order to prevent such a downfall, *sapientia* must be a 'watch tower of counsel' over *scientia*; it must 'check and restrain' her (12.8.13). *Scientia*, being closer to the appetites and the senses, was to be ruled and subdued by 'him' and 'ought to be kept in check' (12.7.10).

155. Ibid., 12.15.25.
156. See Braziel, 'Sex and Fat Chics', 241.
157. Luce Irigaray, *This Sex Which Is Not One*, trans. Catherine Porter with Carolyn Burke (Ithaca: Cornell University Press, 1985), 30.
158. Luce Irigaray, *An Ethics of Sexual Difference*, trans. Carolyn Burke and Gillian C. Gill (Ithaca: Cornell University Press, 1993), 70.
159. Whitford cited in Anne-Claire Mulder, *Divine Flesh, Embodied Word: 'Incarnation' as a Hermeneutical Key to a Feminist Theologian's*

In the weight loss group, like in Western culture, fatness occupies this exilic place. It is an excess or waste that is expelled (exiled) in order to shore up the boundaries of the thin body and to carry the full weight of death and corporeality. Attending the weekly meetings and the daily discipline of slimming are the processes through which women are compelled to exorcize the feminine, and we will see further evidence of this in Chapter 3. That fat is feminine, of course, means that *women's* fat is doubly feminine and so doubly (excessively) dangerous, and this ensures that women's bodies once more become the 'vague conceptual dumping ground'[160] for the maligned body and its sensory experience.

Ancient associations between women and corporeality become moralized in Christian thought through the linkage with sin, and this moralizing connection is repeated in the group as fat is constructed as a virtual confession of Syn. In both cases, the association of corporeality with sin serves to establish the female body as morally culpable and as a seat of irrational sensuality.

One of the most important ways in which Christian theology has marked women's bodies and maligned corporeality is by blaming Eve for the Fall. Depictions of Eve as a sexual temptress, as luring Adam away from perfection, are embedded firmly within early Christian teaching, and serve to position Eve's eating as humanity's original sin and all women as the 'bearers of sin'.[161] 1 Timothy 2.12-14 uses Eve's secondary position in creation and her putative culpability in sin to justify the subordination of women. Drawing on this post-Pauline epistle, Ambrose and Augustine establish the woman as the cause of sin and see in the Genesis narrative the grounds for sexual hierarchy. For Ambrose, the woman is the originator of the man's wrongdoing, not the man of the woman's. For Augustine, Eve rather than Adam is deceived – 'she alone spoke to the serpent, and she

---

Reading of Irigaray's Work (Amsterdam: Amsterdam University Press, 2006), 183. In Irigaray's view, Western thought and culture is structured by the unacknowledged and un-symbolized 'murder of the mother', because the 'man-god-father' has killed her to take power. See Luce Irigaray, 'Women-Mothers, the Silent Substratum of the Social Order', in *The Irigaray Reader*, ed. Margaret Whitford (Oxford: Blackwell, 1991), 47.

160. Carolyn Korsmeyer, *Making Sense of Taste: Food and Philosophy* (Ithaca and London: Cornell University Press, 1999), 35.

161. Rosemary Radford Ruether, *Sexism and God-Talk: Toward a Feminist Theology* (Boston: Beacon Press, 1983), 94.

alone was seduced by him'.[162] According to Augustine, Eve believed the serpent and ate to fulfil her own inordinate desire, whereas Adam knew the serpent was lying but ate out of companionship.[163]

Other early Christian thinkers proffer equally misogynist interpretations of the Eden story. In his discussion of modesty in female dress, the 'lively and verbal'[164] Latin theologian, Tertullian, famously casts all women in the role of Eve. Women are responsible for the Fall, he argues, and ultimately to blame for the death of Christ:

> And do you not know that you are (each) an Eve? The sentence of God on this sex of yours lives in this age: the guilt must of necessity live too. You are the devil's gateway: *you* are the unsealer of that (forbidden) tree: *you* are the first deserter of the divine law: *you* are she who persuaded him whom the devil was not valiant enough to attack. *You* destroyed so easily God's image, man. On account of *your* desert – that is, death – even the Son of God had to die.[165]

Such views have shaped the church's theological anthropology and its theology of sin, not only identifying sin with a fall from a state of integrity to a state of guilt but also identifying women *as* sin. Gluttony has been linked to lust, and control over food aligned with control over sexual desire.[166] Tied to both has been the assumption that lust, the passions and inordinate desire are features of sin particularly associated with women, and this exposes what Brazilian feminist liberation

---

162. Augustine, *On the Trinity*, 12.12.17.

163. This point is made by Rosemary Radford Ruether in her essay, 'Augustine: Sexuality, Gender and Women', in *Feminist Interpretations of Augustine*, ed. Judith Chelius Stark (Pennsylvania: The Pennsylvania State University, 2007), 54.

164. Eric Osborn, 'Tertullian', in *The First Christian Theologians: An Introduction to Theology in the Early Church*, ed. G. R. Evans (Malden, Oxford, Carlton and Victoria: Blackwell Publishers Ltd., 2004), 143.

165. Tertullian, 'On the Apparel of Women', in *Ante-Nicene Fathers*, II.1.1. For Irenaeus, Eve is the cause not only of her own death but also of the death of the whole human race. See Irenaeus, 'Against Heresies', in *The Ante-Nicene Fathers: The Writings of the Fathers Down to AD 325*, ed. Rev. Alexander Roberts and James Donaldson (Grand Rapids: WM. B. Eerdmans Publishing Company, 1981), 3.22.4.

166. Bovey, *The Forbidden Body*, 27.

theologian, Ivone Gebara, observes as a tendency in classical Christian thought to identify women with evil 'as if women incarnate evil'.[167]

Feminist theologians have rightly challenged such misogyny seeing in this a 'malignant image' of male–female relationships and of woman[168] that has infected the whole of the classical tradition and which still retains its hold over the modern psyche.[169] According to Mary Daly, the myth of feminine evil has been pervasive throughout the ages and continues to inform the theological and cultural imagination today.[170] It is hard to dispute her point when we consider that the image of the half-bitten apple appears on every product produced by the American multinational technology company, *Apple*, making them hundreds of billions of dollars each year.[171] Ivone Gebara explains that a similar image of an apple with a bite taken out is displayed in various cities in Latin America to designate places of prostitution or illicit rendezvous.[172] Such symbolic connections between women, food, seduction and permissive sexual conduct demonstrate just how significant the Eve figure is and how good for business. As biblical studies scholar Katie Edwards observes, 'Eve is quite a money-maker. … So long as she can bring in the revenue she will be out there in cinema and magazines with her trusty apple and snake to lure in consumers to take a bite of

---

167. Ivone Gebara, *Out of the Depths: Women's Experience of Evil and Salvation*, trans. Ann Patrick Ware (Minneapolis: Fortress, 2002), 4.

168. Mary Daly, *Beyond God the Father: Towards a Philosophy of Women's Liberation* (London: The Women's Press, 1986), 45.

169. Ruether, *Sexism and God-Talk*, 94–9. Ruether observes that although the Genesis story was certainly not the only story in the ancient world to blame women for evil and is not cited in other parts of the Hebrew Bible as the origin of evil, Christian theologians have consistently treated the story with the utmost seriousness (166). Patriarchal interpretations of Genesis have suggested that Eve's subjugation is a reflection of her God-made inferior nature and a punishment for her culpability for sin. Such sexist theological anthropology, she holds, infects the whole of the classical tradition, from Augustine and Aquinas to Luther and Barth.

170. For Daly, such misogyny aids the non-being of women and justifies male hatred of women and women's hatred of themselves. See *Beyond God the Father*, 45–55, esp. 48.

171. Deborah Sawyer also notes that 'we see … Eve's bitten apple engraved on every iPod across the globe. 'Hidden Subjects', 306.

172. Gebara, *Out of the Depths*, 5.

whatever product she is selling'.[173] The influence of Eve as Christianity's archetypal woman has been felt down the ages and continues to impact contemporary Western and colonial cultures across the globe,[174] informing social attitudes towards women's bodies and appetites.

That women's bodies are especially tied to this symbolic framework of guilt and temptation is especially evident in one August meeting when Mark transgresses the unspoken rule and announces his weight to the group. He weighs seventeen stone he tells us. The silence that follows Mark's disclosure expresses the group's alarm and astonishment at his breach of protocol. Although there is discomfort in the room, no one flinches and Julia, the leader for this particular meeting (because Louise is absent), makes no comment. I wonder to myself whether Julia's reaction would have been different if one of the women had decided to 'out' their size. This, however, is not the only occasion on which Mark breaks the rules. In a separate meeting in August, Louise tells the group that Mark has gained five pounds. In response, he makes a joke about being unable to pass up the opportunity to eat a good Cornish pasty in Cornwall. He then continues to recommend a pub to the group where it is possible to have a giant Yorkshire pudding with sausage, potatoes, vegetables and gravy all inside. Louise is uneasy with his promotion of Syn and quickly tries to move him on, asking him to think about where he might go from here.

On both occasions Mark is undisturbed by his disclosures, despite the way they breach the unspoken rules of the meeting. He is happy to speak his weight, and he is unapologetic about endorsing Syn. Unlike Lisa (above) who succumbs to Louise's demand for remorse, he undermines the canonical assumption that fat is an exposé of shame and guilt by making his own fat unapologetically visible – by 'flaunting' his fat.[175] Of course, this may be a defensive response from Mark – an

---

173. Katie Edwards, *Admen and Eve: The Bible in Contemporary Advertising* (Sheffield: Sheffield Phoenix Press, 2012), 34. According to Edwards, popular culture from the 1990s onwards represents Eve as the archetypal post-feminist who exercises power through 'self-commodification and sexualization' (86). In so doing, such depictions pick up on the 'textual clues' within Genesis that suggest Eve is the more active protagonist.

174. Sawyer, 'Hidden Subjects', 305.

175. Kenji Yoshino discusses 'flaunting' in relation to gay identity. He suggests that the turn of the millennium marks a shift from the requirement to 'pass' (as straight) to a requirement to 'cover'. This is seen, he argues, in

attempt to not appear bothered in public – but it may also be that he feels secure enough in his male body to violate the rules about speaking weight that women feel compelled to obey. His disclosure may infer that Syn is not as serious for him nor guilt as incumbent upon his male body; a point he reinforces in his interview when he tells me that fat does not invalidate men in the same way that it does women. The difference between his behaviour and the etiquette of the women in the group may display how the women more readily accept and internalize blame. It also, however, exposes that the stigma of fat can be defused by bringing fat out into the open, a strategy I develop later in this book.[176] This reveals the dangerous power that flaunting fat presents, especially for women given the way confession is obligatory for them.

Conclusion

This chapter has argued that the Christian notion of 'sin' and its related meanings is translated and used by one commercial secular weight loss community and by ordinary women engaged in the everyday pursuit of slimming in ways that are commensurate with classical tradition. While the diverse authorial knowledges of science, politics, philosophy and health combine to inform discourses about weight, theological systems also play a role, supplying a corpus of meanings that help to gender fat and confirm women's girth as an especial site of danger.

The explicit appeal to the Christian moral language of sin by this secular organization is, in many ways, surprising. At the start of his book on *The Concept of Sin*, Josef Pieper argues that 'we don't hear the word "sin" much anymore', probably because of the 'raised eyebrows' and 'rhetorical "assault"' that might follow. It is only within religious language, he claims, that people speak of sin without embarrassment

---

contemporary resistance to same-sex marriage which signals the demand to cover, distilled in the sentiment: *'Fine, be gay, but don't shove it in our faces'*. In my group, even though Mark is not especially large, he nevertheless flaunts his fat by refusing to apologize. See Kenji Yoshino, *Covering: The Hidden Assault on American Civil Rights* (New York: Random House Publishing Group, 2006), 19. Also see Saguy and Ward's discussion of Yoshino's account of 'flaunting' in their article, 'Coming Out as Fat: Rethinking Stigma', 53–75, esp. 57.

176. In Chapter 6 I suggest that this is a power that can be harnessed towards a distinctly Christian praxis of pride.

and where sin is 'woven into the very fabric of the ordinary language of the believer'.[177] In the group, however, 'Syn' is a term that is clearly and frequently spoken and heard. Although the shift in spelling from 'Sin' to 'Syn' may deflect or at least manage any potential embarrassment arising from employing such a Christian-sounding word in this non-religious setting, and even though the overlay of the seemingly more scientific notion of 'Synergy' helps strip Syn-talk of any reference to God,[178] the language of sin is not obscured or hidden as in other secular commercial weight loss settings. In my group, 'Syn' is referred to openly and its proximity to Christian speech and thought plainly displayed by the original spelling adopted by the company and by the normative meanings members continue to attach to it. By employing the concept in ways that are continuous with dominant theological discourse, the organization follows patriarchal Christian interpretation in making women's bodies carry the burden of guilt. Christian sensibilities – even if partly anonymized – are never erased. It is this combination of overt borrowing from Christianity and tacit concealment of religious sentiment that makes the trope of Syn so successful, enabling the organization to take from the theological treasure chest of meaning while simultaneously obscuring the trope's theological home. This ensures maximum profitability and maximum appeal in a secular context that is often suspicious of religion in the public domain.

177. Josef Pieper, *The Concept of Sin* (South Bend: St. Augustine Press, 2001), 2.
178. I am influenced here by Lynne Gerber who argues that unmarked Protestant discourses continue to influence American secular culture. According to Gerber, the effect of translating Protestant sensibilities into secular discourse is that all trace of religion is erased and the specific locatedness of religious sentiment in historical communities becomes obscured. Instead, dominant religious sensibilities emerge as rational, universal and scientific, but this can never remove the religious sentiment that shaped the secular discourse. See Gerber, *Seeking the Straight and Narrow*, 226–7.

Chapter 2

SYN, SELF-SURVEILLANCE AND TAKING CARE: TENSIONS AND AMBIGUITIES

Chapter 1 considered how the group's Syn-talk resurrects ancient theological associations with danger, disobedience, death and desire and how these work to aid the control of women's bodies. This chapter turns to consider in more detail how traditional theological discourse is modified through the organization's positive narration of Syn and through association with the concept of permission.

In the organization, Syn is encouraged, albeit within certain perimeters, and this means that Syn provides occasion for women to act. Women in the group use the food diary, practise mental methods of recording Syn[1] and produce their own texts to manage Syn. Such techniques of 'Syn-watching', I argue, enable women to become experts at negotiating the tensions between permission and prohibition that structure the Syn system and provide opportunities for women to practise self-determinism. While this may be read as an instance of a 'free market feminism' that cleverly sells women's freedom back to them,[2] attention to the micro-practices of surveillance exposes a more complex account of subjectivity and a broader account of action. The licence attached to Syn invites women to shape intentional selves and foodways and is sometimes embraced by women in ways the plan does not permit. Managing and policing Syn can provide women with opportunities to resist the expectations of the weight loss organization, and while such methods serve to conform women's bodies to patriarchal norms, this does not mitigate the way they simultaneously increase women's capacities. Tensions between discipline and

---

1. By 'mental methods' I refer to the ways in which members come to know and recite and calculate Syn values in their minds.

2. Imelda Whelehan, *The Feminist Bestseller: From Sex and the Single Girl to Sex and the City* (Basingstoke and New York: Palgrave Macmillan, 2005), 155 and Joanne Hollows, *Feminism, Femininity and Popular Culture* (Manchester and New York: Manchester University Press, 2000), 194.

agency performed through body watching techniques in relation to food mirror certain features of historic Christian devotional foodways and ascetic practices. As in Chapter 1, Christian religion emerges once more as an important explanatory aid for making sense of Syn as it takes shape in this secular commercial weight loss setting.

Adapting Theological Discourse: Permission to Syn

The previous chapter began to provide an insight into the contradictory and ambiguous messages the organization produced about Syn. To understand this tension thoroughly, it is necessary to appreciate the emphasis the organization places on the legitimacy of Syn. According to the weight loss guide, Syns 'supply a wonderful safety net, to ensure you lose weight with a mixture of plenty of freewheeling, plus just enough structure and control'; Syn 'takes the guilt right out of eating'. Louise reinforces this point, frequently reminding us that we do not need to deny ourselves the foods we enjoy. A poster in the room advises that Syn is flexible:

> Flexibility is the saviour of many a struggling slimmer.
> Dismiss any rigid diet rules and embrace flexibility.
> Remember flexible Syns.

The flexibility of Syn lies at the centre of the organization's positive narration of Syn. Louise recurrently explains that we are free to choose how to spend and save our Syn allowance, so if we eat lots of Syns on one day, we can always 'pull it back' on the next. The elastic nature of Syn, she counsels, means that we do not have to go hungry or avoid foods we enjoy, and this is experienced by members as a particularly attractive feature of the programme. Explaining why she likes the plan, Jane tells me, 'This one suits me fine because I'm not doing without anything I don't want to do without. Anything I want to eat I can.' Lucy similarly tells me that when eating out, if she wants something from the menu which is high in Syns she will choose it: 'If I want it I'll have it because that's a treat isn't it, and, I'm 'aving it.'

This positive narration of Syn expresses what Kate Cairus and Josée Johnston identify as a 'do-diet' stance.[3] Drawing on focus groups

---

3. Kate Cairus and Josée Johnston, 'Choosing Health: Embodied Neoliberalism, Postfeminism, and the "Do-Diet"', *Theory and Society* 44, no. 2

and interviews with a hundred women in Toronto along with other textual data, they detect a food discourse that presents food choices through the lens of empowerment and health. This discourse reframes restriction as freedom and presents healthy eating 'as a "win-win" choice that need not sacrifice pleasure'.[4] The do-diet, they explain, invites women to consume and is seen in their study by the way women see themselves as positive agentic consumers willingly embracing healthy options. Within this discourse, dieting is stigmatized, aligned with punishing and constricting food practices that deprive women of enjoyment. The do-diet is expressive of neoliberal ideology and modes of governmentality, they argue, because it constructs women as free citizens able to make rational consumer choices and to regulate their bodies for themselves without coercion.[5]

In my group, this discourse takes shape in the organization's positive presentation of Syn which suggests no food is off limits. The poster promoting the flexibility of Syn clearly communicates that while diets restrict and inhibit, Syn sets members free. Syn is a 'saviour'[6] in fact, because it permits women to eat without guilt. Herein we see quite obviously how normative Christian discourse is adapted as Syn is aligned with salvation rather than devastation, with permission, release and embrace rather than with proscription. Syn is about *dos* rather than *don'ts* and makes life easier and better because it delivers members from the suffocating grip of diet regulations. Indeed, according to the website, '"DIET" is a four letter word'.

Such a positive stance guarantees that Syn is not over-conditioned by a Christian logic. The standard theological association of sin with hubris is replaced by a discourse that appears to invite women to listen to their urges and feed their passions. Desire for Synful foods need not be denied, but this does not mean that women can enjoy uninhibited eating. Instead, they must embrace their freedom by imposing their own disciplinary measures. Women are expected to self-govern, and

(March 2015): 153–75. The textual sources they study include healthy eating blogs, magazines and newspaper articles.

4. The authors note that the term 'do-diet' is drawn from one of their textual sources, the Canadian women's magazine, *Chatelaine*. This magazine asks, 'Tired of living in a world of diet don'ts? So are we. That's why we developed the Do Diet, a radical new way to eat that's full of easy dos to get you on the right track' (ibid., 154).

5. Ibid., 156.

6. I will say more about how the group configure salvation in Chapter 3.

this frames Syn within the context of neoliberal governmentality, as Cairus and Johnston observe.

Choosing Syn: A Reassertion of the Neoliberal Enterprising Self

Neoliberalism is characterized by the dismantling of the welfare state, a global free market and global free trade. In this political economy, individual well-being is presumed to be secured through self-interest and consumerism. The enterprising self maximizes its own happiness through the practice of autonomy. Neoliberalism thus extends market rationality to all areas of life[7] – choices about the body are framed as market choices, and citizens figured as rational economic actors. In her discussion of neoliberalism and popular women's culture, Eva Chen describes the subject of neoliberalism as one who 'freely deliberates every action based on a rational cost-benefit calculation'.[8] Here, the individual produces their pleasure and is responsible for their consumer choices; they are 'their own entrepreneur'.[9]

In the weight loss group, women engage in this entrepreneurial business of cost-benefit analysis by making wise personal choices about when to spend Syn and when to save it. They manage their Syn allowance and determine how to consume in ways that maximize 'profit' (ironically read as weight *loss*). The successful slimmer is the woman who eats what she wants while balancing her Syn allowance, producing her own pleasure while reigning herself in at the same time. Effective self-governance demands that indulgence is always tempered by restraint, and this means that the process of spending and saving is a technical one that requires forethought and skill. Samantha saves up her Syns so she can 'pig out' at the weekend when her partner is away. Jacqui balances the liberty of going out at the weekend with more stringent behaviour in the week:

> If I've been bad you know maybe gone out Friday, Saturday night, eating, drinking whatever, you know. I don't have to go out. I can't just go to a friend's house and you know what it's like – a glass of wine and a few nibbles. I have done that and then Sunday, Monday I really try to be strict just so that maybe I can stay the same when I get weighed on a Tuesday.

---

7. Gill and Arthurs, 'Editors' Introduction: New Femininities?', 445.
8. Chen, 'Neoliberalism and Popular Women's Culture', 443.
9. Ibid., 444.

Despite defining her behaviour at the weekend as 'bad', Jacqui here allows herself the nibbles and wine she desires. She does, however, insist that the consumption of these foods must be balanced by strict control if she is to avoid a gain at Tuesday's meeting.

Allowing the self to indulge and then 'pulling it back' to compensate are techniques women learn and perfect. Louise endorses this message by encouraging members to be 'wise' with their Syns. In one August meeting, she invites the group to consider what we think about as 'British' food. 'Fish and chips!' one woman shouts. Louise asks how it might be possible to have a 'chippy tea' that is low in Syn, and the woman proposes that we grill the fish and swop the chips for potato wedges cooked in the oven. Louise is gleeful. It is clear she has another solution. We can still enjoy a chippy tea from the chip shop, she instructs, but we must discard the batter first. In a later meeting in October, Ruth admits that her partiality to crusty bread impedes on her slimming success. Louise invokes the help of the group and asks how it might be possible to still eat crusty bread on the plan. I feel as baffled by this as I did by the chippy tea example, but the solution is similar: we must scoop out the dough from the centre and dispose of it.

In these instances, being wise with Syn requires that members throw bits of food away, just as Gail in the video Kandi Stinson talks about is advised by her 'good' self to throw the rest of the cake she has not yet consumed in the bin.[10] The message Louise communicates is that it is better – less Synful – to waste food than consume it. What is also exposed is that the permission and flexibility of Syn is not without qualification. If women are to eat what they want, then they must modify items by replacing high-Syn ingredients with low-Syn equivalents or by throwing a portion of what they want away. They must become skilled budget holders of their Syn allowance,[11] practising their entrepreneurial freedom in ways that avoid the pitfalls of any type of excess. Although the do-diet stance emerges in the group to suggest that life can carry on as usual without women having to deny themselves of the foods they enjoy, it is quite clear that the permission of Syn is not absolute. In the end, there is only so much 'freewheeling' (to cite the weight loss guide)

---

10. See Chapter 1 where I address this. Also see Stinson, *Women and Dieting Culture*, 127.

11. I discuss the notion of 'Syn' as 'cost' in my article, 'Sin or Slim? Christian Morality and the Politics of Personal Choice in a Secular Commercial Weight Loss Setting'.

women can do before they must abstain and deny themselves what they desire.[12]

The emphasis on freedom and choice then does not remove the need for discipline and control. Instead, women must execute their expert knowledge and decision-making capacities to carefully negotiate the precarious lines between indulgence and restraint. To practise the permission of Syn requires the ongoing work of 'calibration'[13] as women must fashion subjectivities that avoid the risks of being seen as too controlling and fanatical or as too indifferent and relaxed.

Syn, Capitalism and the 'Agonistic' Self

The insistence that women can eat what they want while simultaneously requiring them to repress their desires is reflective of the contradictory structure of economic life under capitalism. According to Susan Bordo, this system produces the 'unstable', 'agonistic' personality: a self torn between 'two mutually incompatible directions':

> On the one hand, as producers of goods and services we must sublimate, delay, repress desires for immediate gratification; we must cultivate the work ethic. On the other hand, as consumers we must display a boundless capacity to capitulate to desire and indulge in impulse; we must hunger for constant and immediate satisfaction. The regulation of desire thus becomes an ongoing problem, as we find ourselves continually besieged by temptation, while socially condemned for overindulgence.[14]

For Bordo, since consumer culture conditions us to lose control at the sight of desirable products, we can only ever respond by matching the

---

12. In *Women and Dieting Culture* Kandi Stinson observes a similar tension. Noting how the organization she joins advises its members that no foods are off limits (130), she reflects that 'it is quite obvious that you can't eat the same way or eat the same foods that you ate before joining and still lose weight' (49). Members can eat a takeaway, but there are still limits built into the programme which require them to restrict their appetites.

13. According to Cairus and Johnston, 'calibration' involves trying to avoid 'being seen as an out-of-control eater on the one hand, or as a controlling "health nut" on the other'. See their article, 'Choosing Health', 154.

14. Bordo, *Unbearable Weight*, 199.

desire to consume with a desire to master our passion for consumption.[15] She claims that bulimia embodies this double bind – displaying both 'a hunger for unrestrained consumption' and 'the requirement that we sober up, [and] "clean up our act"'.[16]

Julie Guthman drives Bordo's analysis further contending that the culture of bulimia is to be read not simply as a tension between competing impulses within the self but as a feature of neoliberal governmentality.[17] Sharing with Bordo a Foucauldian lens, Guthman views governmentality as the result of a set of principles which determine how individuals come to act on themselves. Neoliberal governmentality generates contradictory impulses in individuals. Producing the need to consume and exercise vigilance, this political-economic system compels individuals to participate in society as out-of-control consumers and as self-controlled subjects.[18] It generates 'a political economy of bulimia' and casts 'the perfect subject-citizen' as one who 'is able to achieve both eating and thinness' at the same time. Those who achieve both show on their bodies an ability to manage these competing impulses and produce themselves as responsible, self-disciplined subjects.[19] Whereas thinness marks bodies as deserving because they demonstrate the capacity to manage the dual demands to consume and control, fat expresses poor self-governance and a lack of self-discipline.[20]

In the group, it is women's thinning bodies that become the stages upon which these tensions are played out, and Syn is a device through which women establish themselves as responsible citizens. By skilfully negotiating Syn through their bodies, members prove themselves as rational subjects, able to make free 'marketised choices'.[21] Syn is expressive of the political economy of bulimia that Guthman describes,

15. Ibid., 201.

16. Ibid.

17. Julie Guthman, 'Neoliberalism and the Constitution of Contemporary Bodies', in *The Fat Studies Reader*, 191.

18. Guthman and DuPuis, 'Embodying Neoliberalism', 444.

19. Ibid.

20. Guthman, 'Neoliberalism and the Constitution of Contemporary Bodies', 193.

21. Chen explains that neoliberalism renders choice as a marketized commodity, as 'the active ability to respond to power and the autonomous ability to realize one's potential through one's own efforts and active choice'. Chen, 'Neoliberalism and Popular Women's Culture', 443.

and it is an economy that sits happily alongside the philosophical dualisms of spirit–matter and reason–emotion that characterize the sinful predicament described in Chapter 1. If the theological concept of sin denotes a divided-self or a soul 'torn apart', as Augustine holds, then it continues this association with conflict and agony now, albeit overlaid with neoliberal discourse. Unlike in classical Christian thought, however, Syn actually produces the kind of inner turmoil that Augustine narrates and that is characteristic of consumer capitalism. As a system of permission and prohibition, Syn pulls women in mutually incompatible directions, towards having and not having, encouraging women to eat and abstain, want less but spend more.[22] In order to negotiate this tension, women engage in the skilled work of Syn-watching and self-surveillance. In the rest of this chapter, I investigate the methods women use to police Syn and consider how this disciplinary work allows women to cultivate self-care. Although the organization's embrace of Syn rubs uncomfortably against orthodox theological doctrine, the conflicted project of watching the body continues features of historic asceticism, immersing practitioners within disciplinary relations of power while enabling them to shape their own lives.

Keeping an Eye on Syn: Negotiating Syn through Self-surveillance

Self-surveillance is one of the most important methods by which women negotiate the tension between prohibition and permission built into the system of Syn. Members employ a number of techniques but all pivot around daily rituals of watching, weighing and measuring. This aspect of the plan can provoke anxiety. Not long after joining the group, I sat in my car about to drive to work. As was my usual habit, I took a piece of chewing gum from the pot that sits beside my handbrake before setting off. It only took a few seconds before I convulsively spat out the gum onto the dashboard! I realized I had no idea how many Syns were in the chewing gum and my instant reaction was to eject the potential pollutant from my body before it did its damage. Afterwards, I sat in the car musing about what just happened; about whether something you chew but don't swallow actually has a Syn value and about how my ordinary, trivial routine had suddenly become hyper-significant and a

---

22. Kathleen LeBesco, 'Neoliberalism, Public Health, and the Moral Perils of Fatness', *Critical Public Health* 21, no. 2 (2011): 156.

site of risk. Needless to say, I was late for work but felt determined to investigate the Syn value of chewing gum when I got home.

Patrolling Syn (Syn-watching) in this way is compulsory for members. Participants on the programme are expected to measure milk, weigh cereal, meat, fish (on green days), pasta and rice (on red days) and count Syn. A number of policing methods are employed by members, but the food diary, making mental recordings of Syn and generating bespoke textual sources are three of the most significant.

The Food Diary: Pedagogical Tool and Rationalizing Device

The food diary is provided by the organization as a set of loose rectangular sheets contained in members' starter packs or handed out by Louise in the meeting. All new members are expected to complete the food diary in their first week. When I join, Louise removes a few pages from the stack she is holding and tells me to write down everything I eat; she will look at it next week. Each side of the diary is divided horizontally into four columns. The far left column has a space for members to enter the day and date and contains the start of an emoji – a circle with two dots for eyes, but without the rest of the expression filled in. The face is ready for members to complete as they see fit. The next three columns carry the respective headings of 'Free Food', 'Healthy Extras' and 'Syns' and provide space for members to log relevant items. There is room on each sheet to record three days' worth of eating, although space is tight. When I completed the diary for the first time, I quickly learnt that I would need to reduce the size of my writing significantly if I wanted to fit 'everything' in.

The food diary trains recruits to carefully dissect the contents of meals so that every ingredient for every meal is categorized according to the food groups on the plan. In this way it helps members pay attention to the detail of what goes into their mouths and fulfils the pedagogical function of teaching members how to correctly implement the programme and apply Syn values for themselves. The act of writing helps women internalize and develop specialized knowledge of Syn while confirming that everything consumed 'counts' and must be accurately recalled and remembered. Hevala communicates the importance of writing in her interview:

> I always write what I eat down, always, because I think I don't stay in control of it very well if I don't. So I just have like a little note pad and I just sort of scribble down what I've eaten that day to make sure I've had the right bits of everything.

Hevala uses her own note pad,[23] but she adheres to the method of the food diary by recording everything she eats. Having the 'right bits of everything' expresses how the process provides her with a way to eat a balanced diet. It also, however, displays the way members are trained to methodically dissect and categorize their eating in keeping with the Cartesian logic discussed in Chapter 1. Reproducing foodways on the page helps to sterilize the act of eating. By dissecting meals, members break their food into pieces, into rationally contained parts and into isolated, seemingly unrelated items. The food diary encourages members to approach food first and foremost as Syn, Free Food or Healthy Extras, and thus trains women to make decisions that are governed by these impersonal, technical categories rather than by feeling or mood. This confirms Kandi Stinson's observation that weight loss regimen disassociate members from the emotional aspects of food[24] reducing slimming to a simple matter of education and discipline.[25] Within this mechanical framework, pleasure is never left to roam unchecked.

Writing down Syn is also a way for women to externalize and objectify the food they ingest so that it is spatially separated from their bodies, made visible and available for them to act upon. As such, writing emerges as an important form of abjection. According to Julia Kristeva, the abject is that which transgresses the border, that which we expel because we want to establish and protect ourselves as subjects from the object which threatens to defile.[26] As a practice concerned with abjection, writing down Syn encourages women to regurgitate their food and to expel that which is considered to be unclean, disordered and improper onto the clean, blank page in order to prevent assimilation with it. It mimics the movement of confession already

---

23. Lisa also has a 'little book' in which she records her daily Syns, something Suzanne (her Mum) observes her doing 'religiously'.

24. Stinson, *Women and Dieting Culture*, 210. She recalls how members in her group are encouraged by the leader, Debbie, to 'eat to live' rather than 'live to eat'.

25. Ibid., 161.

26. Julia Kristeva, *Powers of Horror: An Essay on Abjection*, trans. Leon S. Roudiez (New York: Columbia University Press, 1982), 3. For her, 'it is not lack of cleanliness or health that causes abjection but what disturbs identity, system, order. What does not respect borders, positions, rules'. Also see Judith Butler, *Bodies That Matter: On the Discursive Limits of 'Sex'* (New York: Routledge, 1993), 3.

discussed, forming a means by which members can rid themselves of their excess/waste/residue. It also provides an example of the political economy of bulimia previously cited by Guthman.

Maud Ellmann observes this association when she explores the way writing functions in the weight loss practices of US women. According to Ellmann, writing serves as a replacement for eating as women regurgitate every morsel consumed in the form of words. By recording everything consumed, 'the act of composition takes the place of the catharsis of bulimia'.[27] Women reconstitute their food in the written word, she says, even immortalize their food as it becomes '"freeze-dried" upon the page'.[28] Interestingly, Ellmann notes that although it is the slimmer here who forsakes 'fork and knife for pen and ink',[29] we can trace the belief that words substitute for food back to biblical and theological principles. In Deuteronomy 8, the Israelites are reminded that God allows them to be hungry, feeding them with manna to make them understand that 'one does not live by bread alone, but by every word that comes from the mouth of the Lord' (Deut. 8.3). Revelation 10.9 depicts the angel of the Lord telling the narrator to take the scroll and eat it.[30] There are other examples that Ellmann does not list: Jeremiah eats the words of God (Jer. 15.16); Ezekiel is commanded to eat the scroll which contains the message God wants him to give (Ezek. 3.3); Isaiah compares God's message of restoration to food that is 'good' and 'rich' (Isa. 55.2); John tells us that Jesus, the Word of God, is the 'bread of life' (Jn 6.35).[31]

The role of writing in the group resonates with this theological prioritization of words over food. As in these biblical examples, words emerge as types of food because they are sources of sustenance that guide members' actions. Words actually take the place of food since even when women make mental logs of Syn (as we will shortly see), it remains the case that time spent thinking, writing and reading about food is time spent consuming words rather than food itself. Echoing these theological examples, words are placed in control of the flesh and in a reversal of incarnational logic, the flesh made into words.

27. Maud Ellmann, *The Hunger Artists: Starving, Writing & Imprisonment* (London: Virago Press, 1993), 22.
28. Ibid., 23.
29. Ibid., 22.
30. Ibid.
31. Stone, *Practicing Safer Texts*, 11.

The use of writing to keep watch over diet has been given theological expression in various Christian confessional and devotional texts. In the *Life of St. Anthony*, Athanasius retells the story of Anthony the Great, a prominent Christian ascetic among the desert fathers in Egypt, and a figure he describes as providing a 'pattern of discipline'[32] for the life of the monk. According to Athanasius, Anthony was concerned that the recluse should keep a written log of sin so as to keep the body in subjection. Athanasius retells Anthony's advice:

> Let us each one note and write down our actions and the impulses of our soul as though we were going to relate them to each other. ... As then while we are looking at one another, we would not commit carnal sin, so if we record our thoughts as though about to tell them to one another, we shall the more easily keep ourselves free from vile thoughts through shame lest they should be known. Wherefore let that which is written be to us in place of the eyes of our fellow hermits.[33]

Although Anthony imagines the gaze of another, it is clear that his own writing is the watchful eye that polices his impulses and substitutes for the gaze of others he would have experienced had he been living in community. He lauds the practice of self-examination and considers the practice of giving a daily account of the body's actions an important habit for ceasing from sin.[34] For Anthony, control over 'shameful desires' helped keep the passions in check and cultivate obedience to God. Failure to watch the self was a form of 'neglect' that angered God: 'Let us daily abide firm in our discipline, knowing that if we are careless for a single day the Lord will not pardon us, for the sake of the past, but will be wrath against us for our neglect.'[35]

---

32. Athanasius, 'Life of Anthony', in *A Select Library of Nicene and Post-Nicene Fathers of the Christian Church*, trans. Rev. A. Robertson, ed. Philip Schaff and Henry Wace, second series, vol. IV (Edinburgh: T & T Clark/Grand Rapids: W.M. B. Eerdmans Publishing Company, 1978), 1.

33. Ibid., 55.

34. Ibid. Interestingly, according to Athanasius, Anthony emerged from the desert with 'the same habit of body as before, and was neither fat, like a man without exercise, nor lean, from fasting and striving with the demons' (14).

35. Ibid., 18.

Syn-watching in the group obviously emerges in a different sociocultural context. In the ancient world, disease and torture were common realities. Christians had scant control over these circumstances, so controlling the body allowed them to take charge of themselves. In the case of the women, it is an outworking of neoliberal governmentality motivated by the goal of thinness rather than by a hunger for spiritual righteousness. Writing, however, performs a similar disciplinary role as words help patrol members' appetites and enable the mind to take control over the body. It also functions as a confessionary device. One reading of the food diary is that it helps unveil the self so that the truth about the self is exposed on the page. Augustine sees confession in these terms. In *The Confessions*, he provides one of the most famous examples of Christian autobiographical writing. Here, Augustine uses writing to confess and address his own sinfulness, his sexual immorality and his previous involvement with Manicheanism. Reflecting on his own conversion and how he was 'set … free from a craving for sexual gratification',[36] he explains how God causes him to confront himself:

> But, Lord, … you were wrenching me back toward myself, and pulling me round from that standpoint behind my back which I had taken to avoid looking at myself. You set me down before my face, forcing me to mark how despicable I was, how misshapen and begrimed, filthy and festering. I saw and shuddered.[37]

As stated in Chapter 1, Augustine believes that the self deceives itself and sees only what it wants to see. The truth about the self lays hidden beneath its own depravity so confession is necessary in order to draw out sin. It is by knowing one's sins and bearing witness to them that access to the truth about God is made possible. However, unlike members in the group, it is God who causes Augustine to confront himself about the sin he glosses over, supresses and forgets. His self-examination and introspection are orientated towards knowledge and praise of God[38]

---

36. Augustine, *The Confessions*, VIII.6.13.
37. Ibid., VIII.7.16.
38. Augustine, *The Confessions*. He begins this work by exclaiming, 'Great are you, O Lord, and exceedingly worthy of praise. … We humans, who are a due part of your creation, long to praise you.' The instinct of all human persons is to praise God, he insists, and this directs his readers to the heart of his truth-telling quest: his concern is to praise and glorify the Creator. The thought of

rather than knowledge of the self for its own sake. In this respect, his self-writing differs quite significantly from members' written accounts of Syn. As well as performing an explicitly theological function that is missing in the weight loss group, his intention is not simply to 'know thyself' or to follow Socrates in acknowledging that 'the unexamined life is not worth living'; his purpose is to glorify God. Augustine, like Anthony, also confesses to record his inner thoughts and motivations. Members' written records of Syn, on the other hand, simply record the foods consumed, although the emoji attached to each entry allows them to pictorially illustrate their emotional feelings, albeit in a very crude and contained fashion.

The food diary also does not simply tell the truth about Syn. It is a mechanism through which truth is produced and forced out of members' bodies much like the oral confession. When new members join, there is no choice about whether to complete the diary; Louise will check so everyone completes the exercise, possibly because they do not want to be perceived as rebellious so early on in the process. Members are not expected to leave the food diary empty and must divide their eating up into the ready-made spaces provided. As such, the diary compels members to confess themselves in ways the organization prescribes. If participants have gained weight and cannot fathom why, they will be asked either to complete the diary or to fill out a more detailed 'SAS log'.

SAS stands for 'Slimmers against Sabotage'. This more meticulous food diary is intended to diagnose the cause of weight gain. The front of this pro forma requires members to select aims and 'potential danger areas' from two respective pre-given checklists. The back of the sheet asks members to record 'today's food' according to the usual categories of Syns, Free Food and Healthy Extras but now makes them tick against set prompts about whether portions are estimated or measured, whether Syn values are known before eating or found out afterwards, whether food consumed is planned or unplanned, recorded at the time of eating or later in the day. Healthy Extras must be labelled

---

God stirs each person so deeply, he maintains, that 'our heart is unquiet until it rests in you' (I.1.1). Also see Chloë Taylor, *The Culture of Confession from Augustine to Foucault: A Genealogy of the 'Confessing Animal'* (Oxon and New York: Routledge, 2008), 40. According to Taylor, Augustine looks inwards, but he does so in order 'to look up and see God' (30).

as 'a' or 'b',[39] and Free Food categorized as 'speed',[40] 'protein' or 'other Free Food'. The form is not free from judgement as the combined effect of the binary either/or prompts and the more intricate level of detail means that even the slightest departure from the plan confesses the member as culpable for their weight and as guilty of 'self-sabotage'. As a device for reporting foodways, the diary forces members to confess themselves in prescribed ways and so like the spoken confession validates implicit cultural knowledges about weight rather than simply unveiling hidden truths.

Writing, however, is also a means by which women produce themselves. According to Kristeva, in expelling food from the body as abject, the individual spits their selves out because the object of what is expelled can never be entirely separated from the subject who expels it.[41] So in the group, women spit their selves out onto the page, establishing themselves as they abject themselves.[42] The Syn they write cannot be absolutely separated from them as the subjects who expel/write it. As such, writing is a process of self-(r)ejection and self-production. 'And why don't you write?' askes Cixous. 'Write! Writing is for you, you are for you; your body is yours, take it.'[43] Writing is a tool of self-possession that enables women to make their bodies known. It allows their bodies to occupy a place on the page and is a means by which women can constitute (regurgitate) themselves and make their flesh speak. At the same time, the restrictions on the page ensure that women do not write too much or make their bodies too visible; just evident enough to expose their guilt or prove their innocence.

---

39. Healthy Extra 'a' choices are dairy foods that are high in calcium. Members are expected to choose one or two choices from the 'a' category comprising of various types of milk or cheese. 'B' choices not only are high in fibre but also, according to the weight loss guide, 'contain important nutrients for a healthy balanced diet'. 'B' foods vary on red and green days. Members must choose two from the 'b' category.

40. According to the organization, 'speed foods' are 'low in energy density (calories) so they have extra slimming power'.

41. Kristeva, *Powers of Horror*, 3.

42. Ibid., 4.

43. Hélène Cixous, Keith Cohen and Paula Cohen, 'The Laugh of the Medusa', *Signs* 1, no. 4 (1976): 879.

Mentally Logging Syn: Employing the Permission of the Plan to Eat What It Prohibits

Participants do not always write down what they eat. In fact, the tendency to write Syn is only commonplace in the first few weeks of following the plan. Usually from this point on, members make mental logs: 'I don't write them down, I count them in my head,' admits Tracy. Keeping a mental record does not preclude the need to police or record Syn. Lucy, although not making a written log of her Syn, remarks: 'Now I'm thinking in my head, probably, how many Syns have I had today? I go to bed, I lie in bed and think right what have I eaten today? Oh dear, maybe I've had too many Syns!'

In one very important sense, this transition from writing to mentally logging Syn manifests as evidence of an advanced command of the specialized knowledge of Syn and the wider precepts of the plan, rather than being suggestive of a relaxing of members' vigilance. 'I know what they mean. ... I don't sit there with a pencil and paper,' says Ruth; 'It's all ingrained in your head, what you can have,' explains Sarah. Internalized knowledge of Syn thus equips women to make unaided rational judgements about food. At the same time, however, this shift often results in members customizing Syn and in a more flexible – even casual – attitude that ironically resonates with the spirit of flexibility and permission the plan promotes. Suzanne does not always look up the Syn value of foods because she has a 'rough idea' in her head: 'I dunno whether I sort of guess. I suppose I sort of generally know what they are.' She admits that Syn values may have changed but she is happy to stick with her version of the plan; one where her knowledge of Syn is 'general' and 'rough', aligned to a point with 'guessing' and possibly outdated knowledge. When I ask Sarah if she follows the plan strictly, she communicates a similar picture. Although being firm at the start, she now only counts Syn and tends to guess her Healthy Extras: 'I think in my head I have an idea of how much it is. ... I know it's probably over what I'm meant to have but I kind of get used to it.'

Obviously, if Sarah's guessing exceeds the permitted allowance for Healthy Extras, then she will incur Syn that she does not count. The SAS diary would have her understand this as self-sabotage, but she seems less concerned. She tells me, 'I know a couple [of Syns] probably sneak in here and there [but] a little bit extra isn't gonna do too much.' Like Suzanne, she seems happy to make her own (minor) adjustments to the plan by accommodating more Syn than it permits, without apology.

Of course, the adjustments Sarah and Suzanne make to the programme in many ways do not challenge the gendered ideal of the thin female body. Alterations are made but on the proviso that they do not 'do too much' (damage?), and this suggests that weight loss remains intact as the ultimate goal of women's body projects. However, Syn-watching may also provide opportunities for women to trouble the cultural and organizational expectation that fat must be feared and removed. Sarah practises the permission of Syn by refusing to measure the milk in her tea, explaining: 'I don't want to get too obsessed with it; it like control your life. I'd rather it just be there. I'd rather carry on how I'm doing. I'm not in any urgency to suddenly lose.' Although Lisa perfectly embodies the civilized feminine subject of neoliberalism who is not too obsessed or too relaxed, she ties her transgressive behaviour to the fact that she is not in any rush to lose weight. Lisa's embrace of the permission of Syn subsequently appears to sanction a comfortable acceptance of the status quo and to foster a relaxed attitude about fat that would be construed as dangerous by Louise. For Sarah, paying attention to Syn allows her to make deliberate choices that conflict with organizational as well as cultural expectations.

In all of these cases, women's mental logging of Syn affords them opportunities to play with the plan. Syn is transported from the page where it is made visible and fixed in writing, to the invisible and private workings of the mind where it is hard to trace and often customized. Members' preference for mentally recording Syn means that Syn becomes un-policeable and when women refuse to expel their Syn and decide to keep it in – in their minds or in their mouths and stomachs without apology – opportunities for transgression arise.

Women Crafting their Own Bodies of Written Wisdom

The food diary is not the only text women use to police Syn and govern their foodways. Some also set about compiling their own personal collections of recipes, tips and ideas garnered from multiple written sources: from the organization's website and magazine, from the company's published cook books and from recipes shared by fellow members in the group. Sarah prints off recipes from the website to aid her choices; Ruth passes me a handwritten set of instructions for 'the ultimate frittata!' which I take home and use. Samantha extracts salient information from the organization's magazine which she then utilizes to inform her consumer choices in the supermarket:

> The weeks where I've been quite successful … have been the weeks I've sat down on a Sunday or whenever I'm going to go shopping and thought, right, these are the meals and I'll go through the magazine and I'll think right, I'll try that recipe and I'll write it down and I'll use the shopping list and I'll buy it.

Lisa and her Mum, Suzanne, rip out recipes from the organization's magazines that Suzanne has collected and produce their own bespoke 'stack of recipes'. This becomes a tool for Suzanne's other daughter, Veronica, when she visits the family home. Suzanne recalls one occasion when Veronica set about organizing her eating for the week ahead:

> She came and one Saturday morning, 'right, come on, let's see your weekly plan'. I was like 'what you talking about?' She said, 'come on'. So she had her A4, she like split it up [into] days and all that so she went through my freezer and through my cupboards writing a list, a rough list of what there was. 'Right, okay, this is what we've got' and then another piece of paper for a shopping list. She does this every single week. And she was doing like, 'Monday, right, what do you want on Monday off here?' Like with the recipes, like flicking through. And it took about half an hour.

For Veronica, writing becomes a tool that helps her triangulate what food her Mum already has in her cupboards with the received wisdom of the recipes Suzanne and Sarah have collated and with the food she needs to purchase from the supermarket. It helps her organize and order her Mum's week, her cupboards, freezer, shopping list and shopping basket, even the page of A4 that she divides into sections.

As a tool that helps women order their foodways, writing then serves an obvious disciplinary function. Through it, women carve up their appetites and rationalize their desire so that the unruly power of emotion is properly regulated by reason. Women like Samantha, Sarah, Suzanne and Veronica, though, also interfere with organizational materials using these to provoke their own writing – to make lists and charts, or to add their own notes to recipes. They pick out salient pieces of printed or digital matter for their own use and so become decisive selectors and authors of their own authoritative texts, redactors of inherited written wisdom and active in the formation of their own canons. Although time spent thinking, writing and reading about food is once again time spent consuming words rather than food itself, this also directs women towards more decisive and sometimes creative foodways. Speaking about the recipes in the magazine, Sarah, for example, tells me that 'some of them are alright, but the chilli and stuff like that, you need to chuck a hell of a lot more spices in it'. She concludes, 'They normally need a bit more flavour.' Women like Sarah interfere with the received wisdom of the plan to service their own preferences.

The Delight of Self-possession

What these three modes of managing Syn suggest is that spying on the self is not an entirely repressive practice. While conforming women's bodies to the theological and cultural norms discussed in Chapter 1, it also opens up opportunities for women to manoeuvre themselves within this disciplinary setting, to shape their own worlds and, sometimes, to even interrupt or trouble normative conventions. In this sense, Syn-watching provides 'points of resistance'[44] that allow women opportunities to develop and care for themselves.

Syn-watching is also welcomed by women as a pleasurable activity and as a life-enhancing practice. 'I just enjoy doing it,' remarks Jane. Many claim that watching Syn allows them to feel a sense of ownership over their lives and garner new self-awareness: 'It makes you feel more in control of your life,' says Hevala; it leads to 'an expansion in knowledge', says Ruth, and this helps her make more informed decisions about her foodways and to understand why she has gained weight over the years. Women in the group embrace their capacity to police and manage Syn as an opportunity to assert themselves and practise self-accomplishment. 'I'm my own woman,' remarks Ruth proudly when she explains how she now directs her own food choices. Suzanne reflects, 'If I've lost then you feel good about yourself … and think, if I've done that this week I can do the same again next week.' For others, like Tracy, the requirement to watch Syn helps cultivate self-attentiveness and self-reflection that makes her feel more positive about herself, rather than encouraging a flagellation of the self. Time in the group thinking about Syn allows her to have a break from the routine of caring for her young son and to focus on herself: 'I do like to stay to group I mean partly because it's a night off for me. That sounds awful doesn't it, but it's a night just away

---

44. See Foucault, *The History of Sexuality*, 95. Samantha Bartky similarly talks about 'pockets of resistance' in her *Femininity and Domination: Studies in the Phenomenology of Oppression*, 81.

from the bath routine and things like that.' Through Syn-watching, Tracy challenges gender norms as time working on the self enables her to relinquish an aspect of her domestic role and to place her own needs above those of others in her family.

This begins to capture what Michel Foucault expresses as the 'delight' of self-possession and the 'pleasure' of gaining access to the self.[45] For Foucault, this is one of the most important things to understand about power: it does not simply obstruct and limit; it also opens up possibilities and produces subjectivity. According to Foucault, discipline turns power 'into an "aptitude", a "capacity", which it seeks to increase.'[46] Power is creative; it produces new capacities and modes of activity. That is why individuals embrace it:

> What makes power hold good, what makes it accepted, is simply the fact that it doesn't only weigh on us as a force that says no, but that it traverses and produces things, it induces pleasure, forms knowledge, produces discourse. It needs to be considered as a *productive network* which runs through the whole social body, much more than as a negative instance whose function is repression.[47]

In the group, Syn-watching affords women opportunities to work on their bodies, to increase their aptitudes, formulate knowledge and, in some cases, to challenge patriarchal expectations. Women develop capacities for innovation. Helen sees the discipline of having to watch what she eats as an opportunity to 'think outside the box' and practise invention and resourcefulness. Explaining how she feels about the requirement to police Syn, she tells me:

> It doesn't bother me so much but it does mean that you know, you've gotta think outside the box, and think more of okay, what can I eat? What can I get? Um, and you know, how can I, how can I make seven meals out of whatever I've got.

---

45. See Michel Foucault, *The History of Sexuality, Vol. 3, The Care of the Self*, trans. Robert Hurley (London: Penguin Books, 1986), 66.
46. Michel Foucault, *Discipline and Punish: The Birth of the Prison* (London: Penguin Books, 1977), 138.
47. Michel Foucault, *Power/Knowledge: Selected Interviews and Other Writings 1972-1977*, ed. Colin Gordon (New York: Pantheon, 1980), 119.

Lucy comments that 'before [joining the group] I probably ate quite boring stuff you know. So we bought this recipe book from there and … . So, I probably try a few things now that I probably wouldn't have done before.' Others see watching Syn as a chance to reorient their foodways towards more healthy options. Sarah comments that she would 'just eat anything before' she started to police her foodways. She later explains this as involving her 'eating quite a lot of rubbish'. Samantha is 'probably more conscious of what's going in the shopping basket' now that she is watching what she eats. In all cases, Syn-watching is a 'machinery of power'[48] that allows women to cultivate skills in decisiveness and to see themselves as having the capacity to shape their own lives. It provides opportunities for women to re-form past habits, remake themselves and 'convert' to more intentional modes of living.

Challenging the False Consciousness Thesis

Of course, that women become 'good' by practising a daily regimen of control and by skilfully managing the risks of Syn for themselves shows how effectively the capacities women develop are redeployed into the disciplinary work of slimming. The private domains of the kitchen and supermarket are the training grounds where women learn to care and keep their bodies, and this restates a version of the 'feminine mystique'[49] as cooking and feeding work resurface as pathways through which women demonstrate their decency. Food is once more a means of self-fashioning, and feeding work a primary way in which women '"do" gender', providing a means by which women can conduct themselves as 'recognizably womanly'.[50]

The way Syn-watching galvanizes some women to become more experimental with food and to deliberately opt for healthier choices also exposes the ways in which class privilege influences the politics of

---

48. Foucault, *Discipline and Punish*, 138.

49. This notion is famously developed by Betty Friedan to depict how women are duped into thinking their ultimate fulfilment and happiness resides in housework and childcare. See *The Feminine Mystique* (London: Penguin, 1963).

50. Marjorie L. DeVault, *Feeding the Family: The Social Organization of Caring as Gendered Work* (Chicago and London: The University of Chicago Press, 1991), 118.

self-care. In the group, the successful slimmer is expected to have the financial means to cook from fresh, to have well-stocked cupboards and be experimental and knowledgeable about food. She enjoys spending her ('free') time cooking, planning (food) and musing on her body. Seen in these terms, Syn-watching is what Deborah Lupton calls an 'aestheticized leisure activit[y]',[51] a technique that enables women to pursue differentiation, innovation and variety as a deliberate means of improving themselves. According to Lupton, in contemporary Western societies where food is plentiful, variety and innovation in food practices are more important than ever. She claims that food choices are tied up with multiple aspects of subjectivity, including gender and the possession of economic and cultural capital.[52] Watching Syn can be read as one such intentional activity that allows women to accrue cultural capital through the gendered work of cooking and preparing food. That women seek to eat more adventurously and creatively is a pursuit of variety expressive of middle-class privilege and one that ties women again to the domestic sphere.

Awareness of these suspect dimensions of self-surveillance has caused some feminists to refute the claim that slimming can be a legitimate source of enablement for women. According to Kandi Stinson, the suggestion that slimming is an expression of self-care ties women's empowerment necessarily to self-control and weight control specifically, diluting the power it produces.[53] Susan Bordo[54] and Sandra Bartky[55] consider any freedom women experience through slimming to be misplaced and harmful. For Bordo, 'To *feel* autonomous and free while harnessing body and soul to an obsessive body practice is to serve, not transform, a social order that limits female possibilities.'[56] She is clear that dieting functions to produce gender normalization[57] and that any feeling of empowerment that results is illusory, fuelling rather than resisting women's obedience to the market-driven demand for their pounds of flesh. Bartky calls the disciplinary project of slimming

---

51. Deborah Lupton, *Food, the Body and the Self* (London, Thousand Oaks and New Delhi: Sage, 1996), 126.
52. Ibid., 129.
53. Stinson, *Women and Dieting Culture*, 198.
54. Bordo, *Unbearable Weight*.
55. Bartky, *Femininity and Domination*.
56. Bordo, *Unbearable Weight*, 179.
57. Ibid., 184.

a '"set up" [because] every woman who gives herself to it is destined in some degree to fail'.[58] Requiring that appetite be rigorously governed by an iron will,[59] dieting practices produce bodies that are conformed to external norms. She thus argues that disciplinary techniques 'must be understood as aspects of a far larger discipline, an oppressive and inegalitarian system of sexual subordination'.[60]

According to this assessment, the overt aim of slimming is far removed from the covert agenda. It implies that what is 'really' going on when women pursue weight loss is very different to what appears to be happening, even in the minds and lives of women who slim. This, however, significantly obscures and oversimplifies women's expression and experiences of freedom in my group. It also rides roughshod over women's experiences of joy, assuming that feminists have a privileged and more advanced view of the situation. This playing down of freedom overdetermines women as subjects, assuming they are duped by the 'false' promises of the weight loss industry and unable to resist its allure.[61]

Previous discussion in this chapter shows that the women in my group actively participate in the self-governing work of scrutinizing and policing their own bodies. Sometimes this involves the virtual or actual threat of Louise's all-seeing eye or of other women, but techniques of self-surveillance are embraced as opportunities to practise freedom. In this sense, Syn-watching is not entirely repressive. Women in the group

58. Bartky, *Femininity and Domination*, 72.
59. Ibid., 66.
60. Ibid., 75. Similarly for Carole Spitzack, women become both spectacle and spectator in this disciplinary work. They are only made 'free' in this panoptic schema by policing their bodies and by demonstrating submission to the normalizing gaze of power, and this renders any freedom women experience through weight loss 'illusory free choice'. Spitzack, *Confessing Excess*, 45 and 47.
61. Kandi Stinson acknowledges that there are 'fleeting glimpses' of resistance within the weight loss group she attends and observes, seen by the way members pick and choose what suits them and by their questioning of the weight loss programme. We see similar instances in this weight loss group as members select what precepts they will follow and which they will stretch or transgress. She argues that 'we should avoid assuming that women are little more than passive receptors of the messages communicated', although she does not provide much insight into how women question and resist the weight loss plan. See *Women and Dieting Culture*, 199–200.

certainly do not display a docile and uncritical submission to cultural norms that promote thinness as an ideal standard. A number of women resent that Louise spends more time with those who are not 'target members'[62] (and so with members who pay to attend), perceiving in this a way of ensuring their repeat business. Others are concerned about the way fat phobic discourses conspire to judge and vilify fat. Leanne, a mental health nurse, tells me that she is adamant that most diets don't work. She cites statistics and her own personal experience to support this and accuses her workplace of being 'fatist' against her and society of being prejudiced against fat people. She is cynical about the plan and her own investment in it and admits that it has not changed her approach to food nor helped her deal with the emotional reasons why she overeats in the first place.

A number of women also discredit Louise's authority in their interviews or in their comments to me in the meeting room, frequently mocking her reference to water retention as a bogus explanation for weight gain. Others detect that Louise follows a formulaic pattern when she interviews members about their weeks implying that this makes her exchanges robotic. Speaking about the consultants in the organization, Sarah comments, 'They all say the same thing anyway, cos it's obviously all filtered down from head office, this is what, you know, we're gonna do. So the reactions are all the same, the comments are all the same. A lot of the advice is the same.' Helen admits that the organization actually exasperates her body concerns making eating more contentious than it was before she joined the group:

> I think it's kind of replacing one obsession with another. Whereas before I was kind of, you know, not consciously obsessed with food but I would just eat, do you know what I mean, I could quite happily just sit and eat anything and I wouldn't necessarily be bothered. And I did used to have binge, like comfort eating sessions but now, obviously, it's kind of replaced it with the obsession of, oh, you know, I'm actually on green I can't have that, or you know, how many Syns is that?

What these examples show is that many women are conscious of the social conditions that produce the compulsion for thinness and are critical of various cultural and organizational norms. The false consciousness

---

62. The designation 'target member' depicts a member who has achieved their 'Personal Achievement Target' (PAT).

thesis that presents slimming women as docile is inadequate because it fails to sufficiently acknowledge women as critical consumers who use their decision to slim as an opportunity to increase their capacities. Constraint and freedom are both features of Syn-watching techniques and both must be properly acknowledged.

Continuing Features of Historical Christian Asceticism

Before I turn to Foucault to help theorize this further, I want to suggest that Syn-watching understood as a conflicted practice of self-care continues certain features of historical Christian asceticism. In seeing self-surveillance as an opportunity for acting and thinking differently and for cultivating new knowledge and learning, policing Syn comes to reflect an aspect of Christian asceticism often overlooked by feminist theologians, namely, the reorientation and deconditioning of the self. Slimming, of course, also repeats harmful features of ascetic food practices, and I will turn to those in this section also, but tensions between self-care and self-harm and between self-assertion and self-negation are prominent features of women's Syn-watching ways that resonate with Christian ascetic thought and practice.

Breaking the Self's Compulsive Behaviour

In early Christianity, asceticism emerges as a continuation of the 'martyrdom consciousness'[63] and as a voluntary suffering for the faith.[64] If martyrdom provided a means through which believers could be made perfect (through blood), asceticism was a 'daily martyrdom' that continued the image of Christian perfection after the time of persecution.[65] Such perfection was embraced by Christian ascetics as a skilful pursuit, not unlike the work of calibrating Syn. Writing in the fourth century, John Cassian likens the monk to a farmer who toils against gruelling weather conditions to plough the fields, constantly holding before him the goal of a plentiful harvest.[66] For Cassian, the

---

63. Miles, *Fullness of Life*, 20.
64. Gavin Flood, *The Ascetic Self: Subjectivity, Memory, and Tradition* (Cambridge: Cambridge University Press, 2004), 147.
65. Miles, *Fullness of Life*, 20.
66. John Cassian, 'Conferences', in *Nicene and Post-Nicene Fathers*, Second Series, vol. 11, ed. Philip Schaff and Henry Wace, trans. C. S. Gibson (Buffalo:

ascetic life is a skilful life. Just as a soldier uses his expertise to hit the intended target, the ascetic enjoys the end prize of eternal life by cultivating the more immediate *skopos* (goal) of 'purity of heart'.[67] He understands the ascetic life as a life that attends to the body and that practises self-care.

Self-watching in early Christianity is often concerned with fending off the sins of gluttony and lust, as Anthony and Augustine demonstrate, but it is principally a means of reorienting the self's energies. Margaret Miles observes that historical Christian asceticism is rooted in a desire for fullness of life, for lifefulness and aliveness. Ascetic practices are intended to direct the body away from 'deadness' towards participation in the source of life (God) such that Irenaeus claims that 'true life comes from partaking in God', and Origen that 'He does away with the … deadness in us'.[68] She acknowledges that Christian writers frequently fall foul of the suggestion that the body's vitality can be raped for the benefit of the soul and so concludes that 'the old asceticism will not serve us',[69] but she insists that what remains valuable is the vision that the body possessed by the spirit is a body fully alive and already participating in the resurrection life.[70] Asceticism encourages the self to become conscious of its habits and attachments and to break 'the hegemony of the flesh over the body'.[71]

In Christianity, learning, self-knowledge and the reversal of instinctual impulses are all at the very centre of the ascetic life. Christian ascetic practices like solitary prayer, confession, meditation, deprivation of food and sleep, exposure to cold and routine physical work are intended to cultivate the religious self, a self free from socialized patterns of thought and action and free to receive the divine. Miles argues that

---

Christian Literature Publishing Co., 1894). Revised and edited for New Advent by Kevin Knight, http://www.newadvent.org/fathers/350801.htm (accessed 27 May 2018), 1.5. According to Cassian, the 'incessant' and 'diligent labour' of the farmer, like the labour of the trader risking hazards at sea or the military man risking death, was like the toil the monk underwent with 'delight' (1.2), always mindful of the aim of eternal life and leaving behind the 'faults of earlier life' (1.5).

67. Cassian, Conferences, 1.5.
68. Miles, *Fullness of Life*, 33.
69. Ibid., 16.
70. Ibid., 158.
71. Ibid.

fasting, as one important *askesis*, helps the Christian learn to behave differently and to cultivate a new 'organizing centre'.[72] It directs the self's energies away from a grasping after the kinds of pleasures endorsed by dominant culture (e.g. attachment to money, sex, possessions) towards attachment to God. In ascetic practices like fasting, the body trained by culture to seek and receive gratification from sensible objects becomes the tool for breaking such mechanical attraction.[73]

In the slimming group, Syn-watching provides women with opportunities to break with well-established routines, to think differently, to experiment, to become more self-aware and to switch to more intentional food practices. To this extent, it reproduces features of historical Christian asceticism sharing the same contention that confronting the self is necessary as a means of breaking the self's compulsive behaviour. Syn-watching can be read as a practice of self-care that recycles these positive aspects of Christian body policing as it enables women to act to remake themselves. By policing Syn through the food diary, by practising mental methods of recording Syn and by writing and consulting their own bodies of written wisdom, women learn to live and act differently, to see and understand in new ways and to orientate themselves again in the worlds they occupy.

Of course women in the group are not using food to exercise the soul. They are not seeking to cultivate a religious self that renounces the secular values of dominant culture. Their ultimate goal is a transformed outer body that weighs less and looks 'better'; hence, rather than breaking with cultural norms, Syn-watching in many ways helps women conform more closely to them. Ascetic practices within historic Christianity also often take place in social contexts marred by food insecurity and the threat of death[74] and so differ tremendously to the Syn-watching techniques of women in the group where food is available and disease and famine not so apparent. Yet, Syn-watching like the ascetic techniques of historic Christians is a way that women confront ingrained attitudes about food, keep watch over Syn and become skilled experts. It is a care-filled (care-full) practice through which women deliberately shift their mental states and interrupt and examine compulsive behaviour. Like the ancient Christian athletes,

---

72. Margaret R. Miles, *The Image and Practice of Holiness: A Critique of the Classic Manuals of Devotion* (London: SCM, 1988), 96.

73. Ibid.

74. Ibid., 178.

women use their bodies to orient their selves towards aliveness, not in pursuit of bodies possessed by the Spirit of God but to fashion lives that break with accustomed behaviours and which allow their selves to grow and expand.

Self-harm versus Self-care

It is, however, undeniable that such self-fashioning in Christian asceticism often took form in historic acts of self-starvation and self-denial that punished and violated the body. If practices of food restraint helped to cultivate the self, then such practices also frequently repeated the mind over matter dualism by identifying holiness with detachment from the sensible body. Disparagement of the body, appetite and sexuality were key features, exposing the new organizing centre as one aligned more readily with the rational mind able to separate itself from the body's passions. For Cassian, who names gluttony (or 'pleasures of the palate') as the vice from which the remaining seven principal vices stem, the full belly produces 'seeds of wantonness'. When 'choked with the weight of food', the mind is not able to govern its thoughts as it should[75] and certainly will be unable to control lust.[76] Fasting is therefore a way of curbing greed, of placing reason in command of the belly and of defending against the other principal vices. Such insights sometimes caused a great deal of suspicion around cookery. Clement of Alexandria, for example, rendered cooking an 'unhappy art' which led to lavishness.[77] According to him, the flesh must be spurned through prayer and other spiritual exercises so that the body can be detached from the earth, and so the spirit can take flight into the intelligible world:

> So also we raise the head and lift the hands to heaven, and set the feet in motion at the closing utterance of the prayer, following the eagerness of the spirit directed toward the intellectual essence; and

---

75. John Cassian, 'Institutes', in *Nicene and Post-Nicene Fathers*, Second Series. Revised and edited for New Advent by Kevin Knight, http://www.newadvent.org/fathers/350705.htm (accessed 27 May 2018), 5.6.

76. Ibid., 5.11.

77. 'Gluttons, surrounded with the sound of hissing frying-pans, and wearing their whole life away at the pestle and mortar, cling to matter like fire,' he charges. Clement of Alexandria, 'The Instructor', II.1.

endeavouring to abstract the body from the earth, along with the discourse, raising the soul aloft, winged from longing for better things, we compel it to advance to the region of holiness, magnanimously despising the chain of the flesh.[78]

In Christian asceticism, similar tensions between freedom and constraint and self-care and self-harm are evident as in the disciplinary work of women in the group. In both cases, self-harm is an undeniable feature. Although Augustine affirms the physical nature of the resurrected body[79] and its permanent integration with the soul and although he encourages his readers to love the body and 'care for it wisely',[80] he also teaches that the 'perfect peace'[81] enjoyed by the resurrected body is only attained through the (corruptible) body's subjection to the spirit. Anthony, determined to resist the demons in the desert, is said to have 'kept vigil' to such a degree that 'he ate once a day, after sunset, sometimes once in two days and often even in four. His food was bread and salt, his drink, water only'.[82] Weakened by lack of food, he is heartened by 2 Cor. 12.10 and reflects that 'the fibre of the soul is ... sound when the pleasures of the body are diminished'.[83]

The ascetic practices of medieval holy women have been the subject of much theological and feminist attention in recent years, with some equating their attempts at self-mastery through self-starvation with modern forms of anorexia.[84] Insofar as women in my group submit to disciplinary power while simultaneously using self-surveillance to

78. Clement of Alexandria, 'The Stromata, or Miscellaneous', in *Ante-Nicene Fathers: Translations of the Writings of the Fathers Down to AD 325*, vol. II, ed. Rev. Alexander Roberts and James Donaldson (Grand Rapids: WM. B. Eerdmans Publishing Company, 1977), VII.7.

79. Augustine argues that at the resurrection, 'neither the human soul nor the human body suffers complete extinction'. See Augustine, 'On Christian Doctrine' in *A Select Library of the Nicene and Post-Nicene Fathers of the Christian Church*, vol. 11, ed. Philip Schaff (Grand Rapids: WM. B. Eerdmans Publishing Company, 1979), I.21.

80. Ibid., I.25.26
81. Ibid., I.24.25.
82. Athanasius, 'Life of Anthony', 7.
83. Ibid.
84. Rudolf Bell, *Holy Anorexia* (Chicago and London: The University of Chicago Press, 1985).

harness skills in self-management and the ordering of their environment, women also reproduce tensions which have been observed within these ascetic performances. However, it is not simply the harmful effects of medieval holy women's asceticism which are reconstituted by women's Syn-watching techniques.

According to Caroline Walker Bynum, food functioned in multiple and conflicting ways in the lives of religious women living in medieval Europe. Not only was it a source of self-harm but it also enabled women to take their lives into their own hands and control their own environments. It is true, she says, that the mysticism practised by medieval women was characterized by penitential asceticism, especially self-inflicted suffering,[85] but women also used food to shape their own worlds. Given women had more control over food because the preparation and distribution of it was their special concern, food became especially central to women's asceticism in this period.[86] Practices of food restraint were not simply attempts to flee the body and all physicality, she argues, but also exercises which could unite the body with the suffering body of Christ, exercises which enabled a flight into the body as well as a flight from it.[87] The body's suffering in self-starvation (as well as other practices) was a way in which women could fuse with the bodily sufferings of Christ. It was also a way of preparing to receive the Eucharist and feed others.[88] By consuming the host (Christ's body) women were able to taste (eat) God and enjoy (bodily) union with him.

This suggests that for medieval women, the body was important as a site of salvation and deification. Food was also significant because it was by eating God in the Eucharist that women became the suffering body of God that saved. Food and body were both foregrounded. According to Bynum, the subversive power of the mystic's body and of the materiality of food cut across family, religious and institutional power and dominant patriarchal discourses about flesh and female embodiment. Medieval women used food in order to refuse marriage, manipulate their families and escape the dangers of childbirth. Catherine of Siena, for example, rebelled against household tasks by refusing to eat,[89] cut off her hair to make herself ugly, sought disease

---

85. Bynum, *Holy Feast and Holy Fast*, 26.
86. Ibid., 192 and 208.
87. Ibid., 250.
88. Ibid., 220.
89. Ibid., 221.

as an escape from marriage,[90] fed the meat she refused to eat to her brother or cat and used food as a way to define her own life against the traditions, values and trajectories of her family. Through visions and prophetic utterances, women criticized the church and pointed out uncomfortable truths about the world around them.[91] They bypassed priestly mediation by receiving spiritual communion direct from God,[92] claiming direct forgiveness from God and announcing the forgiveness of others. Their fasting became a bargaining tool in some cases, with Catherine demanding God return her mother to life on the grounds of her faithful abstinence.[93] Bynum thus argues that power and authority were functions of medieval women's food practices as they created for themselves saving and serving roles.[94] Rather than destroying their selves, food practices enabled women to shape their own lives – to criticize secular or religious authorities, to claim teaching and leadership responsibilities for which the church provided ambivalent support.[95]

Yet the enabling dimensions of these ascetic practices do not remove their harmful effects. During this period, food abstinence was a way for women to wage war against their flesh, even if they desired bodily union with Christ. It was the *suffering* body of Jesus that women wanted to experience and self-starvation was a means of doing that. The thirteenth-century Italian ascetic, Margaret of Cortona, refused to give herself more than crumbs from the food she received from begging, donating the loaves to the poor instead.[96] Plagued by guilt and shame over a past illicit sexual relationship with a rich nobleman, she is said to have flagellated herself with a knotted rope and punched herself in the face to the point of bruising.[97] Catherine of Siena died at the age of thirty-three as the result of her extreme asceticism. Heavily influenced

90. Ibid., 222.
91. Ibid., 237 and 229.
92. Ibid., 231.
93. Ibid., 234.
94. Ibid., 235.
95. Ibid., 220.
96. Ibid., 142. When ordered to eat by a Friar, Margaret responds by telling him that she has 'no intention of making a peace pact between my body and soul'. Committed to 'tame' her body, she resolves to not stop 'until there is no life left' – cited in Bell, *Holy Anorexia*, 101.
97. Bell, *Holy Anorexia*, 98.

by the desert fathers, she forced twigs down her throat to regurgitate the food she claimed she could not eat. Replacing the consumption of ordinary food with the host and with the consumption of pus from the sick, she condemned her flesh as a 'dung heap'.[98]

Christian asceticism undeniably endorsed sadomasochistic behaviour and sanctioned harm against women. Feminists have understandably seen these pursuits of holiness as dangerous 'self-defiling acts' that encourage self-loathing, hatred of the female body and of other women. According to Mary Daly, asceticism among Christian women is nothing short of 'feminine masochism' because women take pleasure in their own suffering and become complicit in their own 'thinghood'.[99] Deeply embedded within women's psyches and within the social world, this 'sado-ascetic' logic informs women's assessment of themselves causing them to view themselves as guilty and as in need of purification.[100] Such concerns are to be heeded, especially when we consider that Christian asceticism allied women with the sensible world the ascetic must escape. Many of the sayings of the desert fathers identify women with sexual temptation and demons – with the kind of demons Anthony was battling to escape in the desert.[101] Yet, the opportunities asceticism presented for women should not be discounted. According to Rosemary Radford Ruether, the ascetic lifestyle of many women in early Christianity granted them prestige and enabled them to use their wealth to support their own ascetic enterprises. For some, it led to an increase in capacities,[102]

---

98. Bynum, *Holy Feast and Holy Fast*, 168, 172 and 175.

99. Mary Daly, *Pure Lust: Elemental Feminist Philosophy* (London: The Women's Press, 1998), 58–9.

100. Ibid., 57–60. Rosemary Radford Ruether argues that it evidences a compulsion to extract mind from matter and symbolizes women as the locus of death from which the male spirit must flee. See *Sexism and God-Talk: Toward a Feminist Theology*, 79–80.

101. In his telling of the life of Anthony, Athanasius reports, 'And the devil, unhappy wight, one night even took upon him the shape of a woman and imitated all her acts simply to beguile Antony.' Athanasius, 'Life of Anthony', 55.

102. Ruether describes how Macrina, the sister of Basil the Great and Gregory of Nyssa, was a founder of monastic life in her family, while a large number of women from the Roman nobility were founders and leaders of monastic communities; Marcella established a female ascetic community in Rome in the 350s CE; Melania the Elder left Rome in 364 CE and founded a

although it never changed the way leadership was presumed to be the preserve of men. Women practised authority but in consort with self-abnegation. The stigma against their sexuality, Ruether argues, remained inscribed on their bodies.[103]

Of course, the Syn-watching ways of women in the weight loss group are not the same as the ascetic practices of medieval holy women or women in early Christianity. In medieval Europe, for example, food was scarce and famine on the rise. Self-starvation was seen as a defence against gluttony and the ultimate test of self-discipline.[104] In contemporary Euro-American culture, food is mainly available and abundant. The decision to abstain is admired not because food is short but because it shows an ability to control the competing demand to resist and indulge that is endemic to capitalism. Women in the slimming group are not seeking to pursue bodily union with Christ, nor are they starving to bypass marriage or to challenge clerical authority. Both expressions of food restraint, however, are responses to different forms of patriarchal control, whether the coercive power of parents, husbands or religious authorities[105] or the ubiquitous power of the thin ideal. In both cases, the stigma against women's sexuality is confirmed[106] as practices of body policing through food restraint simultaneously immobilize and enable women. Women use food as a tool for the production of subjectivity, using their (gendered) proximity to it as an opportunity to organize their everyday lives, challenge habituated attitudes and behaviours and make autonomous choices that sometimes allow them to play with established norms. Participants may have greater opportunities than their medieval sisters to practise self-accomplishment and influence the contexts they inhabit, but the control of food and body nevertheless affords them access to authority and empowerment in a world still marked by gender inequalities.

---

monastic community for women and one for men; Paula left the East around 385 CE and founded three monastic communities for women and one for men. See Rosemary Radford Ruether, *Introducing Redemption in Christian Feminism* (Sheffield: Sheffield Academic Press, 1998), 34–5.

    103. Ibid., 35.
    104. Bynum, *Holy Feast and Holy Fast*, 2.
    105. Bell, *Holy Anorexia*, 178.
    106. Ellmann, *The Hunger Artist*, 7.

Foucault and Self-care

Foucault's work on technologies of the self can help us theorize these tensions and ambiguities directing us towards an account of self-care that appreciates the complex ways in which discipline and agency interact. Even though the bulk of Foucault's writing is focused on 'technologies of power' that produce docility, he himself admits that he may have paid too much attention to techniques of domination in his earlier work and confirms his mounting interest in the capacity of individuals to shape their own lives and cultivate their selves.[107]

For Foucault, care of the self is a 'technology of the self', a technology which enables people to form and transform themselves and to direct themselves towards their own ends. Technologies of the self concern those practices which 'permit individuals to effect by their own means, or with the help of others, a certain number of operations on their own bodies and souls, thoughts, conduct, and way of being, so as to transform themselves in order to attain a certain state of happiness, purity, wisdom, perfection, or immortality'.[108] Such technologies often function in tandem with technologies of power, he claims, that is, with those technologies which 'determine the conduct of individuals and submit them to certain ends of domination'.[109]

Foucault addresses technologies of the self in relation to a set of practices in late antiquity, practices he sees as being directly rooted in the precept *epimeleisthai sautou*, 'to take care of yourself'.[110] He observes in early Christianity, submission to monastic orders and authorities, the practice of ascetic rituals and confessional self-writing all of which, while inflicting violence on the self, provide opportunities for self-governance and freedom.[111] In ancient Greek and Roman practices of keeping watch over the self, he sees opportunities for individuals to care for the self and to practise what he terms the 'art of existence'. Rather than universal codes of morality being paramount, Greek morality

---

107. Michel Foucault, 'Technologies of the Self', in *Ethics: Essential Works of Foucault 1954-1984*, vol. 1, ed. Paul Rainbow, trans. Robert Hurley (London: Penguin Books, 1994), 225.

108. Ibid.

109. Ibid.

110. Ibid., 226.

111. Jonathan Tran, *Foucault and Theology* (London and New York: T & T Clark, 2011), 96.

revolved around the detailed regulation of the body. The self was like a work of art, crafted and styled through conscious acts. Cultivating the self meant to actively constitute the self by working on the self. It entailed a concern for the self and an attentiveness to daily practices like diet and exercise. Care of the self (*souci de soi*) was an 'aesthetics of existence' providing an occasion to cultivate a beautiful life and to become an ethical subject by having a 'proper, necessary, and sufficient concern for the body'.[112] It required *skill* and as an *askēsis* constituted 'a training of the self by oneself'.[113]

There are problems with Foucault's aesthetics of existence, not least his identification of an artful life with a group of elite male philosophers. For some, this positions his account 'light-years from anything that any feminist might want to endorse'.[114] Feminists have also questioned the usefulness of collaborating with Foucault on the grounds that his emphasis on discipline deprives the modern subject of any agency and authority.[115] However, his analysis of technologies of the self places more emphasis on the capacity of individuals to actively fashion their own identities and so speaks relevantly to the experiences of women in my group. He provides a useful lens for understanding how self-surveillance practices in the group help form women as independent social actors.

For Foucault, the transition from traditional to modern societies has been characterized by a transformation in the exercise of power. Older authoritarian systems were characterized by 'relations of sovereignty'[116] where a feudal lord or monarch would impose compliance through force, while in modern societies, power is exercised by gaining access to the bodies of individuals, their gestures and daily actions. In modern contexts, power is dispersed, no longer located in the person

---

112. Michel Foucault, *The History of Sexuality, Vol. 2, The Use of Pleasure*, trans. Robert Hurley (London: Penguin Books, 1985), 108.

113. Michel Foucault, 'Self Writing', in *Ethics*, 208.

114. Jean Grimshaw, 'Practices of Freedom', in *Up against Foucault: Explorations of Some Tensions between Foucault and Feminism*, ed. Caroline Ramazanoğlu (London and New York: Routledge, 1993), 65.

115. For example, see Linda Alcoff, 'Feminism and Foucault: The Limits to a Collaboration', in *Crises in Continental Philosophy*, ed. Arlene B. Dallery, Charles E. Scott with P. Holley Roberts (New York: State University of New York Press, 1990), 69–87.

116. Foucault, *Discipline and Punish*, 208.

of the sovereign, but everywhere and nowhere, invested in everyone and no one in particular. Power is a ubiquitous relation within which different techniques of power occur. As Cressida Heyes reminds us, this means that, for Foucault, the growth of capabilities and possibilities for flourishing operate in tandem with the intensification of power relations.[117]

Foucault's account of power allows us to acknowledge the increase in capacities women experience in the group – advances in self-possession, self-assertion, self-awareness and self-attentiveness, for example – as features of women's Syn-watching without denying the ways in which these capacities entangle women even more deeply in webs of patriarchal domination. For Heyes, recovering this feature of Foucault's work helps to explain why many women continue to slim despite high failure rates. Women are not 'irrefutably docile' and duped into a state of false consciousness, she argues; they persist with slimming because they experience the process as enabling.[118] As a participant observer in *Weight Watchers*, she sees how communities of women can be mobilized and how observing her self-destructive behaviours might be a useful practice in awareness. Women are given opportunities to celebrate achievement, to experience self-discovery and transformation.[119] Leaflets handed out in meeting, magazine articles, recipe books and website materials, while aiding the primary goal of profit, also help cultivate capacities such as 'working to release negative conditioning, or assuming responsibility for choices about how to live'.[120] She admits that such capacities are frequently recycled back into disciplinary practices, but they nevertheless have the potential to exceed the regime of

---

117. Cressida J. Heyes, 'Foucault Goes to Weight Watchers', 126–49. Also see Cressida J. Heyes, *Self-Transformations: Foucault, Ethics, and Normalized Bodies* (Oxford and New York: Oxford University Press, 2007).

118. In an extended discussion of this within her book, *Self-Transformations*, Heyes questions the assumption that slimming women are somehow less knowledgeable or educated about the social realities lurking behind the ideology of slimness by asking why educated, feminist women who are sceptical about the slender body continue to subscribe to weight loss groups (66).

119. 'It is a feminist commonplace that many women's achievements go unrecognized or are invisible. Losing weight, however, provokes ready congratulation; it is tangible, and can be graphed and tracked.' See Heyes, *Self-Transformations*, 127.

120. Heyes, 'Foucault Goes to Weight Watchers', 140–6.

normalization that produces them. Such skills need not be channelled towards bolstering the thin ideal, she suggests. As such, feminists can embrace the enabling capacities women develop in weight loss contexts without assenting to the intensification of disciplinary power they often require.[121]

Heyes offers valuable insight here. She is right that the capacities women develop in weight-watching techniques need not be deployed in re-positioning the thin ideal as normative because they can be uncoupled from the production of docility. In my group, the practice of self-care through Syn-watching does not produce fully compliant subjects. Women use the permission of Syn to play with the plan in ways it forbids, to relax the boundaries governing Syn and to author their own adjustments without apology. The autonomy and self-determinism women develop and cultivate is not straightforwardly redirected back into the hegemony of thin privilege or into compliance with organizational norms. This shows how, even in the slimming group itself, opportunities for resistance arise. Subjectivity and subjection are never independent of one another, for as Foucault says, 'where there is power, there is resistance', and resistance is never exterior to power.[122]

Rather than signalling a straightforward return to domestic enslavement and a re-articulation of slimming women as oppressed/ duped 'victims', Syn-watching produces a different kind of feminine subjectivity more readily aligned with post-feminism. Rosalind Gill describes post-feminism as a 'sensibility' characterized by an 'entanglement' of feminist and anti-feminist themes.[123] According to her, it shares with neoliberalism a 'current of individualism' which eschews the notion of politics or cultural influence. Every aspect

---

121. Ibid., 146.
122. Michel Foucault, *The History of Sexuality*, 95.
123. Rosalind Gill, 'Postfeminist Media Culture: Elements of a Sensibility', *European Journal of Cultural Studies* 10, no. 2 (2007), 149. Also see Angela McRobbie, 'Post-feminist and Popular Culture', *Feminist Media Studies* 4, no. 3 (2004): 255–64. McRobbie complexifies the understanding of post-feminism as a 'backlash' against feminism famously forwarded by thinkers like Susan Faludi. She suggests that post-feminism invokes feminism to suggest that women can achieve anything now equality has been realised, while simultaneously using this position to suggest that feminism is now defunct. For more, see Susan Faludi, *Backlash: The Undeclared War against Women* (London: Vintage, 1992).

of life is reduced to the personal and women assumed to be free to make choices about their lives, unfettered by inequalities or other power imbalances. For Gill, post-feminism turns 'the personal is political' mantra of second-wave feminism on its head. It mirrors the 'choice biography' of neoliberalism compelling women to frame all aspects of their lives as freely selected to produce personal pleasure and satisfaction[124] and shares with neoliberalism an emphasis on the calculating, self-regulating subject. Such synergies, she argues, suggest that post-feminism is not just a response to feminism but a sensibility partly created through 'the pervasiveness of neoliberal ideas'.[125] That it is women to a greater extent than men who are called to self-manage, to understand their own biographies in terms of freedom of choice, to transform and govern themselves, she suggests, may expose the way neoliberalism is '*always already gendered*'.[126]

Syn-watching proffers an instance of the post-feminist sensibility, testifying to this close affinity with neoliberal discourse. Policing Syn is a post-feminist practice of self-care and one that pushes beyond understanding weight-watching as a 'violent backlash' against feminism,[127] and beyond a re-articulation of slimming women as docile. Women in the group are 'micro-political agents'[128] who embody competing commitments, convictions and demands;[129] they are what Michelle Lazar describes as post-feminist feminine subjects who are

---

124. Gill, 'Postfeminist Media Culture', 154. Also see Michelle Lazar, 'Recuperating Feminism, Reclaiming Femininity: Hybrid Postfeminist Identity in Consumer Advertisements', *Gender and Language* 8, no. 2 (2014): 205–24. Lazar argues that post-feminist discourse is characterized by a 'pronounced sense of self or "I-identity"' (205).

125. Rosalind Gill and Christina Scharff, 'Introduction', in *New Femininities: Postfeminism, Neoliberalism and Subjectivity*, ed. Rosalind Gill and Christina Scharff (New York: Palgrave Macmillan, 2011), 7.

126. Ibid.

127. Naomi Wolf argues that women's obsession with beauty constitutes a 'violent backlash' against feminism. See *The Beauty Myth: How Images of Beauty Are Used against Women*, 10.

128. Patricia Mann, *Micro-Politics: Agency in a Post-Feminist Era* (Minneapolis: University of Minnesota Press, 1994), 32.

129. Mann suggests that post-feminism constitutes a 'bricolage of competing and conflicting forms of agency', as well as 'multiple subject positions'. Ibid., 31, 171 and 207.

characterized by contradiction and ambivalence.[130] Some feminist analysis would suggest that by spending their energies calibrating Syn and using food to cultivate self-care, women in the group are distracted from the structural forces of capitalism, sizeism, sexism and so on that produce and legitimize fat phobia. But some women are not oblivious to these cultural forces, as we have seen, even if they simultaneously acquiesce with them. Rather than effacing the empowerment women experience, we are led to acknowledge that empowerment never operates outside the constraining and gendered conditions of patriarchal discipline. It is true that women's resistance is 'translated eventually into profitable capital and reproductive energy',[131] but empowerment and constraint are both features of Syn-watching. Neither is illusory.

Conclusion

It is not quite as some feminist commentators suggest that secular slimming programmes emphasize the worst aspects of religion, exchanging generosity towards the body for punishing exercises of discipline and deprivation. Although it can be argued that 'the kind of caretaking that … weight-loss groups promote is just the kind that will deliver us into the genocidal working patterns that capitalism loves and our bodies hate',[132] the Syn-watching practices of women in the group are never just unequivocally harmful. Syn-watching is an expression of the Ponopticon scheme[133] as women learn to govern themselves, but within

---

130. Lazar, 'Recuperating Feminism', 221.

131. Chen, 'Neoliberalism and Popular Women's Culture', 447.

132. Isherwood, *The Fat Jesus*, 130 and 128. Deborah Lupton similarly observes that Western societies display a strong link between religion, spirituality, asceticism and dietary regimen, with the Judeo-Christian ethic of renunciation remaining influential in propping up the expectation that restraint will be rewarded. Lupton, *Food, the Body and the Self*, 131 and 137.

133. This is a reference to Foucault's discussion of Bentham's Ponopticon. See Foucault, *Discipline and Punish*, 201–2. Foucault sees Jeremy Bentham's design for the Ponopticon prison as a perfect illustration of the ubiquity of power and the transfer of constraint onto the self-regulating subject. Formed of a central circular tower with wide windows surrounded by an outer ring of multiple cells, the Ponopticon allows the prison guard to watch inmates without ever being seen, while producing in prisoners 'a state of conscious and permanent

this disciplinary anatomy of power women increase their capacities and also use their freedom to resist organizational and sometimes cultural expectations. Women do not refuse disciplinary power but through it actively fashion their own identities. This continues some of the positive as well as negative features of Christian asceticism as women use disciplinary techniques to reorient their lives and shape their own environments. In arguing this, I am not suggesting that Syn-watching is a new feminist *askesis* but that the capacities women cultivate through skilfully negotiating Syn are capacities that feminists should not dismiss. The art of cultivating an intentional existence and of being purposeful about how and what one eats may be a practice of self-care necessary for challenging the cultural conditioning which insists on slenderness as a measure of women's 'goodness' and for challenging the capitalist politics of greed which allows some to eat while others starve. The capacities of innovation, playfulness, self-authorship, self-possession, creativity, self-awareness and self-reflection need not be recycled back into the disciplinary work of slimming. Indeed, as later chapters will show, they may be the very skills women need to resist the hegemony of fat phobia and the thin ideal.

visibility'. Prisoners regulate their own behaviour in the knowledge that they may already be being watched, and so without force govern and watch their own bodies. For Foucault, this epitomizes the workings of disciplinary power showing how discipline produces what he calls 'docile bodies' – 'subjected and practised bodies' (138). Whereas in pre-modern societies good citizens obeyed the sovereign, in modern societies, good citizens govern their own bodies and assume responsibility for the constraints of power. Ponopticism improves the exercise of power by making it more diffuse and subtle.

Chapter 3

SALVATION, 'GETTING RID' AND 'GETTING THERE'

So far, I have explored the way members' beliefs and practices around Syn repeat and reshape theological traditions. I have argued that classical Christian associations with danger, disobedience and disordered desire resurface in participants' Syn-talk to form a gender-coded matrix of meaning that frames women as guilty and that establishes fat as feminine. The notion of 'Syn' in this way follows dominant strands of Christian thought in establishing women's bodies as special sites of danger, irrationality and moral disorder and in confirming the need for the rational will to dominate the unruly appetitive self. Syn, though, is also a positive signifier in the weight loss organization. Understood as a liberatory device that saves women from the gruelling demands of dieting, Syn is marketed as a way for members to embrace flexibility and avoid self-denial. While Syn-watching techniques are examples of the neoliberal political anatomy that ensures compliance to dominant patriarchal norms through self-chosen acts of self-surveillance, policing Syn provides opportunities for women to produce themselves as intentional subjects and to cultivate self-care. Tensions between constraint and freedom resemble some of the complex features of Christian asceticism where harmful practices of abstinence and self-starvation sit alongside an increase in capacities, allowing practitioners to shape their own lives.

In this chapter, I turn to the related theme of salvation[1] and to the redemptive paradigm members construct. While participants do not use the word 'salvation' to speak about losing weight, the company's recycling of the Christian nomenclature of sin means that the Christian

---

1. Some parts of this chapter are taken or adapted from Hannah Bacon, 'Dieting for Salvation: Becoming God by Weighing Less', in *Alternative Salvations: Engaging the Sacred and the Secular*, ed. Hannah Bacon, Wendy Dossett and Steve Knowles (London and New York: Bloomsbury Academic, 2015), 41–51. They are used with kind permission of the publishers.

terminology of salvation is, nevertheless, apposite. Since 'Syn' borrows explicitly from a distinctly Christian theological framework and the word is employed in ways that help shame the presence of fat, the removal of fat naturally takes on meaning as a form of salvation, even in the absence of such overt speech.

Many commentators have observed a connection between the quest for thinness and salvation. In the late 1980s, Roberta Seid argued that American obsessions with weight, diets and fitness adopt the form of traditional religion, supplying a wellness ethic which promises salvation through 'a now-invisible aesthetic and moral structure', one that assumes weight loss and exercise to be 'healthy' and capable of making women happier, more beautiful and more virtuous.[2] The concern to eat right and weight-watch forms part of the contemporary cultural search for 'wellness', she argues, 'a kind of superstate of mental and physical well-being'.[3] This promises not only psychological, physical and emotional transformation but also the birth of an 'other' self – a more successful, happier self with the ability to overcome professional and personal problems.

Seid has not been alone in detecting how the search for thinness connects with the promise of transformation, wellness, health and success. Shelley Bovey has suggested that slimming organizations restate the sinner–saint dyad casting fat people as sinners and marketing weight loss services as offering an opportunity for reform.[4] Naomi Wolf contends that the beauty myth trains women to see beauty as 'heaven or a state of grace',[5] so just as Jesus suffers to bring sinners to new life, so the myth of salvation tells women they must suffer if they want to reach 'the Promised Land' of thinness.[6] Slimming, she suggests, traps women in a 'cycle of purification'[7] where they remake themselves, giving themselves new identities and bodies, only to have their newly manicured selves disappear. Weight loss takes on quasi-baptismal shape as women emerge from their fat transformed, but 'the "new me"

2. Seid, *Never Too Thin*, 10.
3. Ibid., 13.
4. Bovey, *The Forbidden Body*, 33.
5. Wolf, *The Beauty Myth*, 98.
6. Ibid., 101.
7. Ibid., 98.

is washed off with the evening bath,[8] she argues, because the pursuit of thinness is premised on failure and is always elusive.

Since these early contributions, feminists have continued to express alarm at the way the quest for thinness produces a secular salvation myth[9] which encourages women to see beauty and appearance as sources of 'ultimate concern'.[10] Few, however, have engaged seriously with the theological traditions underpinning this quasi-religious rendition of salvation. Instead, emphasis is placed on how this myth of salvation functions to diminish women. For feminist theologian Mary Bringle, the pursuit of thinness reduces the eschaton 'to a matter of appearance and individualized achievement', exchanging eternal life for ephemeral beauty.[11] According to religious studies scholar Michelle Lelwica, it teaches women that salvation depends on sacrifice and submission – 'A woman's "salvation" presumes her shame and requires her self-alienation: her transgression is absolved when she forfeits a sense of agency and a feeling of peace with her own body.'[12] Almost without exception, feminist scholars have claimed that the 'religion' of thinness is built on an entirely vacuous hope, such that it is described by Seid as a 'false religion that does not deliver what it promises'.[13]

In keeping with the previous chapter, I trouble such a uni-dimensional reading of slimming. Plotting the redemptive motifs women develop, I show how these both constrain and empower women and how theological ideas again resonate with the weight loss stories that women narrate. As before, I claim that correlations between the slimming practices and beliefs of ordinary women and Christian patterns of thought and action present Christian religion as an important explanatory tool for making sense of women's weight loss journeys.

Salvation takes on multiple meanings in the group, but especially important are the metaphors of 'getting rid' and 'getting there'. 'Getting

---

8. Ibid., 102.

9. See Lelwica, *Starving for Salvation*, 5.

10. Mary Bringle has argued that if religion concerns the state of being 'ultimately concerned' as Paul Tillich argued, then the amount of time and money spent on slimming suggests that the 'pseudo-ultimate concern of thinness' is a religious pursuit. Bringle, *The God of Thinness*, 27.

11. Ibid., 101.

12. Lelwica, *Starving for Salvation*, 125.

13. Seid, *Never Too Thin*, 19.

rid' identifies salvation not only with a decision women make but also with a course of committed action they take to remove fat and erase excess. As a soteriological motif, this foregrounds the theme of sacrifice highlighted by Lelwica and already discussed in the previous chapter. Common in Christian soteriological discourse, this premises women's self-betterment once more on the practice of self-abandonment and detachment. However, salvation here is not just straightforwardly about self-abnegation as 'getting rid' opens up opportunities for women to participate more fully in society and to grow self-esteem and cultivate social bonds. 'Getting there' identifies the way in which women locate fullness and happiness in an end point when their bodies will be transformed. This shares with Western Christianity an emphasis on pursuing other perfect worlds beyond the present, envisaged now as arrival at a point of positive self-change that guarantees entry into a perfect life-after-fat. This metaphor, though, does not render salvation as a purely private and destructive project, since the journey towards self-betterment is a corporate pilgrimage through which women develop and exchange various forms of capital. If previous chapters have shown that well-established theological ideas about sin live on inside this secular commercial weight loss group, then this chapter demonstrates the notability of certain soteriological motifs and their capacity to sanction as well as trouble the control of women's bodies.

Wellness, Wholeness, Rescue and Escape: Beginning to Plot Soteriological Motifs

Salvation takes on multiple meanings in Christianity. Reconciliation, liberation, justification, deification, satisfaction and sacrifice are among the biblical and theological images that have enjoyed popularity at various stages in Christian history. At the centre of all is an understanding that God's intended good for human beings and the wider world has been distorted and rendered in need of repair. Salvation invariably signals that the world and humanity are in a predicament that requires God's help. As Grace Jantzen reflects, 'To be saved means to be delivered from a situation which [is] problematic or even intolerable; there is a sense of crisis and of rescue from danger.'[14]

---

14. Grace M. Jantzen, 'Feminism and Flourishing: Gender and Metaphor in Feminist Theology', *Feminist Theology* 4, no. 81 (1995): 85.

In the Hebrew Bible, the meaning of salvation is predominantly physical,[15] depicting rescue, escape or protection from concrete circumstances rather than retreat to a spiritual world in a life to come. In Exodus, for example, God saves the people of Israel from the Egyptians (Exod. 14.30); in Isaiah (11.6-9), salvation signals the healing of land and the making of peace with the cosmos; in Zephaniah (3.17-20), it is imaged as the rescue from disaster, oppression, illness and a return to prosperity. Even where an eschatological sense is present, like in Second Isaiah, the salvation imagined suggests the restoration of Israel in its land, not some other-worldly state.[16]

In the New Testament, rescue also takes on concrete form as it comes to be aligned with healing from pain and illness. The Greek verb *sózó* (σώζω) is used when Jesus 'makes well' the woman with a haemorrhage (Mt. 9.22; Mk 5.34) and restores sight to a blind Bartimaus, telling him 'your faith has made you well' (Mk 10.52). It is also used by the disciples when confronted with the stormy waters and fear for their lives, they beseech a sleeping Jesus, 'Lord, save us! We are perishing' (Mt. 8.25). Nevertheless, the verb and its derivatives more regularly depict a spiritual rescue from sin and a restoration of spiritual health. Jesus understands his mission as the 'making well' of sinners (e.g. Mt. 1.21), and forgiveness of sin is imaged as a spiritual form of healing that indicates salvation in Christ.[17]

Salvation also takes on meaning as both a present and an awaited event. Anticipating the imminent return of Christ, Paul speaks about those who are being saved (1 Cor. 1.18; 15.2; 2 Cor. 2.15) as well as those who will be saved (1 Cor. 5.5). Believers experience new status as co-heirs with Christ in the present (Rom. 8.17), but they look forward to the redemption of their bodies in the future (Rom. 8.23). Already saved by grace from their transgressions (Eph. 2.1, 8-9), they are nevertheless required to work out their salvation with fear and trembling (Phil. 2.12). 'Now is the day of salvation' (2 Cor. 6.2) says Paul, but glory is also progressive since 'all of us, with unveiled faces, seeing the glory of the Lord as though reflected in a mirror, are being transformed into the

---

15. Michael D. Coogan, 'Salvation', in *The Oxford Companion to the Bible*, ed. Bruce Metzger and Michael D. Coogan (New York and Oxford: Oxford University Press, 1993), 670.
16. Ibid.
17. Ibid., 670.

same image from one degree of glory to another; for this comes from the Lord, the Spirit' (2 Cor. 3.18).

Despite these different soteriological directions, Paul disputes the Corinthians' theology of realized eschatology seeing their rejection of marriage and their enabling of women to pray and prophesy in the Spirit as an expression of the future kingdom that lay ahead, rather than being indicative of the present.[18] Here, Paul depicts the kingdom as a reality that believers are yet to enjoy. A preference for the future is also detectable in the synoptic gospels and in Acts. Only those who persevere to the end will be saved (Mk 13.13). In Acts 15.11, Peter reassures the apostles and elders that they 'will' be saved just like the Gentiles.[19] According to Rosemary Radford Ruether, this future, other-worldly view of salvation dominates by the close of the New Testament period,[20] and it is this model that has typified and continues to characterize Western Christian thought.[21]

We have already seen in Chapter 1 how members of the group align fat with a threat to health and well-being and how weight loss is deemed to be quite literally life-saving. The organization's 'Let's Beat It Together' campaign presents fat as an illness and danger from which those at risk must be rescued. Further to this, Louise also encourages members to evangelize. In a meeting in September, she hands out a set of flyers advertising the organization and asks us to deposit them in shopping trollies whenever we are next at the supermarket. The reason, she explains, is to try and 'reach' others and gain new members. This displays the proselytizing ambition of the organization as it not only seeks to spread the 'good news' and convert others but also presents the meeting as a type of clinic for those in impending danger. There is

18. Rosemary Radford Ruether, *Women and Redemption: A Theological History*, 2nd edn (Minneapolis: Fortress, 2012), 23. Ruether suggests that through this, Paul sought to shore up gender hierarchies. In rejecting the Corinthian view of realized eschatology, he rejects the view that the hierarchical ordering of male over female and master over slave can be abolished (25).

19. See Coogan, 'Salvation', 670.

20. Ibid., 12–16.

21. This point has been made by a number of feminist and liberation theologians, most strongly perhaps by Rita Nakashima Brock and Rebecca Ann Parker, *Saving Paradise: How Christianity Traded Love of This World for Crucifixion and Empire* (Boston: Beacon Press, 2008). For more, see discussion later in this chapter.

a need to reach others because others are in need of rescue, and joining the community will provide the cure that is needed to save.

In Christian thought, the church has been understood in similar ways. For Augustine, it is Christ's emergency room,[22] offering the medicine of baptism for the disease of sin. Adamant that the Gospels state 'without any ambiguity that unbaptized little ones not only cannot enter the kingdom of God, but cannot possess eternal life',[23] he presents the church as essential to salvation. Working as a priest in what is now northern Algeria at a time when disease and infant mortality were common, he experiences first-hand women running to church to get their sick babies baptized.[24] Salvation has also often been aligned with death, and similar associations resurface in the weight loss group. We have already considered this theme as it relates to sin, but in soteriological terms, salvation is often considered to be wrought through the death of Christ and only fully realized after death in a life to come. The redeemed body is the body that has taken flight from the corruptible body, marred by sin and death, and escaped into a celestial paradise. According to Grace Jantzen, such accounts of salvation display how Christian thought has helped establish a dread of death and fascination with 'worlds of the beyond', feeding a culture of necrophobia.[25] Western modernity is built on this obsession with death, she argues, made visible in the language of war utilized in everyday discourse – in talk of fighting cancer and other 'enemies'.[26]

In the weight loss group, the fascination with other worlds materialises as a longing to experience a life beyond fat. As will become apparent in this chapter, through target-setting members imagine thinner future selves that are birthed by the successful destruction of fat. Languages of war are employed as members are encouraged to 'beat'

22. William Harmless, 'Christ the Paediatrician', 148.

23. See Augustine, *Answer to the Pelagians*, 'Punishment and the Forgiveness of Sin and the Baptism of Little Ones', introduction, trans. and notes Roland J. Teske, ed. John E. Rotelle (New York: New City Press, 1997), III.8.

24. Given the realities of plagues and disease, baptism is understandably depicted in Augustine's theology as 'medication', 'treatment' and 'cure'.

25. Grace M. Jantzen, *Becoming Divine: Toward a Feminist Philosophy of Religion* (Manchester: Manchester University Press, 1998), 129–36, esp. 130.

26. Jantzen suggests that the language of war is ubiquitous in the Western world. We might add the fight against terrorism and obesity as two further examples of 'enemies' we are told to fight in contemporary Western culture.

their fat. Indeed, the 'Let's Beat It Together' campaign communicates that fat (allied with death, disease and illness) must be overcome and destroyed if women are to enter an afterlife (i.e. a life after fat). As is often the case in the Bible, salvation emerges as a material project caught up with making the body better, but this sits awkwardly in the group, as it does in Christian thought and practice, with the competing insistence that salvation is reserved for those who willingly attack their flesh. Repeating the theological tensions discussed already, the dominant account of salvation that emerges presents the body as both a site of care and contempt.

It is also important to note that Western Christianity tends to present salvation as an individual affair concerned with the renewal of the soul. This reflects, in part, the nineteenth-century thought of Friedrich Schleiermacher and his identification of religion with an inner 'feeling' (i.e. a feeling of absolute dependence).[27] The modern turn towards the individual subject has been replicated in liberal and neo-orthodox Christianity,[28] but the Reformation thought of Luther and Calvin has also been instrumental in fixing the individual at the centre of the soteriological enterprise. Their understanding of salvation as a personal faith response to God and as the voluntary assent to follow and trust Christ has had considerable influence on Christian discourse about salvation,[29] and vestiges of this individuated approach resurface again in the redemptive paradigm members construct. Women root their projects of self-change in a personal decision to lose weight, as we will see. Deciding to join the group is a type of personal faith response that

---

27. Friedrich Schleiermacher, *The Christian Faith*, trans. and ed. H. R. Mackintosh and J. S. Stewart, 2nd edn (Edinburgh: T & T Clark, 1999). According to Schleiermacher, knowledge and 'consciousness' of God is located in the inner feeling of absolute dependence which is a feeling available to all.

28. Jantzen, *Becoming Divine*, 94.

29. Luther's emphasis on justification by faith has exerted a profound influence on Protestant accounts of individual salvation. In his commentary on Galatians, he argues that it is 'faith in Christ, which alone justifies – not the law'. See Martin Luther, *Galatians*, The Crossway Classic Commentaries, ed. Alister McGrath and J. I. Packer (Wheaton: Crossway Books, 1998), 86. Calvin similarly holds that salvation is through God alone and that individual faith is necessary for salvation. See John Calvin, *Institutes of the Christian Religion*, trans. Ford Lewis Battles, ed. John T. McNeill (Louisville, Kentucky and London: Westminster John Knox Press, 2006).

involves the mind and intellect in assenting to the precepts of the weight loss plan. Members place their trust in the programme, hoping that it will deliver what it promises. Western culture has been modelled on this individualistic account of salvation, and it sits comfortably alongside the 'atomistic individualism' of Western modernity.[30] This presentation of salvation lingers on not only in the contemporary consumer assumption that bodies must be made better, servicing market forces and the hegemonic thin ideal, but also in the dominant cultural discourse that assumes individuals must take personal responsibility for ameliorating their fat.

According to James Boyce the rise of secularism has not erased the efficacy and power of salvation rhetoric in the modern world. 'Modern history suggests that the disbelief in a saviour might not have removed Western people's deeply ingrained need to be saved,' he argues, but it is simply that emphasis has now shifted to a type of salvation dependent on the forces of consumerism, politics, self-help and technology.[31] In this commercial weight loss setting, the need for salvation is equally pronounced, and the rest of this chapter probes in more detail the theological content of some of these salvation motifs.

Salvation as 'Getting Rid': The Logic of Sacrifice

Underpinning most women's motivation to lose weight in the group is an acknowledgement that they cannot stay as they are, that their excess (i.e. fat) must be removed. Most describe a moment of epiphany when they suddenly realize that self-change is essential. Explaining why she joins the group, Sarah comments, 'There was one day I woke up and I was like, I can't carry on being this big.' Before joining, she had spoken with others and had been told that the plan was easy to follow which made her adamant to act: 'So I was just like, right, I'm going to join!' Tracy describes something 'clicking' in her mind and a realization that failure to act may obstruct her ability to mother well:

> I came [to the group] because I was fed up of being the size that I was, so I wanted to get rid! I think something has to click in your mind so that you're ready to do it, cos if you're not ready then there's

---

30. Jantzen, *Becoming Divine*, 94.
31. Boyce, *Born Bad*, 188.

no point going. And something had clicked and Robert [her son] was … Robert was getting older and um, you know, and running around more and I thought, oh I'm never going to keep up with him if I continue as I'm going. So I thought, well, no; I need to, for myself to feel better, and I thought for the family things as well, you know; just to make me feel better and everything, and that I thought right I need to do it!

For Tracy, there is no alternative other than to 'get rid'. Suzanne similarly explains how a visit to the doctor provides the jolt she needs to join the group. Finding out that she now weighs fourteen stone, she is repulsed into action: 'I couldn't believe it. I was just like, I thought, I just – how have I let myself? I felt ill, I felt horrible, just hated myself'.

For these women, the resolve to remove fat is a conscious decision that shifts their behaviour and changes their direction. Reminiscent of Protestant traditions that emphasize salvation as a personal response and explicit confession of faith, women like Tracy, Suzanne and Sarah locate their wellness in an intentional decision they make to turn their lives around. Salvation is a moment of conversion rooted in an acknowledgement of guilt and repentance. It resembles Christian paradigms in signifying a changing of mind – what the New Testament calls *metanoia* (μετάνοια) – and a gradual shift from past cultures and behaviours to new ways of seeing and being. Conversion here, however, is not simply a 'sudden and dramatic turnaround' like Kandi Stinson observes in her ethnographic study of a slimming group but also a considered course of action.[32] Although Tracy experiences a 'click in the mind', she also reasons that she must act now because she does not want to miss out on being able to keep up with her son as he grows up;

---

32. Stinson, *Women and Dieting Culture*, 124–5. In her fieldwork, Stinson observes how one woman, Lois, associates her dieting conversion with her actual religious conversion. Soon after joining the meeting, Lois tells the group that she no longer needs the oxygen tank she used to be so reliant on because she has been miraculously cured. According to Stinson, Lois sees her conversion as the result of dieting and religious changes in her life. This account of conversion as a dramatic transformation is atypical, Stinson suggests, not only because most people are born into a religion but also because even when they are not, conversion tends to be a rational process and a conscious choice rather than a dramatic experience.

she also wants to feel better about herself. Conversion is rationally and deliberately chosen even if it is also abrupt.

For women like these, the decision to lose weight is also experienced as a form of 'awakening', since it facilitates their self-actualization. According to feminist thealogian, Carol Christ, awakening is similar to conversion, grounding the woman in a new sense of self and reorienting her in the world,[33] but different in so far as it locates the power for self-change within the self. Whereas conversion in male experience connotes a giving up of self and power, awakening connotes the gaining of power and a 'coming to self'.[34] Through awakening, women 'overcome self-negation and self-hatred and refuse to be victims'.[35] In the case of Tracy, Suzanne and Sarah, their decision to lose weight expresses a resolve to take their lives into their own hands and act for themselves. It locates their ability to see and know with themselves rather than with a male authority and to break with patterns of self-hatred. In this way, the decision to 'get rid' is a practice of awakening that facilitates self-care. Yet, the conviction that fat cannot stay nevertheless directs women towards self-erasure and self-negation, traits that Christ associates with the opposite experience of inadequacy she names as 'nothingness'.[36]

I will say more about the theme of conversion in a moment, but what should be clear from the last chapter and from the committed determinism of women like Tracy, Suzanne and Sarah above, is that positive self-change is considered to be necessarily connected to the deliberate ousting of fat from the body. Although slimming encourages a turn to the self, women take hold of their selves by erasing themselves. Reminiscent of early Christian thought and ascetic practice, women conceive that they can only expand their selves by curtailing their fleshy appetites. Sacrifice here does not simply suggest a giving up of foods and of our desire for them but a surrendering of the actual body. By deciding to 'get rid' of fat, women opt to destroy parts of their anatomy. They thus partake in their own dismemberment and deliberately seek

---

33. Carol P. Christ, *Diving Deep and Surfacing: Women Writers on Spiritual Quest*, 3rd edn (Boston: Beacon Press, 1995), 13.

34. Ibid., 19.

35. Ibid., 13.

36. According to Christ, 'nothingness' expresses women's experience of powerlessness, anxiety, self-hatred and lack of self-worth (ibid., 14–18). This feeling of inadequacy is displayed in the way women feel about their bodies and in the belief that a woman 'must diet to rid herself of ugly fat' (ibid., 16).

their own deletion. In this respect slimming is what Melissa Raphael describes as 'a means of burning and consuming the flesh', a process that is inherently funerial' and 'literally, a holocaust'.[37] It provides a way of sacrificing the person as a burnt offering.[38]

Burning Fat

In the book of Leviticus, burning fat is said to be an odour that especially delights God. Forming part of the priestly writings, this text sets out various regulations of Israelite worship, including rules about animal and grain sacrifices.[39] There are specific instructions about how to handle the blood, fat, entrails and the meat of animals, and when discussing the peace offering (Lev. 3.1-17), the purification offering (Lev. 4.8-10) and the guilt offering (Lev. 7.1-10), special attention is given to the burning of internal organs, including the burning of fat.[40] Like all the other sacrificial offerings, the burning of fat on the altar is said to produce 'a pleasing odour to the Lord' (3.5).[41] Blood and fat are to be offered to God and are proscribed for human consumption. Indeed, according to Lev. 3.17, 'All fat is the Lord's. It shall be a perpetual statute throughout your generations, in all your settlements: you must not eat any fat or any blood.'

In her discussion of this proscription in Lev. 3.17, Susan Hill maintains that it suggests God prizes fat so much that he wants it all for God's self. She argues that it is suet fat specifically which is forbidden for human consumption, the fat described in Lev. 3.10 that was a tasty delicacy in the ancient Middle Eastern diet.[42] This is not fat embedded in the meat, she explains, but fat that can be peeled away and which plays a role in

---

37. Raphael, *Thealogy and Embodiment*, 90.

38. For Raphael, although it is important to avoid making 'offensively direct comparisons' between the so-called 'Final Solution' of the Holocaust and weight loss dieting, there is some commonality between their logic, intentions and effects. There is also resonance, she suggests, with the witch burnings where female flesh was burnt to liberate and redeem the soul. Dieting, she argues, is 'a way of living out death' and exposes what she calls 'patriarchy's gynocidal intentions' (89, 90).

39. Hill, *Eating to Excess*, 23.

40. Ibid., 24.

41. Also see Lev. 3.16.

42. Hill, *Eating to Excess*, 26-7.

protecting the internal organs of animals and thus in protecting life.[43] Given the best of the crop and animal are always normally reserved for God and forbidden to humans, she suggests it makes sense to see the suet fat prohibited in Leviticus in a corresponding way, as the best which also should be reserved for God and as a cultic symbol of life and abundance.[44]

For Hill, what is interesting about this prohibition, and what many scholars have difficulty in acknowledging, is that sacrificial fat is valued as a positive symbol of abundance and life. The sacrificing of fat, like the sacrificing of domestic animals, testifies to its worth before God. The prohibition, however, also confirms an important distinction between God and humans: while it is God who supplies humans with food for the preservation of life, it is for humans to respect this. In asserting that it is God who gives the people sustenance to live, the prohibition actually confirms human fatness as emblematic of the misuse of God's abundance. Human fatness represents the dangers of human excess and becomes a marker of disobedience against God.[45] This is the message of Deut. 31.20, she maintains, where God predicts that once brought into the land 'flowing with milk and honey', the Israelites will eat their fill and grow fat, turning to false Gods and breaking the covenant. Human fat is thus ultimately equated with squandering what God supplies for abundant life; it virtually confesses transgression and sin.

In the group, fat is also expressive of Syn and transgressive disproportionate foodways. The sacrificial project of shedding pounds also replicates the message behind the cultic practice of burning fat as the value of the body is expressed through its erasure. If the smell of burning fat on the altar is pleasing to God, then members and Louise are similarly delighted by the sight of lost pounds on the scale. Women do not get rid of their fat because they hold it in high esteem or consider their fat a symbol of life; they seek its destruction because it is abhorrent. But if the sacrificial fat which is burnt is ultimately destroyed by being transmuted into smoke, then women similarly seek to annihilate their fat by making it vanish into thin air. Fat may not be literally burnt, but women still conceive that they can peel it away from their bodies like the fat in Leviticus.

---

43. Ibid., 25.
44. Ibid., 27.
45. Ibid., 30.

Getting Rid of 'Excess Baggage': Thingifying Fat

Louise reinforces this confidence in the detachability of fat by circulating around the group three lumps of lard wrapped in silver foil, each labelled according to its weight ('one pound', 'two pounds' and 'seven and a half pounds'). The first time I experience this is during a meeting in January. Holding the lumps in my hands, I feel unsure about what to do with them. I can't help but ponder how many pieces of lard make up my body. Struggling to hold the larger mass in one hand, my first thought is that I 'carry' so much more on a regular basis. I suddenly feel very heavy. On a separate occasion, Hevala explains to Louise that she has just reached her target weight. She tells the group she is going on holiday so has made a concerted effort to lose that stubborn half pound that was standing in her way. Louise asks if she will be taking the plan on vacation with her, and Hevala says, 'no'. Louise then reassures Hevala that the group will still be there when she returns to help her 'get rid' of any 'excess baggage'.

Both of these instances show how Louise trains members to view their bodies as cultural plastic and to internalize the Cartesian ruse of material detachment. Holding the lard encourages women to perceive their bodies as a collection of pieces that can be disassembled. Louise's reference to fat as 'excess baggage' continues along a similar theme encouraging women to see their fat as some 'thing' external to them that can be passed on, dropped or abandoned, not unlike the lumps of lard themselves. Salvation as the pursuit of weight loss is thus an operation of 'abstractionism': it assumes an individual can step outside of their body long enough to view it from the outside and respond to it objectively.[46] It also reasserts the philosophical and theological mind–body dualism previously discussed following early Christian thinkers in the insistence that salvation can only be obtained by removing the self from the aspect of embodiment that soils its identity. Mirroring the corruptible body that many of the church fathers thought must be left behind in order for the self to enjoy spiritual union with God, fat (as a virtual confession of Syn) is an object that must be abandoned if the authentic, good self is to flourish.

In this sacrificial economy, fat emerges as an extraneous object that members carry. 'You couldn't pick it up now, and I was walking round with it,' says Jane in her interview, reflecting on how 'carrying

---

46. Bordo, *Unbearable Weight*, 2–5. Also see Stinson, *Women and Dieting Culture*, 208.

another four stone around' made her feel like confining herself to the indoors. As an object that can be discarded, it is conjured as something separate from the real self that makes their bodies 'alien' (Jane).[47] In her interview, Leanne tells me she is 'happy with *me*' but loathes her fat; Helen explains that she joined the group because she perceived an incongruity between how she saw herself and how she appeared in photographs. Losing weight provides a way for her to adjust her body to match her self-concept. Integral to the notion of salvation as 'getting rid', then, is an assumption that the authentic person is without fat. Fatness is an 'unlivable' and 'uninhabitable' zone of life[48] that must be escaped if the individual is to become a self, because, as fat activist Le'a Kent observes, 'There is no such thing as a fat *person*.'[49] Giving up or burning fat means to gain selfhood, and this repeats the theological logic of *kenōsis*, insisting that women must lose their selves if they are to save them.

Losing to Gain: No Pain, No Gain!

According to Daphne Hampson the theological principle of *kenōsis* (self-emptying) runs contrary to the valuing of female autonomy at the heart of feminist ethics. She argues that Christian theologians have drawn on Philippians 2 to identify the incarnation with the voluntary self-emptying of the Son of God, and while this principle may be useful for men, it remains to be seen how it might resource a concept of God that is compatible with feminist values.

A similar call towards self-emptying is detectable elsewhere in the New Testament. In the Gospel of Mark (8.35), Jesus instructs the crowd and his disciples that to become his followers, they must 'deny themselves and take up their cross' (Mk 8.35). Those who want to save their life must lose it, and those who lose their life for the sake of the gospel, will save it. Suffering and self-denial are integral to the realization of salvation, and this theme resonates with the meanings members ascribe to slimming. Staying 'on track' is not easy. Hevala tells me that getting to target is 'literally like getting blood out of a stone'. Similar to the way John Cassian imagines the pursuit of eternal life through the metaphor of a farmer toiling against hazardous weather conditions to

---

47. Also see Chapter 1.
48. Butler, *Bodies that Matter*, 3.
49. Kent, 'Fighting Abjection', 135.

plough the fields,[50] women like Hevala experience the journey towards the supreme good of thinness as involving hardship and struggle.

In the New Testament, sacrifice takes on especial meaning in the death of Jesus which is an offering of flesh/death/blood that is said to purify humanity and free it from bondage. This interpretation of the cross has helped to establish self-sacrifice as the highest form of love in Christianity.[51] According to Stephen Moore, Paul's theology in the New Testament has played an important role in securing the link between pain and redemption. Paul defines salvation in terms of 'dying to gain' (Phil. 1.21), a logic modelled through the event of the cross in which believers participate through baptism. In Corinthians, Paul teaches that 'what you sow does not come to life unless it dies' (1 Cor. 15.36). It is only through Jesus's death that sinners are set free from 'the yoke of slavery' (Gal. 5.1). Moore even sees in the synoptic Gospels a 'no pain, no gain' mentality that confirms that salvation goes hand in hand with suffering and struggle; it is what Jesus's predictions of his death in the synoptic Gospels amount to, he argues.[52] It is also what Jesus's statement in John's Gospel suggests when he advises that a grain of wheat must die if it is to bear fruit. Death is a prelude to life, suffering to joy.[53] Moore thus contends that the Canonical Gospels can be read as a 'bodybuilding manual',[54] because the 'no pain, no gain' syllogism is fundamental to bodybuilding philosophy.[55]

These features of bodybuilding, that is, of building the body up, are, however, not so far away from slimming that seeks to shrink the body down. In both cases, it is clear that resurrection requires that there be a crucifixion first. To use Paul's language, one must 'crucify

---

50. Cassian, 'Conferences', 1.5. Also see Chapter 2.

51. Rita Nakashima Brock, *Journeys by Heart: A Christology of Erotic Power* (Eugene: Wipf & Stock, 1988), xii.

52. Stephen D. Moore, *God's Gym: Divine Male Bodies of the Bible* (New York and London: Routledge, 1996), 102.

53. We see this principle carried forward in the Christian tradition, in St. Anthony's counsel to 'Live as though dying daily', for example. See Athanasius, 'Life of Anthony', in *A Select Library of Nicene and Post-Nicene Fathers of the Christian Church*, trans. Rev. A. Robertson, ed. Philip Schaff and Henry Wace, Second Series, vol. IV (Edinburgh: T & T Clark, Grand Rapids, Michigan: William B. Eerdmans Publishing Company, 1978), 91.

54. Moore, *God's Gym*, 102.

55. Ibid.

the flesh' along with its Synful passions to know life in its fullness.[56] The atonement principle of 'ransom' runs alarmingly through this motif as death is the price women must pay for their ultimate fulfilment[57] – they must kill their fat to be rid of Syn. Just as Christ is imaged as scapegoat, buying the freedom of captives and declaring humanity innocent in the judicial court,[58] women spend, save and calculate their Syn in the hope of being declared 'not guilty' by the scale and by Louise. That women actually count Syn – sometimes by placing pennies into a jar – and that Syn itself has a numerical value communicates more explicitly than we might expect the ransom idea that Syn must be 'paid' for.

'Getting Rid' of the Past: Salvation as Conversion

Returning now to the principle of conversion, I want to suggest that this forms part of the sacrificial motif developed in the group. Placed within the context of a 'before' and 'after' logic, getting rid allies the erasure of fat with a triumph over the past.

---

56. This type of masochistic logic has been rightly criticized by feminist theologians for legitimizing abuse and the suffering of innocents. See Joanna Carlson Brown and Rebecca Parker, 'For God So Loved the World', in *Christianity, Patriarchy and Abuse: A Feminist Critique*, ed. Joanna Carlson Brown and Carole R. Bohn (Cleveland: Pilgrim Press, 1989), 1–30. Also see, for example, Brock, *Journeys by Heart*; Brock and Parker, *Saving Paradise*; Mary Grey, *Redeeming the Dream: Feminism, Redemption and Christian Tradition* (London: SPCK, 1989); and Jantzen, *Becoming Divine*. Ivone Gebara sees in the notion of 'salvation' through sacrifice a spiritual valuation of sorrow, suffering and martyrdom. She suggests that the image of Jesus's sacrificial death works in patriarchal society to affect women and men differently, having much more of an effect on those lower down in society and on women and the poor specifically. See Gebara, *Out of the Depths*, 88.

57. Gebara argues that the notion of 'ransom' lives on in the cultural spaces of gyms and beauty parlours. See ibid., 89.

58. Stephen Finlan, *Problems with Atonement: The Origins of, and Controversy about, the Atonement Doctrine* (Collegeville: The Liturgical Press, 2005), 45. In the New Testament, Paul reminds the church in Corinth that they 'were bought with a price' (1 Cor. 6.20 and 7.23).

In one meeting in August, Jane is invited by Louise to pitch for the so-called Woman of the Year award.[59] On the chairs are slips of paper which invite us to name the woman we think is most deserving of the prize. Everyone thinks Jane will win. It is clear she has lost the most weight and members frequently admire her. When invited by Louise, Jane stands to address the group and testifies to how losing weight has transformed her life. She initially joined believing the plan was 'too good to be true', she explains. Her son's fiancée had decided to attend to lose weight before her wedding and had asked Jane to come along. She 'jumped at the opportunity'. She had considered other options like LighterLife,[60] but was concerned about the side-effects of hair loss: she wanted to lose weight, not hair! Since joining she had dedicated herself whole-heartedly to the plan and had lost five stone. She was amazed by her success and didn't quite know how it had happened. The difference in how she felt about herself was unbelievable. When she was large, she was unhappy. She detested her 'horrible weight' which made her feel 'grotesque'. Now she felt good and could shop anywhere. She shows the group a skirt she used to wear when she was larger. Stepping inside, she stretches the waist band away from herself as though to stress its vastness. When asked by Louise whether she used to 'fill' the skirt, she replies with a confident 'yes!' Jane's pride and delight are palpable. She smiles and ends her testimony by urging other women in the group to lose weight now while they are still young.

Jane's oral dividing of her biography into these two distinct periods of 'before' and 'after' is a common feature of weight loss rhetoric and religious conversion. It can be seen in the way Paul transitions from a before self that persecutes Christians to an after self that preaches the Gospel. Indeed, in Christian thought, the conversion of Paul has carried especial significance. Recognized for triggering the global expansion of Christianity, it is arguably the most famous conversion narrative in the Bible. Described in three places in the book of Acts (9.1-30; 22.3-31; 26.9-23), the story is told of Saul who encounters Jesus on the road to Damascus. While on his way to find and punish any Christians, he is blinded by a light and hears Jesus ask of him, 'Saul, why are you

---

59. This award is intended to celebrate the 'member' with the best success story.

60. According to its website, LighterLife is a nationwide UK organization with groups in the UK and Ireland, focused on changing people's attitudes to food as well as what and how they eat. LighterLife, 'About Us', http://www.lighterlife.com/about-us/ (accessed 27 August 2017).

persecuting me?' Jesus tells him to go to Damascus where he must await his calling. His companions guide him there, and Ananias restores his sight, conferring on Paul a calling to be a witness for Christ. He is then baptized and sets about proclaiming the good news of Jesus.

Of course, Paul's conversion marks a shift in his religious persuasion, but he also experiences a change in identity from persecutor to persecuted, cynic to believer. While it is debated as to whether this story describes Paul's 'calling' or 'conversion', what is certainly described is a personal and very direct encounter with Christ which moves Paul from darkness to light, blindness to sight.[61] His conversion is not only a personal response but also a decision to live differently. Paul draws on his own personal encounter with Jesus to justify his status as an apostle and also frequently implores his audience to remember their own conversions when giving direction about how to live. Conversion is thus a seminal moment for him. It signals a decision to follow a different course and culture.

Jane's story reflects some of these features. She too transitions from cynic to believer, and she too experiences her new life as a better way to live. Just as Paul's cynicism is replaced by a confident preaching of Christ to others, so Jane's cynicism is replaced by a new found faith in the weight loss plan which she voluntarily imparts (as 'good news') to others as part of her testimony. If the advice of Paul is to 'boast in the Lord' (2 Cor. 10.17), then Jane proudly testifies to the saving power of the organization. Unlike Paul, she is content to see her body as a sign of her own achievement, positively embracing her success, although she does also imply that her new self emerges quite surprisingly – she doesn't know how her weight loss has happened. Thus, just as God saves Paul, so the weight loss organization rescues Jane. By stressing the need to lose weight now, Jane counsels other women about the urgency of conversion, directing them to the fullness of life that awaits them.

Conversion, Progress and the Narration of Women's Biographies

Conversion for Jane, like Paul, constitutes a progressive narrative characterized by improvement of circumstance. In the group, it allows slimming women to narrate what Ellen Granberg describes as

---

61. Gordon T. Smith, *Transforming Conversion: Rethinking the Language and Contours of Christian Initiation* (Grand Rapids: Baker Academic, 2010), 45.

'a coherent story line'[62] – a story about the self which coherently ties the goal of weight loss to a 'series of positive events' and improvements.[63] Jane's self-narrative moves in a linear progression from her feeling grotesque to her joining the group, experiencing weight loss as something surprising but utterly rewarding and then being able to shop wherever she wants. In many ways this follows the triumphal pattern of conversion that characterizes some religious narratives. According to Arietta Papaconstantinou, Christian conversion accounts are often constituted by 'selective memories, aggrandizing the positive, obliterating the negative, vilifying the predecessor, and advancing in a sweeping movement of progress with few obstacles and no looking back'.[64] The depiction in the New Testament of the 'new' self transformed by the indwelling of Christ and the Spirit follows this kind of pattern. 'Clothe yourselves with the new self', beseeches the author of Ephesians (4.24). Dressed differently, this self has put away the old former self, 'corrupt and deluded by its lusts', and is a self God intends, a self 'created according to the likeness of God in true righteousness and holiness' (Eph. 4.24).[65] This new self fulfils its created potential for good and unbroken union with God. Much like Jane, the new self is a self that breaks free from its old clothes in an upward movement of self-becoming and progress. 'So if anyone is in Christ', Paul instructs, 'there is a new creation: everything old has passed away; see everything has become new!' (2 Cor. 5.18).

Pauline theology, as it came to be interpreted by Augustine and others, saw the fall as abolishing the human capacity to choose the good. For Paul, God sends Jesus into a world of sin and death so that our sinful, corruptible bodies might die with Christ and rise to new life with him through baptism, so we might emerge with Christ free from sin and death (Rom. 6). It is the responsibility of believers to live out this transformation, no longer setting their minds on the flesh (which does not submit to God) but setting their minds on the Spirit (Rom. 8.5-11). Like those who undertake the transforming work of weight loss

62. Granberg, 'Is That All There Is?', 116.
63. Ibid.
64. Arietta Papaconstantinou, 'Introduction', in *Conversion in Late Antiquity: Christianity, Islam, and Beyond: Papers from the Andrew W. Mellon Foundation Sawyer Seminar, University of Oxford 2009-2010*, ed. Arietta Papaconstantinou, Neil McLynn and Daniel L. Schwartz (London and New York: Routledge, 2015), xxv.
65. Also see Col. 3.10.

to fulfil their potential to forge the bodies they want and ought to have, becoming new is about a transition from an old inauthentic life of sin to a new state of being. Conversion in the group repeats the pattern of baptism and is marked by a similar freedom to obey. According to Paul, baptism enables the believer to be inwardly changed, no longer externally governed by the law, but 'obedient from the heart to the form of teaching to which you were entrusted' (Rom. 6.17). In the same way, conversion for women in the group marks a choice women make to obey the plan for themselves; women now act to govern their own bodies as Chapter 2 showed, and this frames submission and obedience in similar terms, as a demonstration of self-governance and righteousness.

The logic of conversion then is a discursive tool that structures women's personal biographies. Its linear and progressive character interprets the decision to 'get rid' as an expression of entrepreneurial freedom that marks the start of a journey towards positive self-change and self-improvement. Set within this system, fat is always an indicator that something has gone wrong. Weight loss conversely is always a corrective to a 'damaged or faulty biographical trajectory'.[66] Jane embodies this pattern of conversion when she stands inside her skirt, the gap between her old and new self symbolized by the vast space between her body and the threshold of her skirt. As well as reiterating the view that fat is a superficial outer layer that encases the inner/thinner self, and in addition to repeating ancient philosophical and theological notions of escape from the weight of the corruptible body already discussed, this also suggests that the reborn body supersedes what existed before. As with Paul, the new self replaces the old. Jane has been set free from her 'horrible weight' that held her down and successfully escaped into a better world beyond, into a life-after-fat. In her interview she tells me that the after-life she now enjoys bears little resemblance to the life she loathed before. When she was large, she did not want to go out. She hated having photographs taken. Now she didn't mind the camera. Now she could run down the street without being out of breath. Now she felt 'fantastic': 'I feel good!' she exclaims. 'If that sounds big headed I'm sorry but it's given me a lot more self-confidence, so yeah I feel good.'

In an essay discussing the importance of developing 'fat histories', Elena Levy-Navarro argues that ubiquitous diet discourse constructs fat people as 'history itself – that is, they are the past that must be dispensed

---

66. Granberg, 'Is That All There Is?', 115.

with as we move towards our seemingly inevitable future progress'.[67] To remain fat is to queer the 'straight' temporal logic of history, she argues, a logic that places the past secondary to the present and the present secondary to the future. Within this straight system, the successful dieter is depicted as a person who has achieved 'maximum longevity', having moved successfully from the past into the present and able to live into the future.[68] She claims that 'in making the fat person into the "before" that must be rejected for the "after", that we only imperfectly become, such discourse would render life uninhabitable for fat people'.[69] The logic is 'apocalyptic' in nature, she suggests, because it signals a complete break with the past even as it implicitly recognizes that work is needed to maintain this disassociation.[70] The temporal sequential logic of 'before' and 'after', ultimately refuses to respect the past, producing a linear view of time that is oppressive.[71]

Of course, Jane's dividing of her personal biography repeats modern assumptions about the inevitability of progress and adheres closely to the related projects of colonialism, capitalism and neoliberalism – fatness is a space that must be occupied (like Jane's skirt) then obliterated for its own civilizing benefit; it is also a predicament that the individual must (pay to) overcome. Immersed within a 'narrative of erasure',[72] fat is consigned to 'an eternal past'[73] and repeatedly expelled from the present in order to protect the present from its defiling touch. Fat is again ejected as 'nauseating bulk waste'[74]/filth/dirt and made placeless.[75] Looking at Jane standing inside her outstretched skirt, it is the absence of fat and the haunting trace of its existence that validates her as successful. Her fat body is evoked so it can be exorcized. This repeats the bulimic logic of abjection that surfaces in women's written and oral confessions, now

67. Levy-Navarro, 'Fattening Queer History', 18.
68. Ibid.
69. Levy-Navarro, 'I'm the New Me', 340.
70. Ibid., 344.
71. Levy-Navarro, 'Fattening Queer History', 19.
72. Kent, 'Fighting Abjection', 134.
73. Ibid., 135.
74. Wolf, *The Beauty Myth*, 191.
75. Douglas describes a number of embodiments as 'placeless' including the indefinable and ambiguous status of the unborn child. See Douglas, *Purity and Danger*, 118.

confirming that it is only when women re-place themselves into tighter, smaller clothes and spaces that they come to exist as persons at all.

Wearing the New Self: 'Passing' as Thin and the Validation of the Saved Self

Clothes are an important material means through which women in the group validate their newly transformed bodies. Just as Jane utilizes her old skirt to prove and authenticate her transition from fat to thin, so many align the formation of a new self with dressing differently. Hevala is more 'experimental' with clothes now that she has lost weight; Sarah feels able to wear more figure-enhancing garments; for Helen, losing weight means that she can now 'get away' with wearing a short skirt:

> When I'm actually out shopping, I still look at the stuff that I used to look at but I don't think, that's not gonna look good I'm a size 16, I think I might be able to get away with that actually, you know. Yeah, that's quite a short skirt but I really like it, you know, and I'm not as big as I was. I do sometimes have to remind myself of that, you know ... . I think in that sense maybe my attitude has changed. I sort of look at stuff and go yeah, you could wear that, rather than oh gosh, no.

It is common for women to consider that losing weight affords them permission to wear clothes they perceive as only suitable for thinner people. Dress is a central way in which women in the group 'pass' as thin, mark their own social acceptance and display their own bodies as legitimate.

Ellen Granberg talks about this as the 'validation of possible selves' – a process of seeking or constructing evidence that confirms that the thinner 'possible self' is being realized.[76] Such validation, she argues, is crucial to identity transformation, justifying the energy invested in self-change and motivating those concerned to continue their weight

---

76. Granberg, 'Is That All There Is?'. Granberg identifies weight loss with Possible Selves theory. 'Possible selves', she explains, 'are those aspects of self which one could become; they include idealized images to strive for as well as negative possibilities one would rather avoid' (110). For her, possible selves provides a useful lens for exploring the meaning of weight loss because it helps identify how the ability to anticipate another self and to imagine the benefits of realizing such an anticipated self can motivate and sustain self-change.

loss efforts.[77] Dressing differently, however, does not simply supply women with external validation, it also fuels levels of self-acceptance: 'I feel happier as I am now,' says Kerry. 'I *can* go out into town and try something on and think well, yeah, it looks ok, you know, rather than not wanting to go and buy anything because I couldn't fit into [it] or I didn't like how I look in something.' Jane tells me that having more choice in clothes shops is 'fabulous' because she no longer has to look for the largest size on the rail. Before she used to have to shop in special shops for larger people, but things are very different now. '*Now* I've got choice and it's just fantastic!'

Rewarding thinner women with greater consumer choice and with access to thin zones of social life obviously provides another instance of the patriarchal consumer ideology that compels women to purchase thinness in exchange for self- and social acceptance. By buying tighter, more figure-hugging clothes, women shore up the hegemonic feminine ideal that defines women through their bodies and sexual appearance; they also prove their normalcy and purchase their body's legitimacy. However, this normalizing dynamic does not mitigate the way access to thin space enables women to build social and cultural capital. Reflecting on her own experience of weight loss as a feminist and social and cultural geographer, Robyn Longhurst claims that 'being slim carries with it some very real rewards'.[78] Despite the obvious disciplinary dimensions, losing weight gives her access to places previously closed to her and facilitates her improved social and cultural well-being. Whereas exercise may have made her healthier, in a society that values slimmer bodies over fatter bodies, it is slimness rather than health which allows her body to become 'ordinary' and to fit in.

In the group, thinning women are able to access public spaces like high street shops and restaurants; they also grow in confidence and self-esteem and report feeling happier speaking to people they do not know. Salvation as a process of getting rid then also allows women to experience genuine social gains. This tension between the politics of normalization and social inclusion is not unique to secular projects of self-change; it also characterizes the healing narratives in the New Testament where wellness/salvation is allied with getting rid of physical and psychological diseases/complaints. Here, Jesus heals the leper (Mt. 8.2-4), people who are blind (Mt. 20.29-34), deaf

---

77. Ibid., 116.
78. Longhurst, 'Becoming Smaller', 88.

(Mk 7.31-34), mute (Mt. 9.32-34) and possessed (Mt. 8.28-34). Some theologians have argued that this renders persons with disabilities invisible through their correction,[79] however healing may not be all that these narratives signal. Although correction may be the 'bottom line of the Gospel stories', a closer look suggests that the act of healing 'is, again and again, subtly connected with different kinds of isolation, different kinds of alienation'.[80] For disability theologian, Wayne Morris, healing in the New Testament often enables restoration of relation and full participation within society. He maintains that many who are healed in the New Testament are invisible in society, ostracized and cut off from community. The demon-possessed man of Lk. 5.1-13 is socially isolated, living on the other side of the lake, and others have tried to restrain him with chains; the woman with haemorrhages in Lk. 8.43-48 spends all her money on a cure and so can be presumed to be poor, like many others Jesus heals; the man who has been ill for thirty-eight years in Jn 5.1-15, who could not get to the pool of water and whose body others step over in order to reach the pool in being healed is made visible and able to participate in society. Such instances, for Morris, render salvation not so much as 'cure' but as 'social and religious participation'.[81] 'The removal of the condition was simply the way that this new saved state was realized'.[82]

Women in the group similarly experience their fat as making them invisible or as disqualifying them from full participation in the worlds they inhabit. Ruth remembers people noticing her when she was younger and thinner and laments that this no longer happens now that she is larger; Tracy thinks her fat gets in the way of her relationship with her son; Kerry recalls how her size made her fear the outdoors and rush

---

79. See, for example, Elizabeth Stuart, 'Disruptive Bodies: Disability, Embodiment and Sexuality', in *The Good News of the Body: Sexual Theology and Feminism*, ed. Lisa Isherwood (New York: New York University Press, 2000), 169–70.

80. Rowan Williams, 'The Theology of Health and Healing – Hildegard Lecture, Thirsk' (7 February 2003), http://rowanwilliams.archbishopofcanterbury.org/articles.php/2111/the-theology-of-health-and-healing-hildegard-lecture-thirsk (accessed 21 February 2017).

81. Wayne Morris, *Salvation as Praxis: A Practical Theology of Salvation for a Multi-Faith World* (London and New York: T & T Clark), 140.

82. Ibid.

to hide when at the pub. Losing weight then emerges as salvific not only because it allows women to fit into normative culture but also because it enables them to be more visible and to grow in confidence, as Tracy comments,

> [My] motivation's probably family probably, and for me, feeling confident really and um … happy how I am. And not sort of, having to feel as if …. I think when I was a lot bigger, I felt as if … I'd just, I'd just sit here in the corner you know and everything. I'm definitely more, um, more at work, I'm more kind of confident, yeah. I mean more within groups. I feel more happy with … You can hold your head high, you know you can walk up can't you. The way you sort of … hunch shoulders and stuff. Yeah I definitely think you get more confidence.

For her, losing weight means she feels better in groups and is able to move her body out of the corner. The opportunities slimming presents for improved self-esteem, greater social inclusion and restored social relationships then should not be underestimated, even if such instances simultaneously assist with conforming women's bodies to oppressive social norms. As in Jesus's healing ministry, the concrete rewards experienced through greater levels of participation are in tension with the disciplinary process that sustains discriminatory attitudes and social systems.

'Getting Rid' of Disfigurement

Some women in the group conceive of their fat as an abnormality that disfigures the body and impedes health or other forms of function. For these women, the past which must be erased so that the 'new' self can emerge out of hiding is a body aligned with disability. Tracy thinks that her fat, if left uncorrected, will make her unable to play with the young son. A poster displayed in the meeting room during the launch of the 'Let's Beat It Together' campaign similarly warns that fat prevents bodies from functioning properly: obesity 'affects our working lives too …. 18 million working days a year are lost due to weight-related illness'. According to these views, fat prevents people from fulfilling their 'normal' function, from moving freely as well as from contributing to society and the economy. This discourse establishes the restoration of functionality through weight loss surgery or through access to weight loss services as just as crucial as medical interventions that correct (other) physical disabilities.[83]

For some women in the group, the reason that fat must be stripped away and discarded is because fat physically disfigures the body, pulling it out of shape and making it abnormal. Reflecting on how she used to look at photos of herself with revulsion, Hevala explains,

> I hated the pictures I saw, I really hated them. My face looked really different because when my face puts on weight it's, erm. I think my eyes get smaller so my cheeks are fatter and it, it just distorts the features of my face that I like the best.

Helen also describes how her fat causes her body to expand beyond its normal limits, making it obscene. Looking at photographs from a work party and a 'night out with the girls', she describes her shock as she observes her 'disgusting' body:

> I was just in tears cos I just looked vulgar, it is disgusting. I mean there's one picture and I'm like … I'm sitting down and my boobs are just like, expanding over the table. There's another picture and my stomach is so large I do look like I'm pregnant. And I was just so shocked by that. It wasn't what I thought I was seeing when I was looking at myself. And I … so I said to Sarah, you know I'm really unhappy.

For women like Helen and Hevala, fat is an abomination. Revolting and embarrassing, it warps the body and turns it into something freakish. That it is the female sexual characteristics of Helen's body that make it so deformed manifests the patriarchal symbolic connection between women's bodies and abnormality and renders the soteriological project of getting rid as one that seeks to erase or at least restrain the female sexual characteristics of women's anatomies. I will say more about that

---

83. See also Department of Health, 'Healthy Lives, Healthy People: A Call to Action on Obesity in England' (13 October 2011), https://www.gov.uk/government/uploads/system/uploads/attachment_data/file/213720/dh_130487.pdf (accessed December 2013). 'At a time when our country needs to rebuild our economy, overweight and obesity impair the productivity of individuals and increase absenteeism' (3). According to this report, obesity and overweight can lead to loss of earnings and the inability to hold down work (16–17).

momentarily. However, what is also clear, and related to this, is that the female body that spills over the table or whose eyes are too small takes up the symbolic position of the monster. When confronted with Helen's remarks it is hard not to be reminded of the unsightly fat body that Ruth imagines 'lurching' through town 'knocking people out with [its] vast size'.

Early Christian theologians often sanctioned similar accounts of bodies that defied 'normality'. Writing in his homily 'On the Love of the Poor', the fourth-century scholar, Gregory of Nyssa, describes the sight of people suffering with diseases such as leprosy aligning those who are disfigured with the monster:

> You see these people whose frightful malady has changed them into beasts. In place of fingernails, the disease has caused them to bear pieces of wood on hands and feet. Strange impressions are left on our paths! ... But we assert that this condition is worse than that of animals. At least beasts preserve, in general, the appearance they had at birth until they die. ... With men all happens as if they change in nature, losing the traits of their species to be transformed into monsters.[84]

Although Gregory uses this example to remind his listeners not to be condemnatory given that they may one day be afflicted by similar diseases, he nevertheless suggests that disfigured bodies are 'strange'. They seem to change their nature and appear almost unhuman. Augustine similarly suggests that those who have extra parts to their bodies are defective and will be restored to a 'normal human form' at the resurrection.[85] Siamese twins will rise as two people rather than as 'one double person'.[86] Each soul will have its own body and 'each will receive his own limbs separately so that all will have complete human bodies'.[87]

---

84. Gregory of Nyssa, 'On the Love of the Poor', cited in Almut Caspary, 'The Patristic Era: Early Christian Attitudes Toward the Disfigured Outcast', in *Disability in the Christian Tradition: A Reader*, ed. Brian Brock and John Swinton (Grand Rapids and Cambridge: William B. Eerdmans Publishing Co., 2012), 51.

85. Augustine, *The Enchiridion on Faith, Hope and Charity*, trans. Bruce Harbert, ed. Boniface Ramsey (New York: New City Press, 1999), 23.87.

86. Ibid.

87. Ibid.

As in the weight loss group, such monstrosities must be corrected, and for Augustine this applies to fatness as well.

In *City of God*, he depicts fatness like Hevala, as a bodily blemish that mars human beauty.[88] In Augustine's view, God's eternal desire is for our bodies to be beautifully proportioned. Just as a craftsperson can recast a statue so that any 'deformity' is lost simply by breaking down the original clay and remaking the object anew, God will restructure our bodies at the resurrection so that any 'deformity' of size is abolished.[89] The potter can reshape a vessel without disposing of any of the original material, and God similarly will re-proportion 'overgrown and emaciated persons' so that 'all that is excessive [is] removed without destroying the integrity of the substance'.[90] For Augustine, like women in the group, fat is a deformity that is separate to the substance of the person, and it is a blemish that will have no place in the perfect future; 'There shall be no deformity resulting from want of proportion in that state in which all that is wrong is corrected,' writes Augustine.[91] Of course, Hevala and Helen wish to dispose of fat rather than re-proportion it in the body as Augustine suggests, but they and other women share a similar belief that the removal of fat will not affect the integrity of the self. The removal of fat simply strips the body of its deformity making it look and be as it should.

'How Are the Dead Raised? With What Kind of Body Do They Come?'

This association between the able body and the resurrected body takes on especial significance in early Christian thought. The question in 1 Corinthians that asks 'How are the dead raised? With what kind of body do they come?' (15.35) was an important one for early Christian thinkers. In an attempt to marry Platonic metaphysics with the notion of a bodily resurrection and to utilize Greek and Roman philosophy to render their faith intelligible and persuasive to their critics, they presented the resurrected body as free from the 'imperfections' of the material flesh.[92] Jesus's healing ministry was considered to prefigure the

---

88. Augustine, 'City of God', in *A Select Library of the Nicene and Post-Nicene Fathers of the Christian Church*, 21.19.
89. Ibid.
90. Ibid.
91. Ibid.
92. For more on this see Candida R. Moss, 'Heavenly Healing: Eschatological Cleansing and the Resurrection of the Dead in the Early Church', *Journal of the American Academy of Religion* 79, no. 4 (2001): 991–1017.

saved state of eternal life with God in heaven, so the fact that Jesus healed those with impairments during his ministry on earth was thought to indicate that God would heal all bodies of their abnormalities in heaven. Hence, the second-century Christian philosopher and apologist Justin Martyr claims that since Jesus restores sight to the blind and hearing to the deaf on earth, so at the resurrection will the body 'rise entire', 'whole' and 'perfect'.[93] Those who experience 'sickness of the flesh' on earth will have their 'dreaded difficulties' healed when they rise again.[94] His contemporary, Irenaeus, contends that the earthly healings of Jesus which restore persons to their 'original condition' prefigure what Christ will achieve in the final resurrection: 'At one time [he healed], as regards each separate member, as it is found in His own handiwork; and at another time He did once for all restore man sound and whole in all points, preparing him perfect for Himself unto the resurrection.'[95] For him, disability is linked to sin,[96] since Jesus's healings are only necessary because creation is 'impaired by wickedness'.[97] The same body that is alive before death rises at the resurrection, just as the same eyes that are blind come to see when Jesus heals them, but the body, like the eyes of the blind, will be 'obtained ... anew in a healthy condition',[98] restored to sight and made 'whole'.

93. Justin Martyr, 'Fragments of the Lost Work of Justin on the Resurrection', in *The Ante-Nicene Fathers: Translations of the Writings of the Fathers Down to AD 325*, vol. I, ed. Rev. Alexander Roberts and James Donaldson, trans. Rev. M. Dods (Grand Rapids: William B. Eerdmans Publishing Company, 1981), IV. Taylor G. Petrey notes that it is scholarly convention to refer to the text's author as pseudo-Justin Martyr because modern scholars debate whether this text can be attributed to Justin. *Resurrecting Parts: Early Christians on Desire, Reproduction and Sexual Difference* (London and New York: Routledge, 2016), 19.

94. Justin, 'On the Resurrection', IV.

95. Irenaeus, 'Against Heresies', 5.12.6.

96. For more on this link within the New Testament and for a discussion of how this subsequently shaped the church's attitude to people with disabilities, see Amos, *Theology and Down Syndrome: Reimaging Disability in Late Modernity* (Texas: Baylor University Press, 2007), esp. 25–38.

97. Irenaeus, 'Against Heresies', 5.12.6.

98. Ibid., 5.12.5.

In the weight loss group, 'getting rid' of fat represents a similar restoration to physical wholeness. Reminiscent of ancient theological views, women consider that the saved body is a body that is 'rid' of its impairment, cured of the visible marks of Syn and transfigured so that it is now without blemish or deformity. The thin body is a resurrected body that emerges from the tomb of fat and from the dark space of Jane's skirt, rid of its physical imperfections. As with Irenaeus, the same body rises as was deformed but without its impairments, although in the case of Jane, the level of discontinuity between her old and new self renders her body anonymous. In her interview, she tells me that a man she used to date failed to recognize her in the supermarket: 'He did not know me, and I'd worked with him for four years or more, and gone out with him for a couple of years and he didn't know me.' Like Mary Magdalene fails to recognize the risen Jesus after visiting the tomb or like the two disciples on the road to Emmaus struggle to recognize the resurrected Jesus as their companion, so the process of transformation that Jane experiences changes her body beyond all recognition, estranging her from her own biography.

'Getting rid', then, is a metaphor of salvation that continues the theological association between the redeemed body and the able body and between fat, deformity and disability. It aligns salvation with the correction of physical abnormalities and defines fat as an abnormality that is distinct from the real self. However, given the physical deformities that women like Tracy and Helen wish to correct are protruding breasts, a pregnant-looking stomach and baby-weight, salvation more specifically requires that women 'get rid' of the female characteristics of their bodies and the maternal features of their physiologies. Put simply, salvation is premised on women 'getting rid' of the female.

'Getting Rid' of the Female: Salvation as a Return to the Past

Lucy thinks her breasts make her look fat and this makes her 'hate' them:

> People like talk to your boobs. Oh look at my stomach, I said, no one looks at your stomach, they look up here [*signals to her chest*]. Big shoulders big boobs. If I had my photograph taken like this [*signals from her waist upwards*], I would look the fattest. I could be the lightest one or the smallest size clothes, but I still look the fattest because I've got massive boobs!

Annoyed that the largeness of her breasts attract attention rather than the smallness of her stomach, she ponders how much her breasts weigh, implying she might be better off without them: 'I wonder how much they weigh – a few pounds? How much do you think they weigh?' For Tracy, it is her baby-weight that constitutes the past that must be purged:

> I think I was quite um, not heavy with Joseph's baby-weight but you do have extra with baby weight and I didn't really do anything after he was born to sort of get rid of that, you know. [You] just get used to wearing the clothes you're wearing don't you and then I started back at work in the September 2008 and … but then it still took me another year, near enough another year to do something about it from there.

This exposes the way femininity is caught up with a bounded identity[99] and how the rejection of the female lies at the centre of what it means to be 'feminine' under patriarchy. Weight loss is a means by which women come to know their place, to internalize that there are boundaries within which their bodies must operate and thresholds their bodies must not pass.[100] It is the sprawling and unbounded nature of the female body which makes it so offensive in these examples, its inability to keep itself in. Helen's breasts breach the threshold of the table, her pregnant-looking stomach breaches the border between self and other and Tracy's baby-weight stubbornly refuses to confine itself to its designated space. Uncontained breasts, baby-weight and a pregnant-looking stomach are all types of trespass that reveal the female body as leaky and uncontainable. These instances show how women's corporeity is inscribed 'as a mode of seepage',[101] representative of formless overflowing excess.[102]

What is also pertinent about the gendered framings of fat in these examples is that unlike the logic of conversion that has women displace

---

99. Hartley, 'Letting Ourselves Go', 63.

100. To borrow from Mary Douglas, we can therefore describe fat as 'matter out of place', as a pollutant that renders the body placeless. See Douglas, *Purity and Danger*, 44.

101. Grosz, *Volatile Bodies*, 203.

102. Ibid., 204. For Grosz this rendering of corporeality constitutes the common way in which women's bodies are coded as bodies that leak and bleed and as bodies subject to their hormonal and reproductive functions.

the past, salvation as a process of getting rid of the female has women return to it. The desire to eliminate any signs of birthing, to return to a pre-pregnancy shape and to reduce or remove breasts identifies salvation with a time before mothering took place or before the female body matured. 'Getting rid' as an expression of salvation then insists on women's arrested development by attempting to 'freeze' women's bodies in time.[103] It is an exercise in time travel as women are 'driven from the present with encouragement to recapture the past'.[104] According to this account, redemption is from 'the disaster of being made woman', as Kim Chernin acknowledges,[105] and it is a project in 'passing' as feminine by effectively becoming male.

Salvation and Becoming Male

In early Christianity, salvation takes on similar meaning as women must become as male if they are to enjoy spiritual union with God and enter heaven. In the apocryphal Gospel of Thomas, Simon Peter objects to Mary staying with Jesus and the other disciples because she is female. Jesus's reply secures the philosophical link between maleness and spirituality: 'Behold, I myself shall lead her so as to make her male, that she too may become a living spirit like you males. For every woman who makes herself male will enter the kingdom of heaven.'[106] For Grace Jantzen, this reflects a whole theological tradition informed by the Platonic assumption that spirituality is the sole province of men. Such a view persisted in the early church, she explains, but what was also irrefutable at this time was that women ascetics were strong women of spirit, 'women whose spirituality could neither be denied nor attributed to their male partner'.[107] This tension led some early Christian thinkers to describe spiritual women as honorary males with 'manly' souls – that

103. Ibid.
104. Wolf, *The Beauty Myth*, 117.
105. Chernin, *The Obsession*, 91.
106. Cited in Jantzen, *Becoming Divine*, 51.
107. Jantzen discusses the example of Perpetua and Felicity, two 'women of spirit' who were renowned for their spiritual depth but who were also consumed by the voyeurism of the male gaze. She explains that both were imprisoned for their faith but both had also given birth. Their maternality operated as a stark reminder of the awkward blend of spirituality and femaleness their bodies presented. See Jantzen, *Becoming Divine*, 50.

is, women with souls that hid 'the sex of their flesh'.[108] She sees the early Christian martyr, Perpetua, as adopting this strategy when she dreams of her own victory in the amphitheatre as a triumph made possible by being 'stripped' and 'changed into a man'.[109] According to Jantzen, the 'sex-change' Perpetua imagines provides her with the confidence and self-assurance she thinks she lacks as a woman.[110]

A similar discourse emerges in the group as women associate the annihilation of their excessive (i.e. female-fat) bodies with a growth in confidence and boldness. Women are not inspired towards actual martyrdom, nor are they concerned to establish themselves as spiritual women, but salvation as 'getting rid' nevertheless depicts a process of sexual transition through which women expand themselves by emptying themselves of their female physiology and by effectively becoming male. Salvation is thus a martyrdom of sorts.

Turning Back Time

Women in the group also imagine younger alternative possible selves. Whereas some seek to return to an actual thinner/younger self of the past, others wish to fashion an entirely new and unprecedented thinner and younger-looking body. Ruth (who is retired) identifies her weight loss with a younger self that used to be popular, nine stone two and with long red hair. She is confident that weight loss can halt the ageing process entirely telling me that the aches and pains she is increasingly experiencing as she gets older are not an inevitable result of the ageing process and can be alleviated by losing weight. Jane produces a younger-looking self that breaks entirely with her past. When Jane pitches for the Woman of the Year award, she receives praise from another woman who tells her that weight loss has 'taken years' off of her. The woman comments that Jane has become almost unrecognizable in comparison to the photo of her former self circulating around the room. Again, we see how Jane's body becomes transfigured beyond recognition, but for her and for Ruth, salvation is a process that invariably signifies a regression into youth.

The association of salvation with paradise lost and with an idealization of the past depicts memories of flawlessness and perfection

---

108. Cited in Jantzen, *Becoming Divine*, 52.
109. Cited in ibid., 50.
110. Ibid., 50–1.

in Eden.[111] According to the Cappadocian Father, Gregory of Nyssa, 'The resurrection promises us nothing else than the restoration of the fallen to their ancient state [… and] a certain return to the first life, bringing back again to Paradise him who was cast out from it.'[112] For him, perfection is located in an eschatological end that is also a return to the beginning. In Jane's case, of course, the return to paradise that rewinds the years is a form of salvation that distorts and erases her history, but for Ruth salvation is about reconnecting with an optimum time in her life when she used to be noticed and stood out. Augustine similarly considers that the resurrected body will rise at its optimum, as it was in its 'prime'.[113] For him, this depicted a body that was 'neither beyond nor under youth, but in that vigor and age to which we know that Christ had arrived'.[114] Reminiscent of the way women like Ruth tie salvation to a nostalgic return to the weights of their youth, he insists that 'every man shall receive his own size which he had in youth, though he died an old man, or which he would have had, supposing he died before his prime'.[115] The body at its prime is a body at the age that Christ reached, around thirty,[116] unblemished and flawless. Augustine is clear that although the body currently lives in time, it must abstain from joy for the sake of the future heaven after which it hopes, for 'by the passage of time we are taught this very lesson of despising time and seeking eternity'.[117] And time is to be despised for good reason, he instructs, for the world is ailing and old. Just as old age brings its complaints, so the world is sick and 'beset with difficulties':[118]

> [Christ] came when everything had grown old, and he made you as good as new. A thing that had been made, been set up, that was going

---

111. Wolf, *The Beauty Myth*, 117.
112. Gregory of Nyssa, 'On the Making of Man', in *A Select Library of Nicene and Post-Nicene Fathers of the Christian Church*, Second Series, vol. 5, ed. Philip Schaff and Henry Wallace (Grand Rapids: William B. Eerdmans Publishing Company, 1979), XVII.2.
113. Augustine, 'City of God', 1–511, XXII.15.
114. Ibid.
115. Ibid., XXII.15.
116. Ibid.
117. Augustine, *On Christian Doctrine*, II.16.25.
118. Augustine, *Sermons*, III/3 (51–94), 'On the New Testament', trans. E. Hill, ed. J. E. Rotelle (New York: New City Press, 1991), 81.8..

to perish, was declining to its end. It was bound to be beset with difficulties; he came, both to encourage you among these difficulties, and also to carry you forward to eternal rest. Don't be eager to cling to an aged world, and unwilling to grow young in Christ, who says to you, 'The world is perishing the world is aging, the world is going to pieces, with the labored, wheezy, breathing of old age. Don't be afraid, *your youth shall be renewed like the eagle's* (Ps 103:5).'[119]

The theological association between salvation and an eternal paradise where change, decay and the passage of time are no more resurfaces in the group as women seek to fashion younger selves and erase all traces of their sexual maturity.

Escaping to the Future: Salvation as 'Getting There'

Despite salvation being imaged as past, present and future event, it is the future which has come to dominate Western thinking about salvation. Salvation is quite literally 'out of this world', taking place in the life beyond the present. Feminists have observed a similar concentration on the future in weight loss culture and have commonly identified slimming with an eschatological vision that defies fulfilment. According to Michelle Lelwica, for example, the power of the slender ideal resides in 'its elusive capacity to represent but forever postpone the wholeness that girls and women variously seek'.[120] For Mary Bringle, the pursuit of thinness has an elusive goal which is endlessly deferred – 'Like the parousia for first-century Christians, even this paltry goal keeps receding,' she insists.[121] The dominant position in feminist research is that slimming is caught up with a false promise of future well-being and the postponement of happiness.

In my group, however, some women do achieve their weight loss goals and speak about arriving at their hoped for destination. Hevala tells me that despite her weight loss being slow, she is content with herself now: 'I am happy with how I am now cos I'm like, I've finally got there and it is nice to know that it's not that easy to stay slim. So it's, it *is* an achievement.' Helen loses the weight she hoped to lose before her

---

119. Ibid. Emphasis in original.
120. Lelwica, *Starving for Salvation*, 60.
121. Bringle, *The God of Thinness*, 101.

wedding; Samantha loses the bloated feeling she used to have and hated. A number of women become target members and enjoy the enabling benefits of their new thinner selves.

Yet, even Hevala (above) acknowledges that staying slim is difficult, repeating the association with suffering and struggle endemic to the economy of sacrifice. For Helen, staying at target is 'impossible', and this is a difficulty Louise seldom helps with:

> When I was at target, I found that really difficult. Obviously trying to maintain is like impossible and the same response is given to everybody: 'Oh well, you know, you've got to up your Healthy Extras but don't up your Syns, and its, it's a bit of you know hit and miss, you've just got to trial and error with this one.' [*Imitates Louise*] And that isn't actually very helpful.

Indeed, for women in the group, while salvation might be realizable it nevertheless remains precarious and fragile because the weight can always go back on. Although at target, Kerry explains, 'I don't want to go back to how I was, to how I looked, to how I felt.' To ensure she does not backslide, she now goes to the gym and has a glass of water and a banana when she returns rather than substituting the gym for a coffee and a slice of cake as she did before.

Reaching an ideal weight, then, brings its own problems, increasing rather than discharging many women's anxieties. Women labour to stay at target and to prevent themselves from 'slipping'. They fear going 'back' or returning to fat and this means that there can be no end or completion to the slimmer's journey. As Lelwica observes, 'Even the most ideal female bodies require routine maintenance.'[122] Louise's weekly commission to 'go forth and shrink' reminds women that the work of weight loss is never done, confirming slimming as a liminal 'status passage'[123] that keeps women betwixt and between the undesirable body of the past/present and the desirable completed happy and fulfilled body of the future.

Weight cycling is a common experience in the group. Suzanne is the longest standing member and despite attending every week has

---

122. Lelwica, *Starving for Salvation*, 61.
123. Monaghan, *Men and the War on Obesity*, 76. According to Monaghan, dieters' bodies are always in a state of limbo, betwixt and between an undesirable and desirable weight.

never achieved her target. Her frequently fluctuating weight causes her some embarrassment. Others experience similar patterns of yo-yoing leading to similar levels of frustration. Lucy remarks, 'I don't know what my target is … cos I'll probably never get there the way I am because I'm putting it on one week and it's off the next.' For Joy, even the experience of gaining one and half pounds makes her feel like she is falling away from her imagined destination: 'I was 9.12 when I started,' she explains. 'I've managed to get eight and a half pounds off, but now I'm back up, seven altogether I've got off. So ideally I'm still not there personally.'

The notion of 'getting there', of arriving at an imagined destination somewhere ahead of time in the future, indicates that women like Lucy and Joy believe there is an end they can and must reach as individuals. Yet this stands in tension with their experience of yo-yoing that conversely signals the difficulty, even impossibility, of arriving. In these narratives, hope in an after-life – in a life-after-fat – sits awkwardly alongside a diminished sense of trust in the self and in the future.[124] While many women believe that the organization allows them the opportunity to reach the end they desire, they nevertheless experience this end as receding.

Of course, Christian discourse depicts salvation variously as the hope of entering the 'promised land', as the realization of the Kingdom of God on earth, as entering into heaven or the life beyond death in full communion with God,[125] but from the early Christian era, salvation tends to be linked with a celestial life beyond the grave and to a future destiny beyond the present. Speaking about heaven, Augustine laments that 'we haven't yet arrived, but we are already on the way, we aren't yet enjoying things there, but we are already sighing for them here'.[126] Aquinas similarly teaches that perfect happiness will only be realized in heaven, 'for then, by a single, uninterrupted and

---

124. Compare this with Stephen Pattison's discussion of the work of Donald Capps and his theological interpretation of shame. Pattison notes how, for Capps, shame arises when the future does not turn out as predicted, leading to doubt about the self and the future. Pattison, *Shame: Theory, Therapy, Theology*, 206.

125. Morris, *Salvation as Praxis*, 4.

126. Augustine, *Sermons III/10 (341-400) on Various Subjects*, trans. E. Hill, ed. J. Rotelle (New York: New City Press, 1995), 400.2.

continuous act our minds will be united with God'.[127] For Aquinas, this is a spiritual vision of contemplative union with God in which the body plays no part.

Such positions resemble the future end some women imagine as being characterized by perfection and ultimate happiness. Helen, for example, joins the group wanting to lose weight for her wedding.[128] She explains, 'I was getting married in 2009, so there was sort of like a vague aim …. It'll give me plenty of time and I can lose loads of weight. And, you know, it will be perfect by the time we get there.' Getting there, although a 'vague aim', portrays an entry into a place where everything will be 'perfect'. Perfection, in Helen's case, is tied up with the fulfilment of heteronormative ideals – with her entry into marriage and her attainment of a thinner body. Together these validate her arrival at a place of ultimate fulfilment which resides in a life beyond the now.

The way Helen disciplines her now body in anticipation of a better future illuminates just how dangerous deferring to an imagined future can be for the well-being of women's bodies. Having lowered her target to accommodate her still shrinking body, Helen discloses to me in one meeting that she now wants to lose even more weight. She joined the group so she would be able to fit into her wedding dress, but having completed that goal and given she is still losing weight, she decides that she 'might as well go for another stone'. One month later, she remarks in a conversation with Sarah and I that sleeping has become uncomfortable because her bones stick out and the bed digs into her.

Helen's ongoing pursuit of weight loss is motivated by a desire to feel happy that never reaches fulfilment. Having lost two and half stone for her wedding, she admits that she is still unable to look back

---

127. Thomas Aquinas, *Summa Theologiæ*, 16 (Ia2æ.1-5), Purpose and Happiness, trans. Thomas Gilby (Cambridge and New York: Cambridge University Press, 2006), 3.2.

128. Jeffery Sobal, Caron Bove and Barbara Rauschenbach discuss the particular association between weight and weddings arguing that weddings provide a unique way of examining the social construction of weight. From their in-depth ethnographic interviews they show that some women opt to manage their weight ahead of getting married by 'taking action' through dieting, conscious that wedding photography immortalizes their appearance. See their essay, 'Weight and Weddings: The Social Construction of Beautiful Brides', in *Interpreting Weight: The Social Management of Fatness and Thinness*, ed. Jeffery Sobal and Donna Maurer (New York: Aldine de Gruyter, 1999), 124 and 131.

at photographs of the day with pride. Although her dress was far too big, she only sees the fat that she later came to lose but hadn't lost by that day:

> I still look back at the pictures and think, but you know, that's quite big, you know, because I did get slimmer than that. So I do still look at them and think, look at that roll of fat, there on the back or whatever, but that's just me nit-picking at my body.

When I ask if she thinks she will ever arrive at a point when she will feel happy with herself, she answers, 'I don't know if there would ever be an end. I'd like to think there would be, but I don't know how low I'd have to go before I thought that, weight wise.' Poignantly she adds, 'for me, it seems to be the smaller I am, the happier I am, which is kind of worrying'.

Indeed, it is worrying because this pattern suggests that only total erasure of her body will produce the kind of happiness and final fulfilment that she desperately seeks – an obedient repetition of the message communicated by the image of the female dancer Louise circulates. Yet, Helen is not oblivious to the seriousness of her reducing habits. Like the classical theologies previously discussed, the future happiness she imagines is allied to a completed body purged of its physical imperfections and is located in a future she cannot yet grasp.

The dangers of this futurizing of salvation within Christian soteriology have been outlined by a number of feminist theologians. Ruether sees in this evidence of the 'Platonizing' of Christianity through which the original historical roots of salvation become increasingly spiritualized.[129] Others suggest that the deferral of salvation to paradise elsewhere threatens to affirm the beyond at the expense of actual history,[130] leading to both a neglect of the present and a de-politicizing and de-moralizing of the challenges, hardships and struggles of this life. Rita Nakashima Brock and Rebecca Parker have presented a damning critique of Western Christianity in this respect, accusing it of removing paradise from today and making humanity's location in space and time a problem. For them, the futurizing of salvation and relocating

---

129. Ruether, *Introducing Redemption*, 63.
130. Gebara, *Out of the Depths*, 124.

of paradise to other worlds foster a restlessness in Westerners making them anxious for home.[131]

Of course, in the group, women seek not only escape into future worlds/bodies but also a return to past perfection, but even this past is a past that is relived in a future history. Whether salvation is behind or ahead, it is seldom in the now, and this fosters a similar kind of restlessness to the type Brock and Parker describe. 'Getting rid', as a redemptive motif, signals that staying in the present – and so in the 'nowness' of fat – is impossible, once more confirming the fat body to a state of exile. As with some features of Christian eschatology, so in the weight loss group, the deferral of salvation to a life beyond the present serves to de-sacralize the material, instil a fear and dread of the maternal body and fuel the drive for mastery.[132] It promotes the same 'earth-fleeting sentiment'.[133]

Beyond Individual Salvation: 'Getting There'
as a Social and Corporate Project

Yet, even if the removal of salvation from the now accommodates women to the lucrative work of endless striving, it is at the same time not solely individualistic nor entirely harmful. Women choose to attend the group rather than follow the plan privately and experience the meeting as an opportunity to build connections with other women through the pursuit of a common goal. Not surprisingly, feminist commentators have looked with suspicion on these kinds of friendships and support mechanisms. Michelle Lelwica claims that slimming clubs prioritize commercial gain over the well-being of members. We might think that the kind of community Weight Watchers offers is positive, she remarks, but 'we must use our critical eye'.[134] Weight loss communities are marketing tools cleverly designed to sustain The Religion of Thinness,

---

131. Brock and Parker, *Saving Paradise*, 417.
132. Jantzen, *Becoming Divine*, 129 and 141.
133. Jacob Waschenfelder, 'Rethinking God for the Sake of a Planet in Peril: Reflections on the Socially Transformative Power of Sallie McFague's Progressive Theology', *Feminist Theology* 19, no. 1 (2010): 91. Also see, for example, Mary Grey, *Redeeming the Dream* and *The Outrageous Pursuit of Hope, Prophetic Dreams for the Twenty-First Century* (London: Dart Longman & Todd, 2000).
134. Lelwica, *The Religion of Thinness*, 212.

and they hook women with 'the hope of meaningful friendships and supportive connections'.[135] Others have been similarly inclined to interpret the relationships forged in weight loss communities as 'transient' and 'anonymous'.[136] For Geneen Roth the friendships women develop help sustain the dangerous message that women 'fit in by hating themselves'.[137]

In my group, this message is one that women learn and transmit. By confessing Syn/fat in the weekly meetings and routinely committing to turning things around, women generate communities of obedience that observe and corroborate thin privilege. However, this is not the only function of community. For some women, attending the group provides opportunities to meet people and generate networks of support that contrast with the loneliness of home. Explaining why she attends the group Kerry reflects:

> Well, you know you're not on your own, you know. And also, it's sort of a way of meeting people. ... They know what you've, what you've been through, cos they've been through it, and um, they know that you can do it to pull it round as well.

This differs starkly from the isolation she describes feeling when her husband worked nights:

> John used to work in printing and there were times when he would work late, times when he would work nights and I was on my own. So I'd go home from work and I knew I was going to be on my own. I would perhaps take fish and chips in for my tea because I didn't want to cook for myself. But as well as that, there would be perhaps a bottle of pop and some crisps and maybe three packets of sweets because ... well, I might fancy that. And by the end of the night I would have consumed the lot.

---

135. Ibid., 215.

136. Daniel Martin argues that relationships among group members in organized weight loss groups can resemble that of 'intimate strangers'. See Martin, 'Organizational Approaches to Shame', 133. Naomi Wolf argues that 'the "supportive" rhetoric of the diet industry masks the obvious: The last thing it wants is for women to get thin once and for all'. Wolf, *The Beauty Myth*, 102.

137. Geneen Roth, *Women, Food and God: An Unexpected Path to Almost Everything* (London: Simon & Schuster, 2010), 28.

Attending group prevents her from feeling alone and so mirrors the comfort she describes receiving from food. It is also an act of care that contrasts with her experience of self-disregard as she struggles to find the motivation to cook for herself when her husband is away.

Hevala tells me that the meeting is a social occasion that enables her to encounter like-minded people and receive support:

> It's nice just from the social thing isn't it, because you're meeting people and getting to know people who've got the same goals in mind and have got ideas about how you can do things to lose weight, or to keep on track. So I think that's why the meeting's good.

She goes on to explain that the sessions help her to feel 'less isolated' and 'like you're more part of something'. In a similar way, Helen comments in her interview that the meeting provides a social time that makes sure she gets out of the house, something she finds especially important when she is diagnosed with a demobilizing condition: 'It was something that I could do, sort of like a commitment that I had to keep to, for myself.' Jane considers that attending the group helps break with her usual pattern by connecting her to other women, thereby departing from the male-centred dynamics of her home:

> **Jane** I've just enjoyed—
> **Dave** [*interrupts*] You enjoy the company, don't you?
> **Jane** The company cos it's the only time I ever see any other females really apart from my sister.
> **Dave** This is a male-dominated household!

In these instances, attending the group helps encourage women out of hiding, out of the home and out of isolation. Certainly this corporate opportunity to disconnect from the realities of the home not only encourages what Naomi Wolf refers to as a 'sedatedness in women',[138] distracting women from the historical and political difficulties of their private lives, but also provides a public space where women can practise their body's legitimacy away from the domestic sphere and value other women's experiences. Women meet new people, forge sisterhoods and rely on one another's empathy. As such, the projects of self-cultivation women follow are not simply self-referential. It is not as Michelle Lelwica suggests that communities dedicated to the pursuit of thinness

---

138. Wolf, *The Beauty Myth*, 128.

fail to provide a sense of belonging that transcends the realm of the individual's life.[139] The selves women craft in my group embrace and respond to the stories of other women.

Of course, this does not negate the disciplinary dynamics of the meeting, but accountability is not just about showing the self to others so it can be judged by them. It also concerns giving the self to others as a gift that can enrich and be enriched by them. Helen speaks about the importance of attending for others:

> Something that I try and tell myself when I am thinking, oh, I don't really want to do it, is well there might be somebody there, you say something and it really helps them. So it's not just about you when you're in the group, it's about everybody else as well.

She reiterates the point later in our discussion,

> I do think it's not necessarily just about you when you're in the group. It's about sharing information, sharing experiences and like I say, you know, somebody might sit there and say actually that's a really good idea and you know, they may have a really good result from it. Um, and also, you know, you get the same back.

Mutual accountability and support is thus not only a means through which women's obedience to thin privilege is secured, it also helps women build genuine relationships with one another. The reciprocity Helen identifies here shows the degree of impact that the social bonds between women have. Most identify listening to others with their own positive self-change, with learning new knowledge and with feeling reassured that they are not alone.

In a discussion of how late modernity in the West has shaped women's lives and notions of femininity, Linda Woodhead argues that women's pursuits of self-generation are not simply self-determined because the sense of valued selfhood depends on 'quotidian interactions with others'.[140] Self-worth is relational, she argues, because it is dependent

---

139. Lelwica, *The Religion of Thinness*, 211. She suggests that the community offered by organized weight loss groups appeals to a feeling of disconnection which is left unresolved due to the gap left by institutional religion.

140. Linda Woodhead, "'Because I'm Worth It!' Religion and Women's Changing Lives in the West', in *Women and Religion in the West: Challenging*

upon 'others' willingness to make space and make time, to listen, acknowledge and recognize'.[141] Likewise, in the weight loss meetings, women listen, acknowledge and recognize one another. They access and exchange resources, including various types of economic, social, political and cultural capital: they share books, recipes and ideas and draw on one another's knowledge, finances and time. Such practices of the self in the context of community provide opportunities for every woman to speak and enable participants to validate their own and other women's worth away from their domestic spheres and without the permission of men.

Certainly, women's interactions serve to encourage one another to get back into the kitchen and supermarket and to focus on their appearance, but the subjectivities women craft in the group resemble what Woodhead calls 'a "part-time" or partial domestic femininity'.[142] These once more can be described as post-feminist subjectivities because they point towards a 'more independent, entitled selfhood',[143] to feminine subjects that have ownership of their own bodies and that feel in charge of how they deploy their bodies as resources. The women believe they deserve to spend time and money on themselves and to occupy space in the public domain without deferring to male authority.[144] The subjectivities women craft through community are also produced in contexts of contradiction that challenge as well as support 'male-referential femininities'.[145] As such, I would suggest that we can embrace a number of features of community modelled in this weight

Secularization, ed. Kristin Aune, Sonya Sharma and Giselle Vincett (Aldershot: Ashgate, 2008), 149.

141. Ibid.
142. Ibid., 155.
143. Ibid.
144. According to Woodhead, this more entitled subjectivity is captured in the L'Oreal slogan, 'Because I'm worth it'. Such a slogan evidences that women now have access to the previously male project of independent selfhood made possible by legislation that has helped ingrain notions of dignity and equality in Western-European culture (ibid., 148). Women can now buy their own property with their own financial resources and can occupy public space legitimately, without deferring to male permission (ibid., 149). The need to make such an assertion of self-worth, however, according to Woodhead, also exposes the fragility of this selfhood (ibid., 152).
145. Ibid., 156.

loss group without assenting to the way they are put to work in the reproduction of disciplinary power. In continuation with the position I outlined in Chapter 2, I propose that we can uncouple these features of community from the hegemony of fat phobia and thin privilege. The cultivation of self-permission; the sharing of stories, knowledge and experience with other women; the building of self-worth through reciprocal exchanges; the making of space and time for other women and the acknowledgement of the validity of other women's experiences are all important features of community that I will later suggest can be put to work in other communal settings to resist rather than acquiesce with the thin ideal.

Church, koinônia and Eucharist

In *The Confessions*, Augustine asks, 'What point is there for me in other people hearing my confessions?'[146] He enquires about his fellow believers, labelling them as a 'curious lot ... eager to pry into the lives of others, but tardy when it comes to correcting their own'.[147] After wondering how it is that others know he is telling the truth about himself when he confesses, he concludes that he and the community to whom he confesses are united in charity and that his confessions may have the effect of saving others from slumping into the despair that says 'I can't'.[148] He acknowledges that those who hear may wish to congratulate him on his progress towards God and to pray for him when they hear about how badly he is doing. 'To people like that I will disclose myself,' Augustine states, because those who listen are motivated by compassion and a 'brotherly mind', not by 'wickedness'.[149] They are 'companions of my joy ... my fellow citizens still on pilgrimage with me'.[150]

This endorsement of community and of the corporate nature of confession resonates with the positive characteristics of community women narrate. Members are compassionate rather than judgemental (on the whole), willing to assist others and aware of the importance of others in their own weight loss journeys. Women both serve and

146. Augustine, *The Confessions*, X.3.3.
147. Ibid.
148. Ibid., X.3.4.
149. Ibid., X.4.5.
150. Ibid., X.4.6.

are served by one another, and this sharing is a source of hope and companionship.

Of course, a similar modelling of reciprocity and mutual sharing has been prominent in shaping Christian thinking about what it means to be the church. In Christianity, the church features prominently as a community of believers gathered in response to the gift of God in Jesus.[151] It is a community of disparate people united by hope and trust in God, a community who share a common life and purpose. The church is a pilgrim church, presently 'at home in the body' and 'away from the Lord' (2 Cor. 5.6) but 'longing to be clothed with our heavenly dwelling' (2 Cor. 5.2). As Augustine puts it, the church is a 'heavenly city' on pilgrimage in the world,[152] the City of God living in the world but always a 'stranger'.[153]

The weight loss community takes on similar significance as a gathered people of resident aliens who are on their way towards their ultimate hope. They too are a pilgrimage community on the move and in transit. Both food and fellowship characterize this community resonating with the corporate and Eucharistic dimensions of the church. According to the New Testament, the church is the context within which salvation is 'worked out' (Phil. 2.12).[154] It is a community in which members are accountable to one another and confession and forgiveness comprise features of its life together. The church is a corporate body characterized by fellowship and communion, features that are glimpsed by the Greek term *koinônia*.[155] The book of Acts identifies the communal life of

---

151. George H. Tavard, *The Church, Community of Salvation: An Ecumenical Ecclesiology* (Collegeville: The Liturgical Press, 1992), 11.

152. Augustine, 'City of God', 15.15.

153. Ibid., 18.1. Augustine distinguishes the City of God from the city of this world. While the City of God is made present in this world, its home is in heaven. Both cities have different origins: 'These two series of generations accordingly, the one of Cain, the other of Seth, represent the two cities in their distinctive ranks, the one the heavenly city, which sojourns on earth, the other the earthly city, which gapes after earthly joys, and grovels in them as if they were the only joys' (15.15).

154. Christiaan Mostert, 'Salvation's Setting: Election, Justification and the Church', in *God of Salvation: Soteriology in Theological Perspective*, ed. Ivor J. Davidson and Murray A. Rae (Farnham: Ashgate, 2011), 134.

155. Gerald O'Collins, *Jesus Our Redeemer: A Christian Approach to Salvation* (New York and Oxford: Oxford University Press, 2007), 202.

believers with a devotion to breaking bread. It is a central feature of the image of the church as the body of Christ, working in unity to witness to the grace of God.

In the group, salvation is also 'worked out' in community and the processes of confession and absolution are integral to its corporate life, as we have seen. Women share the same hope and a common purpose, and food is similarly a means through which fellowship is shared and solidarity forged. Just as believers in the church might ingest the body and blood of Jesus in order to participate in his body and share in the redemption of God, women partake of the food tasters which demonstrate the effectiveness of the weight loss plan, in the hope that they will assimilate with its wisdom. By eating the tasters, women ingest the precepts of the plan and trust that their bodies will be transformed. Bread and wine are ironically categorized as Syn by the slimming organization, but the weight loss community, like the faith community, eat what is considered to be salvific. In both cases, food is a crucial site of salvation. Just as Augustine imagines his fellow believers praying for him and approaching him with 'brotherly' minds, participants consider fellow members to be sources of reassurance and motivation. In this sense, women become food for one another, giving their time and bodies for each other's encouragement and support, but without dismissing their own needs. The logic of sacrifice runs deep in the group, but salvation as a corporate, fleshy, communal project encourages women to return to their bodies, to food and to the bodies of others, at the same time as it instructs them to leave their fat behind.

Conclusion

Christian ideas about salvation offer an important hermeneutical tool for understanding the redemptive motifs that surface in the weight loss group. Although reference to 'God' and 'salvation' are absent, mainstream Christian ideas about salvation which have helped shape our Western cultural imagination lurk anonymously in the background. The redemptive paradigm developed in the group encourages both an escape from the body, corporeality and food and a closer connection with them. This tension not only helps construct the agonistic personality and supports the modern projects of consumer capitalism and neoliberalism but also suggests that there are salvageable features of slimming and the related classical soteriologies that resonate with it. The corporate and corporeal nature of salvation places the body centre stage. Moreover, associations between salvation and projects that build women's self-esteem, that enable women to narrate their own lives and influence their own environments, that build solidarity with other women through fellowship and through the sharing of stories and experience and that allow women to practise a new cultural habit are important features of the redemptive paradigm developed in the group. These contrast with harmful features of slimming discourse and related Christian soteriology that prioritize the future and other worlds, foreground death and sacrifice as a route to salvation, align fatness with incompleteness and emphasize the need to be reborn as another body. The remaining chapters use the recoverable components of women's Syn-talk and salvation narratives to inform and shape alternative accounts of these theological themes in the hope that they may direct women towards greater aliveness in a fat-phobic world.

Chapter 4

RETHINKING SIN: SIZEISM, THE VICTIMIZATION OF FOOD AND THE DIVIDED SELF

The last three chapters have traced and explored the various meanings the slimming group and organization ascribe to Syn and how weight loss takes on significance as a form of salvation. The next three chapters use the experiences of the women and my own critical reflections on them to push these theological categories in new directions. My emphasis shifts from charting how slimming resonates with aspects of historical Christian thought to redefining sin and salvation in light of my ethnography. Certain features of classical theology are retained, but much is also troubled or rejected in light of the case study discussed in the first part of this book. My reflections on the way the group's salvation narratives resonate with well-established Christian ideas now provide me with clues for how to theologically develop these categories. By amplifying the aspects of women's Syn and salvation narratives together with related theological traditions which have been shown to be worthwhile and by modifying or rejecting those aspects which have been shown to engender harm, I construct practical theologies of sin and salvation which speak back to Christian thought and weight loss culture. In so doing, I argue that Christian theology can make a meaningful intervention into contemporary debate about fat and that faith-based practices can be sites of revolution. While this chapter returns to the notion of 'sin', Chapters 5 and 6 focus on the practical meanings of 'salvation' and on how certain activities around alimentation and weight might challenge the vilification of women's bodies and appetites.

Sin and salvation remain controversial concepts in feminist theology. Evoking Daphne Hampson's argument in *Swallowing a Fishbone*,[1] Kathryn Greene-McCreight suggests that 'one of the fishbones of

1. Daphne Hampson, *Swallowing a Fishbone? Feminist Theologians Debate Christianity* (London: SPCK, 1996).

classical Christianity on which feminist theologies often choke is the doctrine of sin'.[2] In her view, this Christian principle is especially problematic to feminists because it jars with the Enlightenment belief in progress and the perfectibility of humanity. For Mary Daly, nothing less than the castration of Christianity will suffice if feminists are committed to the Second Coming of women and to their development as subjects. This must necessarily involve 'cutting away ... the myths of sin and salvation', she insists,[3] for both are symptoms of the same disease of 'supermale arrogance'. Seen in the Christian story by the way salvation relies on the ultimate male superhero (Jesus), this arrogance has the effect of locating women's wellness and fullness in their deference to a male saviour, rather than in their own self-discovery and 'woman-consciousness'.[4]

Feminist theologians are right to be reluctant when it comes to embracing the language and logic of sin. The Augustinian concept of 'original sin' as an innate defect presents human beings as fundamentally bad, and this can do nothing for women who so often have been made to feel like their bodies are inherently flawed. It fails to give sufficient value to women's capacity to act and determine their own lives – a point that must be retained if we are to value women's experiences of agency in the group. However, equally unhelpful is to unequivocally endorse the perfectibility of humanity, not least because reflection on the weight loss group demonstrates how the pursuit of progress and perfection resources patterns of body dissatisfaction among women. Such insights must be taken seriously when thinking theologically about the categories of 'sin' and 'salvation', I suggest. This requires giving theological expression to the tension between freedom and constraint evidenced in the weight loss group. The theological tropes of sin and salvation should help us to relinquish the pursuit of perfection while acknowledging women as agential subjects who have the capacity to shape their own environments, all without ignoring the ways our bodies, lives and actions are simultaneously constrained by external forces.

Feminist theologians are also right to be suspicious of salvation motifs that locate salvation in one man and encourage women to swap

---

2. Kathryn Greene-McCreight, *Feminist Reconstructions of Christian Doctrine: Narrative Analysis and Appraisal* (New York and Oxford: Oxford University Press, 2000), 56.

3. Daly, *Beyond God the Father*, 71–2.

4. Ibid., 71.

self-discovery for self-abnegation and suffering. I reject as an inadequate theological expression of God's love the logic of atonement that premises redemption on the blood and killing of an innocent. We have already seen how the ransom metaphor aligns with the sacrificial projects of women who crucify their fat to rid themselves of Syn, legitimizing once more the theological position that says women are saved through suffering and through their own voluntary acts of crucifixion. Given this, it seems to me that if Christian theologies and actions are to defend the fullness and livingness of all women, we need descriptions of sin and salvation motivated by kindness and a passion for reconciliation, not by war and an obsession with death.

The theological proposals I offer in the following three chapters seek to attend to these practical concerns. I begin in this chapter by returning to the notion of 'sin' and suggest a set of related meanings that are informed by the analysis and critique of Syn-talk already provided. Patterns and insights garnered from my time inside the group become instructive for shaping an expansive theological description that respects the lives of the women while having application beyond this setting. As Serene Jones argues, the concept of 'sin' must be allowed to 'travel widely' so that it engages with the nuances of ordinary women's lives.[5] In this chapter, it is the lives of ordinary women inside the weight loss group that inform the theological meanings I develop. My theological offerings are thus resourced by these women but they also travel beyond the confines of the group to speak into a wider culture where fat is vilified and thinness sacralized.

Sin, I suggest, describes that which disrupts our God-intended, original createdness for relation, aliveness and flourishing, and can be appropriately named as 'sizeism', the 'victimization of food' and the 'divided self'. Such designations deliberately return to insights already garnered from women's experiences inside the group, but these are now reframed within an analytic feminist theology of sin. In critical dialogue with the feminist hamartiology of Rosemary Radford Ruether, I propose that sin gives expression to a number of distorted ways of relating to food, fat and the 'bodyself'.[6] It not only pronounces a negative judgement that such relations violate God's intentions but also performs a positive and

---

5. Jones, *Feminist Theory and Christian Theology*, 112, 114.

6. Carter Heyward presents the notion of the 'bodyself' to depict the body and self as one integrated unit. See, for example, *Touching Our Strength: The Erotic as Power and the Love of God*, 8.

rhetorical function, orienting women towards the cultivation of hope. The notion of 'sin' is a useful and useable cultural resource, I argue, and offers a distinctly Christian way of speaking about the distortions that are worn on women's bodies in weight loss contexts. In a cultural setting where fears about food and fat abide and are resourced in part by the Christian notion of 'sin', the theological challenge is to name sin 'for our time' and for 'our situation', to borrow from Sallie McFague, mindful that 'the "old" ways, the old solutions, will not do for us'.[7]

Sin as a Distorted Way of Relating

Sin is a concrete reality experienced in everyday life. It takes material form because it is rooted in the complex nexus of social relations rather than being an abstract theological idea or spiritual condition. The term depicts ways of relating that diminish bodies and which prevent bodies from thriving. As McFague argues, 'Sin and salvation are earthly matters, fleshy, concrete and particular matters having to do with disproportion and well-being *in relation* to the forms of God's presence we encounter in our daily, ordinary lives: other bodies.'[8] Sin is both historical and relational. It conveys that things are not as they should be because as humans, we invest in destructive patterns of behaviour that thwart our capacity to live respectfully alongside other bodies. Sin, then, is a form of 'distorted relationality',[9] to use Rosemary Radford Ruether's description, and it is this account of sin that I wish to draw upon.

Dialoguing with Rosemary Radford Ruether

Ruether's definition of sin has been incredibly influential in feminist hamartiology. She is not minded to think about the particular

---

7. I borrow this terminology from Sallie McFague who argues that the Judeo-Christian imperialistic depiction of the God–world relationship must be reimagined for our time where the threat of nuclear holocaust is real. See *Models of God: Theology for an Ecological, Nuclear Age* (Philadelphia: Fortress Press, 1987), especially the 'Preface', x.

8. Sallie McFague, *The Body of God: An Ecological Theology* (Minneapolis: Fortress, 1993), 114.

9. Ruether, *Introducing Redemption*, 71; Ruether, *Sexism and God-Talk*, 174.

distortions that are worn on women's bodies as they engage in the slimming process, but her position gives theological expression to the way we have seen dualisms damage women's relationship to food and fat in the weight loss group.

Ruether rejects the classical view that understands women's subordination as integral to the order of creation and as made worse by Eve's disobedience. Instead, she names such theological constructs as examples of sin that undermine God's creation and distort human nature.[10] According to Ruether, the equality of women is the true will of God, so there is a theological mandate for defending and affirming the full humanity of women and their equal status as *imago Dei*. When thinking about sin, she does not begin with the classical Christian view that defines this as a condition of alienation from God. Convinced that such an account is 'either meaningless or highly misleading to most people today',[11] she starts instead from the concept of alienation from one another. In this view, sin depicts a violation of the mutual and life-giving relations intended by God that nourish life on earth. 'Life is sustained by a biotic relationality in which the whole attains well-being through mutually affirming interdependency,'[12] so sin is a distortion of this inter-relationality. For Ruether, it is only when we understand our alienation from one another that we can understand how this becomes manifest in larger systems of social power that are 'sick-making and violent'.[13] She is clear that distorted relations between ourselves and others give birth to destructive patterns and organizational systems that not only destroy society but also violate the environment and earth as well.[14] It is only by glimpsing this 'expanded' understanding of alienation, she argues, that we can start to see how sin is expressive of our alienation from God. If God is the 'living matrix of matter/ energy' which holds the whole planet together in mutually interacting relationality,[15] then when we exploit other humans, the earth and non-

---

10. Rosemary Radford Ruether, 'Gender and Redemption in Christian Theological History', *Feminist Theology* 7, no. 21 (1999): 104.

11. Ruether, *Introducing Redemption*, 70.

12. Ibid., 71.

13. Ibid., 70.

14. Ibid.

15. Rosemary Radford Ruether, 'Dualism and the Nature of Evil in Feminist Theology', *Studies in Christian Ethics* 5, no. 1 (1992): 35.

human animals, we separate ourselves from God as 'the very source and sustaining matrix of life itself'.[16]

In Ruether's view, then, sin is a distortion of mutual, interdependent relationship. She suggests that this is more in keeping with the Hebraic understanding of God and evil that sees God as relating lovingly and directly to the people of Israel and to nature. This tradition identifies evil with unjust relationship between peoples, she argues, and with the related effects this has on the earth.[17] It is not rooted in a primordial Fall that all human beings subsequently inherit from birth. Seeking to recover aspects of this tradition, she maintains that humans are born with an equal capacity for good and evil, so sin belongs to the sphere of human freedom.[18] Specifically, sin is a misuse of freedom and a violation of the basic relations that sustain life.[19] It is what she calls 'culpable evil' and points towards not only personal but also collective culpability in creating exploitative patterns of relationship that diminish the self and others. In this way, Ruether holds that the concept of 'sin' confirms both personal and social responsibility in changing the status quo,[20] for although it is not easy to demarcate the region of what we can influence, the fact we are able to change things once thought to be unchangeable means that we should not downplay our ability to act.[21]

The Three Dimensions of Sin

There are three dimensions of sin, according to Ruether: the 'personal–interpersonal' dimension, the 'social–historical' dimension and the 'ideological–cultural' dimension. When one individual or group claims absolute rights and power over another, exalting themselves

---

16. Ruether, *Introducing Redemption*, 70.

17. For more on this, see Rosemary Radford Ruether, *Gaia and God: An Ecofeminist Theology of Earth Healing* (New York: HarperCollins, 1992), 205–14.

18. Ruether, *Introducing Redemption*, 71.

19. Ruether, 'Dualism and the Nature of Evil', 37.

20. Ibid., 36. Ruether goes on to argue that sin – as culpable evil – is distinct from mortality, since we have no control over the limits of life. 'Mortality is not our fault, nor is escape from it within our capacities,' she argues. She thus stresses the need to distinguish between 'tragedy and sin' and between evil and 'the turbulence of nature beyond our control and the limits of life in the mortality of all organisms' (36).

21. Ibid., 36–7.

at their expense and to the detriment of others with whom they are interdependent, this is an instance of interpersonal sin.[22] For Ruether, the system of sexism[23] provides an example of sinful intersubjective relationships as men have historically exalted themselves and claimed an absolute right to power over and against women. Patriarchal masculinity has developed in men a confidence in their own power over women and others, she believes. This confident control has only been preserved by men masking their latent insecurity and by projecting such insecurity onto women so that it can be punished.[24] Indeed, male right to power has only been established by 'projection' and 'exploitation',[25] she claims – by making women the cultural carriers of the rejected qualities of their embodiment and by exploiting women on the basis that they represent all the qualities that have been devalued. Sin is a form of idolatrous pride whereby 'the powerful one falls in love with a phoney picture of himself as powerful, and the powerless one falls in love with the image of herself as powerless'.[26] According to Ruether, this has resulted in a distortion of male and female humanity and a 'ravaging' of relationship between men and women.[27]

Yet, the interpersonal–personal dimension of sin is not exclusive to relations between men and women. Although Ruether's earlier work identifies sexism as original sin, she is clear in her later reflections that the same cycle of violence is found in all forms of dominating relationships including those shaped by classism, racism, anti-Semitism and militarism. These distorted modes of relation are also rooted in the insecure self as repression of the other functions in the same way to mask the self's fear of vulnerability and dependency.[28] Sin also concerns the way individuals are separated from themselves, describing 'distorted

---

22. Ruether, *Introducing Redemption*, 71.

23. In *Sexism and God-Talk,* Ruether describes sexism as the 'gender privilege of males over females' (165).

24. Ruether, *Introducing Redemption*, 72–3.

25. Ruether identifies these as 'two interconnected but distinguishable aspects [of] the ideology of the "other" as of lesser value'. *Sexism and God-Talk*, 162.

26. Derek Nelson, *What's Wrong with Sin? Sin in Individual and Social Perspective from Schleiermacher to Theologies of Liberation* (London and New York: T & T Clark, 2009), 149.

27. Ruether, *Sexism and God-Talk?*, 178.

28. Ruether, *Introducing Redemption*, 73.

relations within ourselves that cause not only abuse of our bodies, but also isolation of certain parts of ourselves from other parts'.[29]

The 'social–historical' dimension of sin communicates that such distorted ways of relating are learnt and inherited modes of behaviour. According to Ruether, exploitative interpersonal relations are buttressed by social and historical structures of evil that are 'distorted on the side of alienation and violence'.[30] Borrowing from the biblical tradition, she argues that systemic systems of domination are 'powers and principalities' that precondition our choices:

> These powers and principalities are precisely the heritage of systemic social evil, which conditions our personal choices before we choose and prevents us from fully understanding our own choices and actions. Sexism is one of these powers and principalities of historical, systemic, social evil that conditions our choices as males and females from before our birth.[31]

Sin, then, is often experienced as un-freedom and as a type of bondage, she claims,[32] 'as a power that defines and controls us and that we feel powerless to change, even when we become aware of it as wrong'.[33] Sexist, racist, classist and militarist social systems shape us from birth, informing the world in which we live and influencing personal and social action; it can, therefore, be hard to understand ourselves as social agents in this 'atmosphere of evil'.[34]

Ruether shares with the tradition of original sin the view that sin is inherited, but for her, sin concerns the historical reproduction of skewed social relations rather than the transmission of a congenital disease through carnal lust, as Augustine had it.[35] She contends that even though historical systems of evil interfere to shape our actions and attitudes, this does not render us powerless for 'we are not left without

---

29. Rosemary Radford Ruether, 'Women and Sin: Response to Mary Elise Lowe', *Dialog: A Journal of Theology*, 39, no. 3 (2000): 234.

30. Ruether, *Introducing Redemption*, 70.

31. Ruether, *Sexism and God-Talk*, 181–2.

32. Ruether admits that the notion of 'bondage to sin' is implicit rather than explicit in her work. See Ruether, 'Women and Sin', 233.

33. Ruether, *Introducing Redemption*, 74.

34. Wiley, *Original Sin*, 175.

35. Ruether, *Introducing Redemption*, 74.

a trace of our "*imago Dei*".[36] Our capacity for good connects us to our 'authentic existence' and 'true "nature"',[37] to 'our capacity for healthy and life-giving relationality'.[38] Humans are born with two tendencies, she says, a tendency to just and loving relationships and a tendency to exploitative, unjust relationships.[39] Although we are birthed into a world that makes it far easier to engage in hostile relations, we are not left without the ability to follow our good tendency or without positive examples of loving right relation provided by others and modelled by Jesus.[40]

The final dimension of sin Ruether outlines is the 'ideological–cultural dimension'. This concerns the way oppressive social systems are supported by ideologies that feed the hegemonic culture. In such social contexts, exploitative relations appear natural and as divinely ordained. According to Ruether, many social institutions conform our bodies to these sick-making forms of relationship. Among them are the family, school, church and the media. All socialize individuals and groups to accept their allotted place within systems of violence.

Learning from and Critiquing Ruether: Sin in the Context of Slimming Culture

Ruether's account of sin has much to offer. Perhaps most importantly, she identifies how the pitting of male against female, human against non-human, mind against matter breeds exploitative structural patterns that then shape our beliefs about what constitutes the normal. Drawing on the experiences of women in the weight loss group, we can extend this view of sin to name the distorted ordering of human relations that pits the good-thin-rational-orderly (symbolically masculine) body against the bad-fat-irrational-disorderly (symbolically feminine) body. This dualism preconditions women in particular to wage war against their fat, to vilify fatness as a defect in themselves and others and to see thinness as normal. It also orders the 'good' sensible (thin) eater over the 'bad' irrational (fat) eater. Both are extended but related expressions

---

36. Ibid.
37. Ibid., 70.
38. Ibid., 74.
39. Ibid.
40. Ibid.

of 'the good-evil, superior-inferior dualism'[41] Ruether's account of sin addresses.

Ruether also effectively expresses the relational nature of sin reminding her readers that we are all social beings. This position would be supported further by an understanding of God that sees human relationality as expressive of divine community and interrelationality, and the Trinity provides a wonderful resource for this.[42] Indeed, a turn towards the Trinity would help defend against a common criticism of Ruether which charges her with erasing God's transcendence. Mary Elise Lowe claims that Ruether 'seems to make God dependent upon the world by over-emphasizing God's immanence in the world';[43] Alistair McFadyen similarly sees in feminist hamartiologies like Ruether's a tendency to 'make God so immanent to the dynamics of "right relation" or selfhood that any meaningful distinction between them threatens to collapse'.[44] In both cases the fear is that God's otherness is not preserved. Some also worry that her appeal to mutual life-giving relations is too vague, lacking a clear sense of what constitutes a positive mode of relationship.[45]

By invoking a Trinitarian image of God we are drawn to think of God in much more personal terms and in a way that preserves God's otherness without compromising God's togetherness with the world. I have argued elsewhere that communion, friendship and openness characterize the nature of God's love as Trinity and are the expression of mutual love and life and of a liveliness which is overflowing and dynamic.[46] Notwithstanding its sexist ideology, the Trinity offers

41. Ruether, *Sexism and God-Talk*, 163.

42. For more on this, see Hannah Bacon, *What's Right with the Trinity? Conversations in Feminist Theology* (Farnham and Burlington: Ashgate, 2009).

43. Mary Elise Lowe, 'Theology Update: Woman Oriented Hamartiologies: A Survey of the Shift from Powerlessness to Right Relationship', *Dialog: A Journal of Theology* 39, no. 2 (2000): 122.

44. McFadyen, *Bound to Sin*, 164. Ruether strongly disputes this charge, however. In her response to Lowe, she clarifies that she does not see her understanding of God as one of dependence on the world. 'Transcendence is about God being radically free from our distorted systems of sin and our justifying lies and at the same time being closer to us than we are to ourselves.' See Ruether, 'Women and Sin', 235.

45. See, for example, Nelson, *What's Wrong with Sin?*, 158.

46. Bacon, *What's Right with the Trinity?*, 79. Also see Leonardo Boff, *Trinity and Society*, trans. Paul Burns (Eugene: Wipf & Stock, 1988), 4, 32.

a model of co-equality that confirms the Creator as God, Christ the Redeemer as God and the Spirit Sustainer as God.[47] Each has their own work to achieve, but there are not three gods because each is so open to the others and so present with the others at all times, that we can speak of a union where there is only one love, one act and one will.[48] As Jürgen Moltmann recognizes, the unity of God is a unity of persons (or subjects) in relationship expressed in the doctrine of *perichoresis*.[49] To image God as Trinity is to say that God is never alone and that God is typified by a yearning for relation, always beckoning the other to come close. When we speak of God's relating we speak not just about how God acts but also about who God is,[50] for 'God is nothing except in relation'.[51] This communal image of God provides a vision not only of mutual relationship within the Godhead but also of a reciprocal I–Thou encounter between God and ourselves as bodies.

A Trinitarian understanding of God allows us to locate our own relating within the context of God's relating. To relate well is to relate as God relates, so when we practise loving mutual forms of relation we live into the Trinitarian image of God. Since the Trinity does not depict a duality in God, it does not reduce human forms of ethical relating to the heterosexual couple or to other binary pairings. The communitarian ethic corresponding to the Trinitarian community suggests that we live into the image of God when we live in openness and community with all other human beings and all other creatures in ways that respect their unique particularity. Of course, to say that our mutual companionship images the Trinity is not without problem because the

---

47. I borrow this language of Creator, Redeemer and Sustainer from McFague's, *Models of God*. This constitutes one way in which we might meaningfully speak about the Trinity, but it is not the only way.

48. Also see Boff, *Trinity and Society*, 84.

49. Jürgen Moltmann, *The Trinity and the Kingdom of God: The Doctrine of God* (Munich: SMC, 1981).

50. As Cynthia L. Rigby puts it, 'God's loving and relating are not only something God *does* but also something God really *is*.' See her essay, 'Scandalous Presence: Incarnation and Trinity', in *Feminist and Womanist Essays in Reformed Dogmatics*, ed. Amy Plantinga Pauw and Serene Jones (Louisville and London: Westminster John Knox Press, 2006), 63. Also see Bacon, *What's Right with the Trinity?*, 79.

51. Carter Heyward, *Our Passion for Justice: Images of Power, Sexuality, and Liberation* (New York: The Pilgrim Press, 1984), 142.

notion of *imago Dei* has historically privileged qualities like reason and the intellect that have been shown to operate negatively in the weight loss group. Yet, being in the image of the Trinity communicates the radical message that we are intended for community and for a form of relating that is not exploitative.[52] Humans sin through relating in ways that violate their capacity for mutual, loving and just relationship with one another and with themselves. This means that sinfulness is not an inevitable innate state, as Augustine held. Rather, it is something that permeates all human existence; sin is 'a symptom of the unavoidably relational nature of human existence through which we come to be damaged and damage others'.[53] As the damage we do to ourselves and to others when we try to avoid our relational nature, sin depicts our brokenness or 'brokenheartedness', as Rita Nakashima Brock describes it[54] – our vulnerability – not how evil and wilfully disobedient we are. Sin against self and others is a relational tear rather than an ontological defect, and it is something to be healed rather than punished.[55]

Thinking about God as Trinity allows us to follow Ruether in understanding the world as a biotic relationality (where the whole attains well-being through mutually affirming interdependency) without erasing God's otherness. In this panentheistic model of the God–world relationship, the world exists *in* God rather than *as* God. The Trinitarian God is the power that holds the whole planet together in mutually interacting relationality, yet God is always more than these interdependent relationships because even though the world does not exist apart from God, God's reality extends beyond the world. 'There is, as it were, a limit on our side not on God's,' as Sallie McFague puts it. Understanding God in these terms suggests that distorted forms of relationship that harm others and the planet also harm God because the whole of creation and history are integral to the divine experience. 'God, having created the world, also dwells in it, and conversely the world

---

52. Many theologians and feminist theologians promoting a so-called social Trinity argue this and suggest that inequalities in church and society offend the Trinity. See, for example, Bacon, *What's Right with the Trinity?*, Catherine Mowry LaCugna, *God for Us: The Trinity and Christian Life* (New York: HarperCollins Publishers, 1991); Boff, *Trinity and Society*; Moltmann, *The Trinity and the Kingdom of God*.
53. Brock, *Journeys by Heart*.
54. Ibid., 7.
55. Brock also makes this point. See ibid.

which he [sic] has created exists in him [sic]', explains Moltmann.[56] Hence, sin against other people, animals and nature is sin against the body and flesh of God.[57] This Trinitarian account allows us to preserve God's difference while refusing to separate our modes of relating from God. It also claims that God as Trinity is never without flesh – not only the flesh of Christ but also the fleshiness of our bodies and the world.

Ruether may not root right relation in a Trinitarian model of God, but she does skilfully hold together individual culpability with social conditioning. For her, sin has both a personal and a systemic side, and this provides a theological way of rendering the tensions between personal freedom and constraint already identified in this book as a central feature of slimming and Syn-watching. In many ways, Ruether echoes Foucault in reminding us that we never exercise our own freedom outside of the constraining forces of social relations. 'There is no evil that is not relational,' she suggests,[58] because even the most personal acts take place in social and historic contexts. We must avoid any temptation to engage in 'false individualizing'.[59]

This appositely departs from the theological position echoed in the weight loss group that says sin is a purely private and inward-looking affair. It also challenges Augustine's pessimism and lack of confidence in the self by preserving a belief in our equal capacity for good. Ruether affirms human freedom and our ability to choose that which fosters

---

56. Jürgen Moltmann, *God in Creation: A New Theology of Creation and the Spirit of God*, trans. M. Kohl (London and Philadelphia: 1989), 98. Petr Macek understands Moltmann's panentheistic conceptualization of God as suggesting two kinds of indwelling: God's indwelling in the world which is divine and the world's indwelling in God which is worldly. See his essay, 'The Doctrine of Creation in the Messianic Theology of Jürgen Moltmann', *Communio Viatorum* 49 (2007): 167.

57. McFague, *The Body of God*, 114.

58. Ibid.

59. This is a shared concern of feminist theologians wanting to take seriously the social side of sin. Carter Heyward, for example, criticizes the liberal theology of Paul Tillich for presenting estrangement as an inner struggle and so for failing to acknowledge human angst as a social, material condition characterized by alienated social relations. For more, see her essay, 'Heterosexist Theology: Being above It All', in *Feminist Theological Ethics: A Reader*, ed. Lois K. Daly, Robin W. Lovin and Douglas F. Ottata (Louisville: Westminster John Knox Press, 1994), 174–5.

a loving relationship, echoing the sense of freedom and power women in the group experience as self-making. Such a notion of 'sin' preserves women's capacity to resist the hegemony of fat phobia while refusing to pretend that it is possible to detach from the painful realities of this distorted world. Sin is the freedom to act, even in social contexts that condition our behaviour. It provides a theological way of holding together the reality of women's entanglement in fat-hating, thin-loving culture with the capacity to resist and fashion change. Such an account of sin allows us to acknowledge with Ruether that 'the boundaries between freedom and fate are fluid',[60] but to reaffirm that human responsibility forms part of the extended web of social power that conditions our behaviour.

According to Ruether, *metanoia* indicates the birthing of a new culture. Described by her as 'soul-making',[61] as a 'change of mind' and as a process of enhancing our capacities for good, both as individuals and as communities, it depicts a personal and social movement towards more just and loving relations. Ruether is clear that 'there will be no millennium when it is established "once-for-all"',[62] but this does not deter her from asserting that social systems which exploit and diminish individuals and groups can be reshaped and oppressive structures transformed.[63] In a similar way I want to suggest that sin allows us to frame fat phobia and fears about food as learned behaviours that although entrenched can be challenged. We can live with the inescapableness of distorted relationality (sin) and our inevitable and complex location in it – what Kathleen Sands names as 'tragedy'[64] – without seeing ourselves as powerless to change any of it. Sin depicts our power to act in a fallen world.

Critics of Ruether may worry that she presents sexism as the root of all evil. While I do not share this view, it is easy to see how some reach this conclusion. In *Sexism and God-Talk*, she locates the beginnings of human alienation in 'group egoism', where groups of individuals in the earliest communities protected their own status by oppressing others. This was a collective rather than individual dichotomizing of

---

60. Ruether, 'Dualism and the Nature of Evil', 36.
61. Ruether, *Introducing Redemption*, 74–5.
62. Ibid., 39.
63. Ibid., 37.
64. Kathleen M. Sands, *Escape from Paradise: Evil and Tragedy in Feminist Theology* (Minneapolis: Fortress Press, 1994).

the self–other relationship,[65] she argues, and one in which the males of tribal groups defined the collective self against the other as female.[66] Mary McClintock Fulkerson accuses Ruether of presenting sexism as a universal sin that has been passed on unaltered throughout history. She also claims that it 'renders male-female relations as the primary site and form of sin's brokenness'.[67] In my view, however, Ruether is not guilty of this charge. Even in her early work, she suggests that group egoism sets itself against a range of 'alien groups', including 'women, other races, nature, and so on',[68] and this point only becomes more and more pronounced as her scholarship develops. She accuses Fulkerson and others of not paying attention to the range of her work, and I think this challenge is fair.[69]

From this critical review of Ruether's hamartiology, it does seem to me that her approach can be extended in ways that allow us to name as sin certain distorted ways of relating that resonate with the case study outlined in the first part of this book and which speak meaningfully to our contemporary situation where fears about food and fat are prolific. First, if sexism, racism, colonialism, militarism and heterosexism breed relations of domination that violate women's flourishing, then sizeism can be seen as accompanying these as an intersecting distortion of right relation. To label sizeism as sin makes explicit and judges as contrary to God's intentions the way we vilify fat in our own relations with one another and with ourselves, acknowledging at the same time that theological and religious as well as social, political and economic systems work to shape our attitudes and actions. Second, sin describes a distorted relationship with food that points to a ruptured connection with our love of food, with other bodies who eat and produce it and with the planet that gifts it. It depicts exploitative ways of relating to the body and to our food which are encouraged in slimming culture. Third, sin describes a condition of self-alienation that is facilitated by sizeism and by the victimization of food. Borrowing from the Pauline–Augustinian tradition the notion of 'the divided self', I suggest that sin

---

65. Ruether, *Sexism and God-Talk*, 163–4.
66. Ibid., 162.
67. Mary McClintock Fulkerson, 'Sexism as Original Sin: Developing a Theacentric Discourse', *Journal of the American Academy of Religion* 59, no. 4 (1991): 667.
68. Ruether, *Sexism and God-Talk*, 163.
69. Ruether, 'Women and Sin', 235.

speaks to the way fears about food and weight pull women in mutually incompatible directions, tearing our bodies apart. Sin in all three instances is a fracture in relationship that has 'personal–interpersonal', 'social–historical' and 'ideological–cultural' dimensions.

A Distorted Relationship to Fat: Sizeism as Sin

Sizeism includes fatism (anti-fat beliefs and behaviours) and fat phobia[70] (fear and hatred of fat and fat people). It also comprises the unabated privileging of thinness. Among many women in the group, the fear and hatred of fat encourages self-loathing and a restlessness in the present. Louise's universal commissioning of members to 'go forth and shrink' confirms that women can never cease from the project of thinning and that fat is uninhabitable. Many women consider it wrong to feel happy with putting on weight; some run out of the meeting through fear that their fat will be publically exposed; others deliberately avoid going out in public because they dread being judged for their size. Such instances indicate the damaging ways in which sizeism takes shape in women's lives.

As a harmful arrangement of relationship that prizes thin bodies over all other bodies, sizeism takes the thin subject as normative and measures all other bodies against that standard. It is a colonial system because it norms all bodies through the 'imperial paradigm',[71] by imposing the white, Western, able-bodied, middle-class feminine ideal on all women, without exception. In this neoliberal and imperialist system that overlooks difference, the presumption of thinness – what we might call 'compulsory thinness' – functions as a threat. Just as French feminist and philosopher Monique Wittig considers that compulsory heterosexuality threatens that 'you-will-be-straight-or-you-will-not-be',[72] compulsory thinness warns 'you-will-be-thin-or-you-will-not-be'. Fat invalidates a person and women especially through association with the sensible realm of the passions. Just as Ruether identifies about sexism, sizeism erects divisions between people and encourages us to

---

70. For a fantastic discussion of fat phobia, see Cooper's, *Fat and Proud*, 17–66.

71. Lelwica, Hoglund and McNallie, 'Spreading the Religion of Thinness'. Also see Chapter 1.

72. Monique Wittig, 'The Straight Mind', *Feminist Issues* 1, no. 1 (1980): 107.

think in binary oppositions. In this structure of domination, the variety of human body shapes is reduced to the two opposites of 'fat' or 'thin' and the hatred of fat exposed as being integral to the cycle of violence that destroys life-affirming relationship with our bodies and with the bodies of others. This foundational binary opposition judges as deficient all bodies that fail to occupy the narrow space of thinness, fuelling and sustaining what Sallie McFague refers to as 'pletherophobia' – a fear of different kinds of bodies.[73]

Sizeism then refuses any positive symbolization of fat. It is an expression of fat oppression defined as discrimination against fat people,[74] but does not only manifest itself through the victimization of fat people. In an extension of conventional meaning, I understand sizeism as depicting a far-reaching terror of fat that strikes fear, guilt and self-hatred into the lives of a multiplicity of people, especially women. In the weight loss group, sizeism affects and continues to govern the behaviour of women who reach their ideal weight. It manifests in the assumption that fat – whether actual or perceived, miniscule or substantial – is untenable and to be dreaded, and that weight loss is an unquestionable good for all women independent of size. Sizeism expresses the complex and multiple ways in which the stigmatization of fat affects differently sized bodies, rendering as unliveable the lives of variously sized women who do not pass as thin.[75] It is what fat activist Charlotte Cooper calls 'a power system in which we are all losers by various degrees',[76] and like sexism, racism, homophobia, classism and other distorted systems, is caught up in the web of social power relations and hierarchies that marginalize particular social groups.[77]

The personal–interpersonal dimension of the sin of sizeism expresses a distorted pattern of social relations where thin bodies claim priority

---

73. McFague, *The Body of God*, 53.

74. Laura Brown and Esther D. Rothblum, 'Editorial Statement', in *Overcoming Fear of Fat*, ed. Laura Brown and Esther D. Rothblum (New York: Routledge, 2015), 1.

75. Deborah Lupton, for example, argues that fat people are not the only people impacted by anti-fat obesity discourse. She notes how mothers of young children are also subject to 'moralizing and guilt-inducing imperatives' in health policy and media representation on 'childhood obesity'. Deborah Lupton, *Fat* (London and New York: Routledge, 2013), 89.

76. Cooper, *Fat and Proud*, 33.

77. Ibid., 32.

over all other bodies and where our relations with one another and with ourselves are defined by this dualistic split. In this system, fatness is vilified in similar ways to how Ruether describes the denigration of nature within patriarchy; it is imagined as passive and irrational, as 'dead stuff' that is 'totally malleable'.[78] In the group, women relate to their fat in this way, as an object that is carried extraneous to the self that can be dropped at will. Synonymous with the sensuous 'bad body',[79] fat is aligned with the sensible feminine and with the sensible appetite that must be dominated by reason. This exploitative relationship to fat thwarts our created intention as creatures made by God for mutually affirming interdependent relationship because it frustrates our capacity to live in peace with our fat and to value not-thin bodies as equivalent human persons. According to Ruether, the domination of women and the earth equates to a denial of our dependency on mothers and nature and to an attempt to sterilize their potency.[80] The attempt to dominate fat expresses a similar 'culture of deceit',[81] failing to acknowledge our dependency on fat for survival. 'Fat represents life', says fat activist Marilyn Wann; it keeps the body warm, protects the internal organs from injury and stores energy the body can use.[82] Indeed, like the fat in Leviticus discussed in Chapter 3, fat protects life and makes life possible. The sin of sizeism describes the masking and maligning of this dependency as we imagine we can live successfully without these bits of our bodies, assuming that the body can only live fully when fat has been fully removed. Extending the cycle of violence that distorts relations of interdependency between self and others, sizeism exposes a refusal to acknowledge the finite limits of our embodiment.

Women and men are located differently in this unequal system of power. We know from earlier chapters that sizeism can be described as another instance of 'sexism in action'[83] and as tightly bound up with

---

78. Ibid.

79. Ruether argues that in Western dualism, the sensual 'other' is pitted against the rational, controlling 'us' in order to justify relations of domination and power. See 'Dualism and the Nature of Evil', 32.

80. Ruether, *Gaia and God*, 200.

81. Ibid.

82. Marilyn Wann, *FAT!SO? Because You Don't Have to Apologize for Your Size* (Berkeley: Ten Speed Press, 1998), 14.

83. Brown and Rothblum, 'Editorial Statement', 1.

gender inequalities.[84] However, we also know that the gendering of fat is tied to other structures of domination, including classist, racist, heterosexist, imperialist and (as I have argued) Christian theological and religious systems.[85] The colonial, Eurocentric, middle-class, able-bodied, heteropatriarchal account of femininity that norms women's bodies in the weight loss group ensures that the bodies of certain women – of Helen (who is disabled) and Hevala (who is Middle Eastern) – are especially stigmatized. Moreover, it is clear that women are not simply passive victims in a corrupt system but also active in the victimization of one another and agents that practise their freedom in ways that sometimes resist sizeist expectations. The dynamics of domination are complex then: women not only collaborate in the norming of other women's bodies and in the exploitation of their own but also resist organizational and cultural scripts.

The 'social–historical' dimension of the sin of sizeism retains from the Augustinian–Pauline tradition the view that evil is not simply the sum of individual decisions. Sizeism is an inherited sin; it is an enculturated attitude and set of assumptions about weight and fat that distort our relationship with others and with ourselves. As Ruether rightly informs, 'We do not start with a clean slate,'[86] and in Euro-American culture, sizeism colours our choices, attitudes and actions. It is transmitted through political, economic, medical, legal, linguistic and religious/theological systems that privilege thinner bodies and discriminate against fatter ones. Fat phobia is manifest in weight-based prejudice that sees fat people, and fat women in particular, experience higher rates of household poverty and receive less annual income than thinner women.[87] In education and the family, anti-fat sentiment is

---

84. Bringle, *The God of Thinness*, 109.

85. Elisabeth Schüssler Fiorenza's notion of 'kyriarchy' gives expression to the ways in which oppression is both multiple and multiplicative and so provides a useful tool here. According to Fiorenza, structures of domination are multi-structural forming part of a kyriarchal system of power that operates 'not only along the axis of gender but also along those of race, class, culture, and religion'. For more, see *But She Said: Feminist Practices of Biblical Interpretation* (Boston: Beacon Press, 1992), 122 and 177.

86. Ruether, *Gaia and God*, 142.

87. Steven L. Gortmaker, Aviva Must, James M. Perrin, Arthur M. Sobol and William H. Dietz, 'Social and Economic Consequences of Overweight in Adolescence and Young Adulthood', *The New England Journal of Medicine*

often learnt as second nature.[88] Reports suggest that some teachers have lower expectations for fatter children[89] and that school environments can be sites of 'ongoing prejudice, unnoticed discrimination, and almost constant harassment' for fat students.[90] Sizeism is passed on in education about food and cookery, in the assumption of the weight loss group that eating well means to consume with thinness in mind. Jamie Oliver's 'Ministry of Food' provides a further example of this, as his eight-week cookery programme intended to mobilize local communities to cook more and prepare more nutritious meals, fails to disentangle health and the love and enjoyment of food from the pursuit of thinness. A poster in the window of the Ministry of Food hub in Bradford (UK) uses the acronym 'SLIM' to convey its message:

–Save money
–Learn to cook
–Invest in your health
–Making cooking fun

This mantra would sit comfortably in the slimming club's meeting room since it shares the assumption that nutrition and eating well are synonymous with being slim.[91]

Of course, health and medical institutions also participate in the sin of sizeism when they espouse fat phobic attitudes, when unchecked biases among health professionals cause some fat people to fear

329 (1993): 1008–12, http://www.nejm.org/doi/full/10.1056/NEJM199309303291406 (accessed 1 May 2017). According to this study that examines the relation between overweight among 10,039 adolescents and young adults and their social and economic status seven years later, previously 'overweight' women earned $6,710 less per year than women who had not been overweight and had higher rates of household poverty.

88. See Rina Rossignol's description of her own upbringing in 'Fat Liberation (?) Assumptions of a Thin World', 5.

89. NAAFA, 'Education', https://naafaonline.com/dev2/the_issues/education.html (accessed 1 May 2017).

90. National Education Association, 'Report on Size Discrimination', http://www.lectlaw.com/files/con28.htm (accessed 1 May 2017).

91. See 'Jamie's Ministry of Food', http://www.jamieoliver.com/jamies-ministry-of-food/ (accessed 5 May 2017). I saw this poster in the window of the Ministry of Food hub in Bradford on 10 August 2016.

going to the doctor because weight becomes the primary issue in the consultation room, independent of the health complaint.[92] The assumption that fat is the direct result of poor diet, overeating and a lack of exercise has been consistently challenged by fat acceptance campaigners and scientists who argue that the anti-obesity position relies on a poor and often over-generalized interpretation of data, and I will say more about this in Chapter 6. Linguistic systems also play a role as discourses and languages about fat contribute to the shaming of fat bodies. The 'f' word is employed as an insult that resources patterns of name calling in the public media, successfully maligning a myriad of differently sized bodies.[93]

To view sizeism as a social and historical sin means we can follow Augustine in seeing ourselves as being prone to sin, since immersion within sizeist culture makes women more likely to acquiesce with it. As Wann suggests, 'Every person who lives in a fat-hating culture inevitably absorbs anti-fat beliefs, assumptions, and stereotypes, and also inevitably comes to occupy a position in relation to power arrangements that are based on weight.'[94] Sizeism, however, is not a universal sin because it depends on its continual transmission by social forces and has not been transmitted unmodified throughout history. Historian Peter Stearns observes that it was only between 1890 and 1910 that middle-class America started its battle against the bulge and reversed what he calls a 'generation-long plumpness fad'. Prior to this doctors had recommended solid weight in response to nervousness. Shifts in fashion, fat-control devices and a growth in public comment on fat were instrumental to this social change, he explains, as were changes to do with women's equality, sexual and maternal roles.[95] Sizeism then is not inevitable, a point also supported by the way the thin ideal fails to have universal application across all cultures.[96]

92. Rossignol, 'Fat Liberation', 8.
93. See Wann, *FAT!SO?*, 18–19.
94. Marilyn Wann, 'Foreword', in *The Fat Studies Reader*, xi.
95. Peter N. Stearns, *Fat History: Bodies and Beauty in the Modern West* (New York and London: New York University Press), 10. Also see Hillel Schwartz, *Never Satisfied: A Cultural History of Diets, Fantasies and Fat* (New York: The Free Press, 1986) and Abigail Saguy, *What's Wrong with Fat?* (New York: Oxford University Press, 2014), 28.
96. Rebecca Popenoe, 'Ideal', in *Fat: The Anthropology of an Obsession*, ed. Don Kulick and Anne Meneley (London: Penguin, 2005), 10–11. Anthropologist

Fat phobia is a social structure composed of both a 'cultural schema' and 'material resources'.[97] Whereas the cultural schema in contemporary wealthy Western societies defines thinner bodies as morally, medically, sexually and aesthetically desirable and fatter bodies as not so, economic and political material resources from state governments, other agencies and organizations support and direct this schema, including medical establishments, pharmaceutical companies (who produce diet drugs) and weight loss organizations.[98] Commercial slimming clubs, like the one at the centre of this book, are part of the fat phobic climate of evil that transmits distorted ways of relating to fat, establishing fatness in binary opposition to normality. They feed off the culturally enforced body insecurities of women in particular, but I want to make a distinction between slimming organizations and the distorted arrangement of sizeist human relationships they promote and sustain. Like Ruether, I maintain that sin is not a 'something' but a form of broken relationship that belongs to the sphere of human freedom. It depicts the way we use our freedom to exploit and victimize ourselves and others, and it is these distorted social relations that breed wider destructive patterns in society that constitute sin.[99] Weight loss organizations do promote exploitative ways of relating to the body, confirming fat as a thing that must be destroyed. They also teach women to measure their worth in relation to the frequency of their own defleshing, but this is not all that commercial slimming companies do. They are also environments where women can practise more loving forms of relating to their bodies and to other women. Given this, slimming clubs cannot be absolutely branded as evil, nor women's participation in them straightforwardly judged as sin.

Rebecca Popenoe describes living among desert Arabs on the border of Nigeria in the 1990s and finding that women from diverse ethnic groups actually wanted to be fat. The Nigerian nurses she worked with would weigh themselves putting clothes on rather than taking them off in order to increase the number on the scale.

97. Saguy and Ward, 'Coming Out as Fat', 54–5.
98. Ibid., 55.
99. Ruether, for example, argues that the system of sexism as a system originating with humans and perpetuated by humans 'is not just the sum of the individuals. Precisely as a system it becomes bigger than any of us or all of us *as individuals*.' See *Sexism and God-Talk*, 182.

The 'ideological–cultural' dimension of sizeism concerns the way fat hatred meets us as common sense and normal. In this hegemonic realm of meaning, fat oppression and fat shaming are presented as natural and theologically justified as good. Fat is unambiguously a confession of sin – sloth or greed – and exposes a woman's guilt. We have seen Christian hamartiology lend important support to the ideological assumption that weight loss is normal and right. Such assumptions form part of the cultural schema many women are born into, a sizeist schema which, according to Saguy and Ward, is 'virtual' as well as actual because it exists as traces in our memories and is not always conscious.[100] This schema assumes that not-thin people are to blame for their size, that fat is synonymous with bad health, sloth, ugliness and with eating too much and that those who say they are happy with their fat must be lying. As an ideology that functions to normalize prejudicial attitudes about weight, sizeism is an example of the way we frequently experience dynamics of domination as 'benign, not brutal; natural, not perverse'.[101]

A Distorted Relation to Food: The Victimization of Food as Sin

As well as speaking meaningfully about a distorted relation with fat, 'sin' describes a distorted relationship with food. Nigel Slater is one of my favourite TV celebrity chefs, and in his third volume of *The Kitchen Diaries*, he shares his concerns about what he sees as the 'current victimization of food' – a tendency to 'divide the contents of our plates into heroes and villains'. According to Slater, making something to eat is an 'art' which should be a 'lifelong joy'. 'Good food' should not be fetishized but something we 'take in our stride'.[102] Victimizing our food by labelling it 'good' or 'bad' risks sucking the life out of eating through shaming us over our food choices. He worries where this will lead: 'If this escalates historians may look back on this generation as one in which society's decision about what to eat was driven by guilt and shame rather than by good taste or pleasure,' he warns.[103]

---

100. Saguy and Ward, 'Coming Out as Fat', 55.
101. Heyward, *Touching Our Strength*, 57.
102. Nigel Slater, *A Year of Good Eating: The Kitchen Diaries III* (London: Fourth Estate, 2015), xiii.
103. Ibid., xiv. Interestingly, Slater retains the language of 'good' food despite criticizing the way foods are categorized as heroes and villains, but good food

In the slimming group, food and foodways are polarized as 'good' or 'bad', 'right' or 'wrong' depending on their proximity to Syn. For women, the panacea to the predicament of fat and the 'bad' foodways that produce it is 'sensible' eating, a mode of consumption that is obvious, possessed by anyone with intelligence and which confirms that certain foods and eating behaviours must be avoided, modified or tightly regulated to avoid a gain on the scale. This way of eating forgoes taste for the sake of staying on track. To eat sensibly is to make food choices based on a rational consideration of Syn and one's weight loss goals. It is determined by a person's ability to rationally order their appetite so that the desire for pleasure (that is taste) does not overcome the desire for thinness.

Of course, it is much easier to follow Slater's advice and take 'good' food in our stride and embrace it as a life-enriching aspect, if we have the economic means to do so. He speaks from a position of privilege, but his words begin to express a distorted way of relating to food which correlates with observable patterns in the weight loss group. Like the predicament he describes in British foodways, many women attribute instrumental value to the food they eat, rendering it good insofar as it is able to service the goal of weight loss. Sensible eating is thus expressive of what Deborah Lupton terms the 'food/health/beauty triplex', where food is categorized according to how slimming or fattening it is and how it contributes to producing the slim ideal.[104] In the group, it is Syn that troubles women rather than calories per se as Lupton conceives, but as an instance of this wider nexus of distorted social relations, women find it hard to think about food without deliberating its slimming potential. This fuels a struggle over food that even thinner women find themselves trapped in, and it has the same effect as Slater fears: it drains the life out of eating.

Naming the victimization of food as sin theologically expresses a separation and estrangement from the joy of food. As an instance of personal–interpersonal sin, it describes a way of relating to food where we demean the physicality of food and deny the body pleasure. We may eat to get thin and so ascribe our food instrumental value and see eating more as a means to an end. The 'market and machine logics' of advanced

depicts items that are pleasurable and nice to taste rather than foods chosen because of guilt, beliefs about certain foods being 'bad' or in the hope that they will produce weight loss.

104. Lupton, *Fat*, 70 and Lupton, *Food, the Body and the Self*, 138.

capitalism assist in this system by reducing food to a commodity,[105] encouraging consumers to see it simply in terms of calories and nutrients that need to be in the right proportion. According to Norman Wirzba, this view identifies food as fuel for our machine-like bodies – 'Though some food may taste better than other food, there is little about it that should give us pause for wonder or reverence.'[106] Without such wonder and reverence, he claims, food becomes a 'thing' that we feel entitled to own and (ab)use to achieve our desired end.

In this setting, it matters little how we treat food in the pursuit of the ultimate goal of thinness. The weight loss organization encourages women to victimize food when it guides that edible items can be thrown away and taste forfeited if it means that women avoid 'self sabotage'. If the ultimate goal of thinness is the supreme good, then the primary purpose of food is to assist the project of weight loss. When food is victimized, the plight of the environment and animals and the ethics of food production and distribution are trivialized because our ultimate concern is 'getting rid' and 'getting there', and one must avoid any distractions. The use of food to construct a thinner self then encourages various forms of forgetfulness – amnesia about our dependency on food, about our reliance on the planet that yields it, on the workers that produce it and on other eaters who also need food to survive. According to Wirzba, today's global food economy is marked by 'injustice, estrangement and bewilderment'.[107] For him, we are a people in 'exile' who do not know how to live joyfully, peacefully and sustainably, or in ways that foster mutual flourishing and delight.[108] Instead, we eat in ways that violate the earth as our life-giving and life-sustaining home, harming the body of God's world and other bodies that live in it. The state of exile, he suggests, describes how we are cut off from the realities of how our food is grown, how systems of food production are degrading the land, animals and other people.[109]

Sin, understood as the victimization of food, expresses not only an alienation from the pleasure of food where people, and women in particular, eat without delight but also a separation from those

---

105. Norman Wirzba, *Food & Faith: A Theology of Eating* (New York: Cambridge University Press, 2011), xvi.
106. Ibid., xii.
107. Ibid., 71.
108. Ibid., 72.
109. Ibid., 71.

involved in the production of food and from others who do not enjoy food security. It depicts a forgetting of our dependency on others and a forgetting of the way we are vulnerable to one another. When we eat in exile we eat without connection or affection, experiencing food as an object of convenience or as a threat that must be vanquished. We also forget that we are dependent on food as a source of life.

All sides of the victimization of food – the estrangement from pleasure, the disconnection from others in the global food economy and the refusal to acknowledge our dependency on food for life – are expressive of distorted relations we are born into. This is the 'social-historical' dimension of sin. The family, medical establishments, health care organizations, public policies, education providers and (as I have shown) inherited Christian ideas about sin all help to scare us about food.[110] The global free-market economy encourages amnesia towards the plight of others and ensures that only those with the financial capital can choose to eat ethically. Built on the inattentiveness of consumers it also affords 'freedom' only to the rich. Supermarkets display attractive and inexpensive food, discouraging consumers from thinking too much about the plight of animals, the exploitative wages and conditions of those producing food or about the amount of plastic that goes into landfill. Trade and production are wedded to market mechanisms that privilege the wealthy. As individuals and communities we are entangled in global capitalism and within complex webs of food production and supply that taint us without our knowing. Anna Fisk describes the trappings of this system when she reflects how a decision to buy and drink a coffee can see us passively consent to the exploitation of coffee

---

110. A recent article in *The Guardian* suggests that millennials are plagued by the search for 'extreme perfectionism about food' and that it is adding to their stress levels. Whether through dieting, 'clean eating' or yoga, the striving for healthiness and perfection can produce despair about never being good enough. The result is that many young people and girls especially feel guilty 'just for enjoying a chocolate bar'. Sarah Marsh, 'All That Striving for Healthiness is Making Millennials More Anxious than Ever', *The Guardian* (11 March 2016), https://www.theguardian.com/commentisfree/2016/mar/11/striving-for-hea lthiness-makes-us-unhappy-millennials (accessed 30 August 2017). Also see https://www.aviva.co.uk/media-centre/story/17307/younger-generation-bu rdened-with-anxiety-and-lonel/; http://www.apa.org/news/press/releases/s tress/index.aspx. Marsh describes 'millennials' as those who are aged between eighteen and thirty-three.

growers in majority-world countries. Even our best efforts to buy fair trade goods can result in us contributing to corruption and violence somewhere else in the world, she argues. For Fisk this means that in the minority world, 'repentance' or turning around is practically impossible because it is so difficult to untangle our personal responsibilities from the faceless evils of global capitalism.[111] As such, it is important to recognize that the victimization of food, like the sin of sizeism, involves tragedy and human culpability. Ruether refers to the 'tragedy of finitude of the human perspective' but when it comes to food, we can lament the particular ways in which the limitation of our human location makes us unable to visualize the sequences of destruction set in motion by our alimentary choices.[112]

As an historically inherited condition, the victimization of food trains women in particular to fear their tastes. In the wealthy West, it also produces 'confused eaters',[113] eaters who are baffled about what is pleasing to consume, who daren't eat in case what they think fosters health turns out to make the body sick or fat. This confusion is frequently generated and displayed in the public media; it is seen in the conflict between the new drinking guidelines presented by the Chief Medical Officer for England that suggest any degree of alcohol poses a risk to health and new research from Harvard University that links the drinking of wine to the prevention of cancer and memory loss.[114] This is the 'paradox' of food that characterizes today's global food economy.[115] It is a paradox that keeps women estranged from the pleasure of eating and which is reflected in the contradictory account of Syn forwarded by the weight loss organization.

As with sizeism, this conception of sin maintains that slimming organizations constitute one of the material resources that direct and sustain the cultural schema of food victimization, contributing to the atmosphere of evil that predisposes women to fear their tastes and eat in exile. Yet, given this slimming group also provides

---

111. Anna Fisk, *Sex, Sin, and Our Selves: Encounters in Feminist Theology and Contemporary Women's Literature* (Eugene: Pickwick Publications, 2014), 129.

112. Ruether, *Gaia and God*, 200.

113. Wirzba, *Food & Faith*, 74.

114. See Saffron Alexander, 'Is a Glass of Wine a Night Healthy?', *The Telegraph* (3 March 2016), http://www.telegraph.co.uk/food-and-drink/wine/is-red-wine-really-healthy/(accessed 8 September 2016).

115. Wirzba, *Food & Faith*, 74.

a setting where women can pursue their own pleasure sometimes in ways that permanently alter the weight loss plan, slimming cannot be simplistically identified as sinful, nor commercial weight loss companies branded as evil. The ideological–cultural dimension of the victimization of food makes our discomfort over food appear normal and intelligent. According to this hegemonic world of meaning, being apprehensive about food is wise, especially in light of the obesity 'epidemic'. In fact the rigorous policing of our food and weight given they are necessary companions in this sizeist schema, proves that we are upstanding citizens with a concern for the well-being of our bodies and society. The curtailment of desire avoids the snare of sin and is venerated as a practice of holiness. The hegemonic power of the victimization of food means that we eat in exile often without realizing, so accustomed are we to scrutinizing our foodways based on a sizeist bias. Destructive dimensions of food economies remain hidden when food is victimized, making it difficult for us to see our exilic condition as a problem.[116]

A Distorted Relation to the Self: Sin as the Divided Self

Sizeism and the victimization of food mutually support one another. Both are expressive of a third form of distorted relationality which is a feature of the contradictions of modernity. The 'divided self' is a description of sin that borrows from the Augustinian–Pauline tradition the notion of a self at war with itself. This, however, does not depict a self that is inherently depraved or congenitally wounded but speaks instead about a self that is conditioned to enact its own dismemberment. According to Lisa Isherwood and Marcella Althaus-Reid, the slicing of women's bodies is a 'pervading theological praxis with direct consequences for women's bodies and lives'.[117] The cut, sliced and mutilated bodies of women is a feature of modern capitalist society that Christianity has

---

116. Ibid.
117. Marcella Althaus-Reid and Lisa Isherwood, 'Introduction: Slicing Women's Bodies: Christianity and the Cut, Mutilated and Cosmetically Altered Believers', in *Controversies in Body Theology*, ed. Marcella Althaus-Reid and Lisa Isherwood (London: SCM, 2008), 1.

sanctioned and even helped produce, they argue, not least through acts of 'theological dismemberment' that split mind from body.[118]

In the weight loss group, the image of the female dancer divided into fourteen parts symbolizes the sacrificial act of dismemberment that women are expected to perform on themselves. Equally, the soteriological motif of 'getting rid' confirms that women can only be complete by erasing themselves. Women must not only learn to relate to their bodies as pieces but also dismantle them one section at a time in the pursuit of fullness. The 'deadly weapon of dualism'[119] Isherwood and Althaus-Reid locate in Christian thought materializes in this sacrificial economy and practice of dismemberment.

Paul's anthropology of the divided self expounded in Romans 5–7 has been an important feature of this deadly weapon, splitting the old self 'in Adam' from the new self 'in Christ'. This logic has been shown to take on renewed form in the weight loss group as getting rid becomes a means of detaching the self from the corruptible body and from all things female. Given the way this binary supports a separation from pleasure and the appetitive self, the Augustinian–Pauline account of the divided self will not do. Rather, I propose that this motif speaks of a self that is in turmoil because it refuses to receive its feelings. Caught in the 'double bind' encouraged by neoliberal consumer capitalism, women like those in the group anxiously grasp at asceticism then at the pleasures of consumption.[120] The sin of self-division thus speaks of a distorted relation to our bodyselves that has women, in particular, pull their bodies in opposite directions. This is an agonistic self 'torn apart in its distress',[121] to reuse Augustine's words, a self at odds with its desires, cut off from peace and self-acceptance, anxiously seeking escape or erasure. Mary Daly is right that 'the task at hand is [the] healing of the divided self, which means breaking the idols that have kept it torn apart'.[122] In a culture obsessed with thin, these idols are many, but they include the colonial skinny ideal and the harmful theological and cultural association of food and appetite with sin.

---

118. Ibid., 2.

119. Ibid.

120. This is the dual imperative Lupton names as the 'continual dialectic' of consumer culture in *Food, the Body and the Self*, 153.

121. Augustine, *The Confessions*, VIII.10.24.

122. Daly, *Beyond God the Father*, 81.

As a distorted relation to ourselves, the divided self is a personal–interpersonal sin because it speaks not only of a disconnection with our own bodies but also of bifurcations in our corporate body as we fail to relate justly to others. It is a distorted condition characterized by a number of dualisms that 'break our collective body' and that 'shatter us, one by one'.[123] Isolating certain parts of ourselves from other parts,[124] we forget to see our bodies as our home, as us,[125] and fail to see the self and body as a single unit (as the 'bodyself'). We approach our bodies and fat as though from the outside, as objects we 'carry' and need to 'get rid' of. In the battle between our outer and inner selves, we fantasize that we can exit our flesh and forget our finitude. We devote our energy to ensuring our stomachs are ruled by reason while at the same time trying to align our bodies and appetites with the neoliberal assurance that we do not need to deprive ourselves. Caught between a rock and a hard place, the divided self is separated from the aliveness and livingness that is God's intention.

The 'social–historical' dimension of the sin of self-division stresses that it is a social condition that we are born into. Sin is again a form of 'bondage' as women experience entrapment within a perpetual state of inner turmoil. However, as women we are not powerless victims of the system. We are positioned variously and complexly within it as victims and victimizers, as complicit in our own and other women's self-division and as vanquished by external powers and principalities. In its 'ideological–cultural' form, the sin of self-division presents the slicing of women's bodies and the fraught and divided nature of the agonistic self as normal. Theologically, the combative stance against the body comes to be prized as righteous and viewed as a spiritual virtue. Those who excel in this enterprise are like the spiritual athletes of the past, well-disciplined and skilled in the art of detachment. Aided by the contradictions of consumer capitalism and by patterns of social conditioning repeated in the family, church, the global media and commercial weight loss environments, the divided self quietly disappears under 'the radar of the construction of the normal'.[126]

---

123. Heyward, *Touching Our Strength*, 7.

124. See Ruether's description of sin in 'Women and Sin', 234.

125. For more on this, see Elisabeth Moltmann-Wendel, *I Am My Body: New Ways of Embodiment* (London: SCM Press, 1994), 1–34.

126. Althaus-Reid and Isherwood, 'Introduction: Slicing Women's Bodies', 2.

Conclusion: Evil and Sin

Naming these three historical, concrete realities as sin on the basis of women's ordinary lives and wider reflection on affluent Western culture is to propose a theology of sin that is rhetorically sensitive to the women in the weight loss group.[127] Women here are competent social actors who are also trapped in webs of disciplinary power. The concrete descriptions of sin outlined above give theological expression to this tension by attending to the personal-interpersonal, social-historical and ideological-cultural dimensions of sin. In this model, sin locates women's freedom and agency in a wider web of power relations that condition our behaviour but that we also have some capacity to resist.

The language of sin here does not operate to unilaterally judge individual women because sizeism, the victimization of food and self-division are social conditions that are bigger than any individual. As Marjorie Suchocki puts it, 'Sin is not a contained act, but an extended event in an interdependent world.'[128] As such, these instances of sin are also instances of evil because they describe material and cultural distorted relations of power that are outside of our direct control. Indeed, evil refers to impersonal systems of power that are distorted by exploitative patterns of relationship. As descriptions of evil, sizeism, the victimization of food and the divided self then point to damaging cultural and linguistic patterns, to 'habits of language'[129] and to institutional practices that encourage exploitative ways of relating to food, fat and the bodyself. To judge women for acquiescing with these would be to fall into the trap of 'false individualizing' noted by Ruether. As I argued earlier, sin depicts the damage we do to ourselves and others, not how 'bad' we are. It suggests a relational tear and so requires healing, not judgement. This, however, does not mean that women are devoid of any responsibility. Responsibility points towards our 'capacity for change',[130] however, rather than straightforwardly assigning fault. It confirms that we are not without the ability to resist.

---

127. I am influenced here by Jones, *Feminist Theory and Christian Theology*, 110.

128. Marjorie Suchocki, *Fall to Violence: Original Sin in Relational Theology* (New York: Continuum, 1994), 45.

129. Jones, *Feminist Theory and Christian Theology*, 123.

130. Ruether, 'Dualism and the Nature of Evil', 36.

I have argued that sin is not the great equalizer. One difficulty with the notion of 'original sin' is that it suggests that all persons are identically guilty. In recovering aspects of this concept it is crucial to avoid this trap since it repeats the imperialist neglect of difference and the neoliberal ruse that all women are equally free (and so compelled) to act. Women are variously situated in the sins of sizeism, food victimization and self-division because they embody a diversity of identities. Women are not just born into sexist contexts. Race, culture, class, disability, sexuality and age are among the sites of difference in my group that intersect with and help construct distorted ways of relating to food, fat and the bodyself. Levels of agency then depend on the particularities of women's identities and embodiments and so will differ between women. Certain women will find it easier to resist sin than others so agency must be "rhetorically scaled" to meet their differing situations.[131]

Sin fractures our relationship with God. Rather than being simply ethical categories that speak of crimes against our bodyselves or against the bodies of others, the designations I have offered in this chapter are expressive of tears in our connection with the very life force that gives us breath. Sin names those realities in which the livingness of women is diminished, and this is sin because God is a 'living God' and we are children of the living God (Rom. 9.26). Elizabeth Johnson observes how this phrase runs through the whole Bible identifying 'the Source of life as dynamic, bounteous, and full of surprises'.[132] Living means not dead, and as living water is 'fresh, alive, flowing', the appellation of the living God conjures up a God who is 'full of energy and spirit, alive with designs for liberation and healing' and alive with mystery and surprise.[133] The confession that God is a Trinity of persons means that when we relate lovingly to our fat, food and selves, we live into the image of this relational God, and I will say more about this when discussing salvation shortly. If the Trinitarian God is the power that holds the whole planet together in mutually interacting relationality, then the distorted forms of relationship identified as sin in this chapter which harm self, others and the planet also harm the flesh of God.

---

131. Jones, *Feminist Theory and Christian Theology*, 123.

132. Elizabeth Johnson, *Quest for the Living God: Mapping Frontiers in the Theology of God* (London: Continuum, 2007), 4.

133. Ibid., 4.

4. Rethinking Sin

Christian sin-talk can make a plausible intervention into secular speech about weight. The designations I have offered turn the Christian symbol of sin back on itself, naming as sin distorted relations with our fat, our food and our bodyselves that classical theologies of sin have helped resource. Sin communicates that the world is not as it should be, propelling us towards repentant action in search of the fullness of life that God desires for us. If God has a stake in human happiness and flourishing and if the livingness and aliveness of bodies is intimately connected to the livingness and glory of the Trinitarian God, then the life-diminishing realities of sin are located within the hopeful grasp of God's grace. Knowledge of sin drives us to pursue alternative futures, and in the next chapter I argue that food practices can be important ways of doing this. If sin is a distorted way of relating that divides us from the pleasure of food, then salvation is the work of healing and reconciliation that joins our eating and feeling back together.

Chapter 5

RETHINKING SALVATION:
A (RE)TURN TO 'SENSIBLE' EATING

Food plays a major role in the Bible. Early Christian interpretations of the Eden narrative identify food and women's eating with danger and shame, and we have seen how this theological position resurfaces in women's narrations of Syn. However, this is not the only depiction of food in the Christian story. One of the most significant ways in which food is presented in the Bible is as a gift from God. In Exodus, God provides manna for the people of Israel in the wilderness (Exod. 16.1-36), an act of divine feeding that nourishes and sustains the people for forty years.[1] In Psalm 104, God's abundant giving of food to the whole of creation is lauded. Surveying the heavens and the earth, the waters and springs, birds, tress and mountains in a way reflective of Genesis, the text exclaims that 'all look to you to give them their food in due season' (Ps. 104.27-28). The message is that God provides food for birds and animals making the flourishing of all life possible, not just human life.[2] God's gifting of food is also seen in the New Testament when Jesus prays that God give the people their 'daily bread' (Mt. 6.11). It is seen too in Jesus's self-designation as the 'bread of life' (Jn 6.35) who, like the manna in Exodus, is sent from heaven but 'for the life of the world' (Jn 6.51) rather than for the nourishment of the people of Israel alone. According to the Gospels, Jesus feeds the hungry multitudes from meagre loaves and fishes (Mk 6.30-44; Lk. 9.14; Jn 6.10; and Mk 8.9; Mt. 15.39) and, at the Last Supper, presents

---

1. For more on the manna story, see Andrea Bieler and Luise Schottroff, *The Eucharist: Bodies, Bread, Resurrection* (Minneapolis: Fortress, 2007), 99. Also see Montoya, *The Theology of Food*, 122–42 for a discussion of how the manna narrative is continued through the New Testament.

2. Don Schweitzer, 'Food as Gift, Necessity and Possibility', *Religious Studies and Theology* 20, no. 2 (2001): 1–19.

his own flesh and blood as food and drink. According to John, this enables Jesus and those who eat to abide in one another (Jn 6.56). In these stories, food is a nourishing gift given by God and leads to life; it is a means through which the superabundance, love and sharing of God are revealed.[3]

Cherishing food as a gift from God is an important starting point when responding to the victimization of food identified as sin in the previous chapter. Jesus's ministry also shows the significance of food and eating for healing distorted relationships in communities. This chapter draws on these and other theological resources in order to argue that eating can be an important redemptive act that joins our fragmented bodies back together. It returns to the notion of 'sensible eating' developed and emphasized by members in the group and sanctioned by dominant theological tradition, investing this now with new meaning. Rather than supporting the rationalization of food which promotes abstinence from pleasure as paradigmatic of 'good' foodways, I develop a theology of 'taste' and 'touch' which recovers the principle of permission enacted by the women in the group but which disrupts the economy of sacrifice integral to the group's conjuring of Syn and salvation. Sensible eating, I argue, can be one way of repentantly turning away from sin towards our own aliveness and God's fullness. To eat with sense is to eat our way towards salvation.

The Fleshiness of Salvation

Salvation is a form of action, a mode of doing that emerges from a refusal to let sin have the last word. It unmasks and ruptures the dominant hegemony of food victimization together with the sexual phobias that establish food as a threat, while positively celebrating food as a gift from God to be relished and enjoyed.

Ivone Gebara's image of redemption provides a useful starting point for thinking about what salvation might mean in a world where food is victimized. As a postcolonial Catholic Brazilian liberation theologian, she reconceives the meaning of salvation in response to a number of questions, most notably, 'What salvation (or salvations) do women need? What do women actually experience as salvation?'[4] Salvation, she

---

3. Montoya, *The Theology of Food*, 123.
4. Gebara, *Out of the Depths*, 109.

insists, only takes on meaning in relation to the daily lived experience of ordinary women[5] and is driven by practical concerns:

> Salvation will not be something outside the fabric of life but will take place within the heart of it. It springs from the expected and the unexpected, from the near and the far, from the known and the unknown. ... Salvation is what helps us live in the present moment, even when it feeds a dream of greater happiness.[6]

For Gebara, salvation is whatever makes women thrive and survive. It is not identified with the crucifixion of one man or with the related ideological stance that suffering is inherently good, a view that she believes sanctions the oppression of women and the poor. ('One cross cannot contain all sufferings or all crosses,' she incisively reflects.[7]) For Gebara, salvation is the struggle against the cross which we take up alongside other women and men similarly committed to saying 'no' to violence and dehumanization. It is a communal project within which the cross exists as a mundane reality rather than a centrepiece or spiritual path to emulate.[8] Immersed as a mundane part of the community and everyday life, the cross symbolizes the ongoing reality of suffering.

However, accompanying the cross, according to Gebara, are 'everyday resurrections', instances where women recover life, hope and justice even when these experiences are fleeting.[9] On these occasions, resurrection is lived in the here and now rather than simply anticipated after death. It situates ourselves in the concrete histories of our bodies and is a 'dynamic movement' towards love and fulfilment. Redemption is found in tangible instances of joy that nourish our bodies and lives:[10] in music that calms the spirit, in a glass of beer, a piece of bread or a cup of coffee shared with friends.[11] These kinds of 'mini-salvations' or

5. Ibid.
6. Ibid., 121.
7. Ibid., 120.
8. Ibid., 115. Gebara recounts how in Latin America, the symbol of the crucified Jesus is often surrounded by people, plants and animals and suggests that as such it 'loses its exclusive centrality in order to appear as an ordinary element of life carried by everyone'.
9. Ibid., 121.
10. Ibid., 125.
11. Ibid., 124.

'micro-salvations',[12] she claims, do not substitute for the political and theological project of securing a better life for all, because the private and public, individual and collective accompany one another. Yet salvation can never be once and for all because 'no sooner it comes than it is gone'.[13] Firmly rooted in the limits of our flesh, our bodies provide the first (although not necessarily last) word about salvation and hope.[14] Like a glass of water that quenches thirst only for thirst to eventually return, salvation is temporary and fragile.[15] It is a daily process that we must begin afresh each day.

Gebara's rich and colourful account drives home the proximity of salvation to the throbbing pulse of daily life and to our fleshy encounters with food. I share her view that the cross does not offer an endorsement of suffering but expresses the realities of pain in a fractured world. Her refusal to separate the personal from the political compels us to consider how personal action can shape new futures that extend beyond the individual. She helpfully prizes salvation from the traditional association with escape already criticized and locates redemption squarely in the mundane and ordinary. Such an emphasis on the fleshy day-to-day is the only place to begin thinking about salvation if it is to speak meaningfully to the corporeal enterprise of slimming.

Beginning with the flourishing of bodies in the ordinary day-to-day is continuous with the ministry of Jesus in the New Testament. When Jesus heals the sick, he acts to help those who are despised and alienated in society to live and flourish. As such, he reveals God's inclusive kin-dom[16] and roots salvation in bodies, history and time. Similarly, I suggest that salvation concerns liberative action in the here and now and the restoring of right relation. It is not about sacrifice, debt, emulating crucifixion or reframing suffering as fundamentally good. This logic has been shown to function dangerously in the slimming group and to support a capitalist system that makes money out of women's

12. Ibid., 125.
13. Ibid.
14. Ibid.
15. Ibid.
16. I borrow the term 'kin-dom' from Isasi-Díaz who explains that this replaces the sexist and hierarchical emphasis on reign and rule suggested by the term 'kingdom' with the image of family and community so central to Latina culture. See Ada María Isasi-Díaz, *La Lucha Continues: Mujerista Theology* (Maryknoll: Orbis Books, 2004), 236, footnote no. 1.

defleshing. Marcella Althaus-Reid suggests that if the divine–human and God–world relationship is based on a debt economy, then there can be nothing alarming about the amount of people sacrificed by global capitalism.[17] In the weight loss industry where the burning of female fat is a pleasant odour that pleases the markets, the debt metaphor does little to challenge the structures of evil that train women to forfeit taste for the sake of erasing their flesh. However, if God desires 'steadfast love and not sacrifice, the knowledge of God rather than burnt-offerings' (Hos. 6.6), then salvation must be reimagined away from this sacrificial metaphor. Salvation, I contend, is the pursuit of reconciliation and healing in the here and now in response to the distortions that mark our relationships, including our relating to food, fat and the bodyself.

Such an earthly account of redemption does not supplant Christian eschatology, nor does it suggest that salvation is the work of people alone. Instead, it insists with Ada María Isasi-Díaz that we participate in the future exactly by altering the now.[18] Redeeming the present performs the Christian call to shape and realize God's future together. This is a prophetic eschatology that stands against fatalism and which hopes beyond all hope that the world can be changed. Instead of conceptualizing God as locked outside of human history or as determining everything that occurs, I envisage God as working for transformation in this world with the help of human agents.[19] Isaiah 65 provides an inspiring vision of this, making clear the historicity of the new heaven and new earth. This passage shows that the inequalities that offend Yahweh are committed in real geographic spaces (hills and the mountains) (Isa. 65.7) and that God's reward will also happen in

---

17. Marcella Althaus-Reid, 'Queering the Cross: The Politics of Redemption and the External Debt', *Feminist Theology* 15, no. 3 (2007): 294. According to Althaus-Reid, the debt narrative can also never be palatable for Christian feminists concerned about global debt because the multitude of human sacrifices involved in redemption only imitate the bloody road taken by a tortured god dying on a cross. 'The point is that no economy of freedom and no alternative *Basileia* or Kingdom of God can happen while Christ continues to be associated with an economy of debt, as in the case of redemption, which has serious cultural and economic limitations' (298).

18. Also see Isasi-Díaz, *La Lucha Continues*, 225.

19. This is also how Emilie M. Townes describes prophetic eschatology in *In a Blaze of Glory: Womanist Spirituality as Social Witness* (Nashville: Abingdon Press, 1995), 122.

time, in 'the here and now of Israel'[20] (cf. Isa. 65.10). It is this world that will be changed since people will eat, drink and rejoice (Isa. 65.13), build houses and live in them, plant vineyards and consume their fruit (Isa. 65.21), enjoy the work of their hands rather than labouring in vain (Isa. 65.22-23).

Salvation rendered this way constitutes a 'practical eschatology' and 'lived hope' wherein human conduct and Christian action help remake history.[21] It continues the call to 'do something about it' summoned by women in the group but without demanding that women reinvest their time and energy in dismembering their fat or separating their minds from their emotions. As a practice of hope, salvation encompasses the call 'to live *now as if*, to cite Letty Russell, *as if* 'the new creation is already present in our lives (1 Cor. 7.25-31)'.[22] Forgoing an endorsement of paradise as other-worldly, this instead tasks the faithful with the redemptive work of transforming history with God at our side. It calls for a certain obstinacy. Stubbornness in relation to hope is a key component of building and living God's future, comprising of our determination to persist despite the cycles of violence that condition us to attack our bodies and the bodies of others. The practice of hope requires imagination and risk – the imagination to visualize alternatives and the willingness to risk getting it wrong and to live differently in the now. This is a practical imagining of the kin-dom of God and one that believers must live into rather than simply passively anticipate. It requires an ability not only to see the world through new eyes but also to make the world anew through our bodies. To borrow from Monica Coleman, salvation is 'meaningful work' that contributes to the quality of life and to care of the self.[23] It describes the concrete struggle for life – for 'liveable lives'[24] – in the here and now.

20. Isasi-Díaz, *La Lucha Continues*, 228.

21. Jürgen Moltmann, 'Liberating and Anticipating the Future', in *Liberating Eschatology: Essays in Honor of Letty M. Russell*, ed. Margaret A. Farley and Serene Jones (Louisville: Westminster John Knox Press, 1999), 190.

22. Letty M. Russell, *Human Liberation in a Feminist Perspective – A Theology* (Philadelphia: The Westminster Press, 1974), 42.

23. Monica A. Coleman, 'Sacrifice, Surrogacy and Salvation', *Black Theology: An International Journal* 12, no. 3 (2014): 210.

24. According to Butler, the question underpinning the notion of a liveable life is this: 'What things need to be done, what conditions fulfilled, in order for life to become life?' See Judith Butler, *Undoing Gender* (New York: Routledge, 2004), 39.

The descriptions of salvation I develop in this chapter and in Chapter 6 do not offer a once-and-for-all solution to the forms of sin I have already outlined. To do so would be to collapse salvation into a 'utopian impulse'[25] that is naive to the limits of what is possible. Following Gebara and Ruether, I contend that salvation is the ongoing, daily pursuit of more just and loving relations rather than a fixed end or millennium where everything is suddenly fixed. Salvation is not simply about changing our minds about sin. It is a performative practice that involves the whole body in intentionally living out alternative realities in contexts of sin that continue to limit us. Given women are positioned variously in relation to sin, salvation will take on multiple forms and be informed by the specific identities and embodied experiences of the women concerned. The proposals I make in these two chapters aim to be rhetorically sensitive to the lives of women in the slimming group at the centre of this study.

Salvation as a Queer Performance

The concept of 'performativity' is an important one. In the 1990s, queer philosopher Judith Butler made a central contribution to feminist theory by suggesting that gender was a performative identity. Reflecting on the cultural imposition of normative heterosexuality, she argued that gender was best understood as a series of acts we perform in compliance with tacit social scripts. While it may look natural on the surface, 'it has no ontological status apart from the various acts which constitute its reality'.[26] Gender is not a stable identity which gives rise to certain behaviours but is produced through a 'stylized repetition of acts'.[27] It is through conscious and unconscious repetitions of behaviours that gender is produced.

To understand salvation as a performative practice means to understand sin as a reality that materializes through a concealed process of repetition we perform as normal.[28] The victimization of food and fat and the cultivation of an agonistic personality are behaviours we

---

25. Jones, *Feminist Theory and Christian Theology*, 131.
26. Judith Butler, *Gender Trouble: Feminism and the Subversion of Identity* (New York and London: Routledge, 2007), 185.
27. Ibid., 191.
28. Judith Butler, *Bodies that Matter: On the Discursive Limits of 'Sex'* (London and New York: Routledge, 2011).

learn through cultural training. Like gender, they are modes of doing rather than being. That does not mean they are illusory or somehow not real; it simply means they are produced rather than inevitable or inherent. As scripts we perform, the sins of sizeism, the victimization of food and self-division can be subverted and undone because the material surfaces of sin are permeable and up for negotiation. While the scripts of compulsory thinness, food victimization and self-division shape what our bodies do, they do not contain what is possible. 'For something to be compulsory shows that it is not necessary,' says Sara Ahmed; 'One does not have to do what one is compelled to do.'[29]

Salvation as the Performance of Embodied Alternatives: Jesus's Ministry of Food

Turning specifically to the way food practices might heal the distortions of sin, I want to draw on a number of theological resources, beginning now with Jesus's ministry of food. Jesus's foodways provide a good example of how eating can be a sensuous counter-cultural activity that challenges inherited cultural and religious norms and habituated behaviour. Although the purity laws of the Hebrew Bible depict some foods as unclean, in the New Testament Jesus declares all food clean teaching that the real danger of defilement lies in evil thoughts and actions which filter from the heart rather than in food that goes into the stomach.[30] Jesus's ministry is an embrace of others that uses food to challenge social conventions. He eats with social outcasts, mostly as a guest, and accepts the hospitality of so-called sinners. Lisa Isherwood notes that although the Gospel of Luke links the hospitality Jesus receives from those outside the law to their repentance, the other Gospels do not. This, she maintains, illuminates the real 'scandal' of Jesus – that he eats and drinks with the wicked and tells them that God especially loves them. The radical, counter-cultural logic of Jesus's foodways not only

---

29. Sara Ahmed draws on the notion of 'compulsory heterosexuality' to argue that the repetition of scripts which suggest heterosexuality as an ideal coupling shape our bodies and actions. By orienting us towards some objects and not others, compulsory heterosexuality affects how we live, but if something is compulsory it must be also possible to resist. See Sara Ahmed, *The Cultural Politics of Emotion*, 2nd edn (Edinburgh: Edinburgh University Press, 2014), 145.

30. Mk 7.18-19.

positions him as a guest and stranger at the table of so-called 'wicked' hosts, which in the culture of the time would depict Jesus as vulnerable and dependent on them,[31] but also suggests that God's kin-dom is a reign where the outcast is welcomed and loved. As Isherwood puts it,

> By accepting the hospitality of the wicked Jesus in his own body preaches the way that Yahweh operates to save, to bring in his reign, namely through inclusion rather than exclusion, through extravagant, reckless generosity in which all debts are cancelled.[32]

By accepting the welcome of the vulnerable, by eating with sinners and by encouraging his hosts to feed the sick and the poor, Jesus confirms the equal dignity of all persons at the table.[33] He performs an 'embodied alternative'[34] to the social norms of his day, using His body to make room for others who are outcast and despised.

Also pertinent about Jesus's ministry of food is that hospitality is not simply about feeding family and friends but about restoring those on the margins of society to participation in community life. In Mt. 25.31-46 Jesus teaches that those who feed the hungry, welcome the stranger and visit the sick actually feed, welcome and care for him, practising God's hospitality to those in need.[35] This embodied alternative would not have been popular in a culture where the sick, the lame, the mentally ill and others were viewed as unclean. Jesus's body – his eating and drinking – ruptures hegemonic cultural habits, and this is meaningful work continued by the early church who similarly use food to challenge social status and to generate social bonds. Meeting in households where hospitality was central, the first believers shared meals as a way of learning to live together and value one another in the face of cultural and economic divisions.[36]

---

31. Also see Christine D. Pohl, *Making Room: Recovering Hospitality as a Christian Tradition* (Grand Rapids; Cambridge: William R. Eerdmans Publishing Company, 1999), 5.

32. Isherwood and Stuart, *Introducing Body Theology*, 60.

33. Pohl, *Making Room*, 6.

34. Lisa Isherwood, 'Sex and Body Politics: Issues for Feminist Theology', in *The Good News of the Body*, 33.

35. Ibid., 23.

36. Pohl, 'Hospitality and the Mental Health of Children and Families', *American Journal of Orthopsychiatry* 81, no. 4 (2011): 482–8. Jesus's hospitality

Jesus sees the meals he eats with sinners as symbolic of the future heavenly banquet where hunger will be gratified.[37] According to Mark (14.25), Matthew (26.29) and Luke (22.15-18), for example, Jesus tells those gathered at the Last Supper that he will not eat and drink again until he eats and drinks at the eschatological meal. His eating and drinking point forwards to a time when all will eat and drink in the company of God. By eating, that future is brought into the now. Isaiah describes this future as a banquet where 'the Lord of hosts will make for all peoples a feast of rich food, a feast of well-matured wines, of rich food filled with marrow, of well-matured wines strained clear' (Isa. 25.6). This is a feast meant for enjoyment, and it is a feast meant for all. The eschatological banquet that is implied is no ordinary meal. As Norman Wirzba argues, feasts and banquets 'are about celebration and merriment, both of which, from a utility point of view, are unnecessary'.[38] Jesus's food ministry anticipates and makes present this joyful, celebratory meal that will see humans participate in the justice of God through food and laughter in the company of others. His food practices are productive because they create this alternative, making present a world where food is not just a utility but the locus of God's life and sharing and a source of human and divine rejoicing.

According to the Bible, Jesus's enjoyment of food does not go unnoticed. The New Testament tells us that Jesus came eating and drinking (Lk. 7.34; Mt. 11.19), a personal characteristic and feature

extends the tradition of hospitality outlined in the Hebrew Bible. According to Christine Pohl, in ancient times, the practice of hospitality would have been essential as a form of mutual aid. Without it, travellers and strangers would be vulnerable, left without shelter or protection. 'Hospitality involved welcoming strangers into personal space', she explains, 'usually one's home but also one's community, and offering them food, shelter, protection, and respect' (482). In the Old Testament, hospitality communicates God's concern for the vulnerable. The Israelites must remember that they were once strangers and slaves in Egypt and that God tended to their needs, and so they must similarly protect the stranger, widow, poor, orphan and the resident alien (Deuteronomy 24).

37. Isherwood and Stuart, *Introducing Body Theology*, 61. Also see Montoya, *The Theology of Food*, 141. Examples cited here by Montoya include Isa. 25.6-10; 55.1-4; Amos 9.11-15; Jer. 31.10-14; Mt. 8.11; Mk 2.11; Lk. 6.21; 12.35-48; 13.28-30; 14.7-24; 22.28-30; Rev. 19.5-10.

38. Wirzba, *Food & Faith*, 228. Ecclesiastes even reminds us that 'feasts are made for laughter; wine gladdens life' (Eccl. 10.19).

of his ministry that wins him the reputation of being 'a glutton and a drunkard, a friend of tax collectors and sinners!' (Lk. 7.34). For Susan Hill, this places him squarely in the company of the rebellious son in Deuteronomy who, being similarly accused of being 'a glutton and a drunkard', is condemned to punishment and death by stoning (Deut. 21.18-21). So radical is Jesus's eating ministry, she argues, so different to John the Baptist's fasting tradition that it appears to have the potential to kill him[39] – such is the danger of embracing embodied alternatives it would seem. In Jesus's ministry, eating is a site of sensuality that holds together physical pleasure and a joyful encounter with food with building communities that welcome the stranger and value all bodies as passionately loved by God. Through eating and drinking, Jesus challenges the religious and cultural dictates of his day.

Of course, we cannot speak about Jesus's foodways without mentioning his feeding of the hungry multitudes from a few loaves and fishes.[40] This story should be read in the context of a long biblical tradition of God giving food as a gift for the sustenance and nourishment of the people, a pattern I began to sketch at the start of this chapter. It finds its place alongside the gifting of manna from heaven and Jesus's self-designation as the 'bread of life'. In all these examples, food leads to life rather than death (as is the typical interpretation of Eden) and is a means of participating in God's goodness. According to Christine Pohl, when Jesus feeds the masses, he is the host who provides sustenance and welcome. Designating himself as the 'bread of life' (Jn 6.35), Jesus depicts himself as both host and meal. He is the bread and living water that feeds the hungry and quenches the thirsty (Jn 7.37).[41]

These bread stories, however, start to expose a difficulty with the theological framing of food as gift: namely, that it potentially returns us to the view expressed in the weight loss group and echoed in some features of classical Christian tradition that food is valuable primarily for meeting human need. In their discussion of the Eucharist as 'gift exchange', Andrea Bieler and Luise Schottroff argue that when God rains down manna from heaven, it is to give the people of Israel enough nourishment to get through the day. When Jesus feeds the multitudes

---

39. Hill, *Eating to Excess*, 36–8.
40. Mk 6.30-44; Lk. 9.14; Jn 6.10 and Mk 8.9; Mt. 15.39.
41. Pohl, *Making Room*, 30.

with loaves and fishes, it is enough to fill each person (Mk 6.42).[42] Jesus as the bread of life is sufficient for all. These manna stories communicate that food as gift is about God giving people ample to fill them. The 'economy of grace', they argue, runs contrary to the 'market economy' of limitless consumption and accumulation, a lesson the people of Israel learn when they try to store up the manna which ruins as a result. Whereas in the former God gives enough to fill everyone, in the latter 'the strong and the healthy are to consume, to have an excess and to throw it away'.[43]

While this theological picture challenges the 'market and machine logics'[44] of advanced capitalism localized in distorted patterns of relating to food in a weight-obsessed culture, what is missing is an affirmation of desire. If food is for necessity alone, for meeting human need for nourishment only, then the logic of the organization that identifies Synful eating with eating foods which are not necessary is sanctioned, along with the theological suspicion of pleasure that supports it. The sensual and embodied nature of Jesus's food ministry clearly provides a challenge to this. However, given this feature of the manna stories, we may need a more rigorous endorsement of pleasure. To that end, I want to turn to the wisdom of Qohelet.[45]

---

42. Bieler and Schottroff, *The Eucharist*, 77–80. Also see Jayne Steele, 'Chocolate and Bread: Gendering Sacred and Profane Foods in Contemporary Cultural Representations', *Theology and Sexuality* 14, no. 3 (2008): 321–34. Here Steele claims that in Western culture, bread (unlike chocolate) 'summons the notion of need before desire' (328). Like Bieler and Schottroff, she argues that Jesus's feeding of the five thousand 'concerns need, not desire'. While bread suggests need rather than desire, fruit and sweetness summon the notion of 'desire' and 'want'. Christianity, she believes, has helped to mark out the sacred from the profane by gendering food such that sweetness is viewed as feminine and as synonymous with temptation and desire. It is Eve's sweet tooth that gets her into trouble and which sees her 'straying into the paths of profanity' (323–4). Don Schweitzer similarly claims that when food is discussed in the Bible, the focus is not so much on the food itself as on God as the giver of food and on food as a necessity of life. See Schweitzer, 'Food as Gift'.

43. Bieler and Schottroff, *The Eucharist*, 77.

44. Wirzba, *Food & Faith*, xvi.

45. There are other theological resources that can help with this. The Songs of Songs provides a radical celebration of pleasure and sexuality which has been discussed by Lisa Isherwood in her feminist theological reflection on fat

'There is Nothing Better for People under the Sun than to Eat, and Drink, and Enjoy Themselves'

Qohelet is a likeable figure. His reflections on life and human existence exude for me a kind of realism: wickedness occupies the place of justice (Eccl. 3.16), the righteous perish while the wicked prosper (7.15), power resides on the side of the oppressor (4.1). It is hard to argue with the insights of this teacher. Qohelet is also a radical figure because he embraces an unreserved celebration of pleasure and the joy of eating and drinking in particular: 'There is nothing better for mortals than to eat and drink, and find enjoyment in their toil. This also, I saw, is from the hand of God' (2.24-25). Qohelet reaches this position not long after his initial dismissal of the pursuit of pleasure as vain (2.11). Eating and drinking, he now contends, are gifts from God given for enjoyment, a fitting response to the futilities of toil, wisdom and worry.[46] Repeated again in 3.12-13, Qohelet observes that 'it is God's gift that all should eat and drink and take pleasure in all their toil' (3.13).

According to Ken Stone, the identification of eating and drinking with divine gift is significant. Also important is the way 3.12-13 defines doing what is good as a practice of pleasure rather than just as a moral activity. To do what is good, he claims, means to experience good, to enjoy oneself.[47] It signals physical enjoyment. This rendering of the goodness of pleasure is reiterated again in 5.18 and enjoyment from eating and drinking lauded further in 8.15. For Stone, it is in the final chapter that Qohelet reaches his ultimate conclusion, swapping the language of observation for the language of command:[48] 'Go, eat your bread with enjoyment, and drink your wine with a merry heart; for God has long ago approved what you do' (9.7). Eating and drinking are endorsed by God as an experience of pleasure and in 9.9 this is extended to sexual pleasure[49] where Qohelet challenges his initial conclusion

and by Ken Stone. I have also used this text to theologically reframe desire. See Isherwood, *The Fat Jesus*, 41–5; Stone, *Practicing Safer Texts*, 90–111; Hannah Bacon, 'Expanding Bodies, Expanding God: Feminist Theology in Search of a "Fatter" Future', *Feminist Theology* 21, no. 3 (2013): 309–26.

46. Stone, *Practicing Safer Texts*, 137.
47. Ibid.
48. Ibid., 138.
49. Stone suggests that the NRSV translation that says, 'Enjoy life with the wife whom you love' is more accurately translated 'with a woman whom you love' given there is no Hebrew word exclusively for 'wife'. With the insertion of

(in 2.11) that such pleasure is just as vain as all his other quests for fulfilment. Now sexual enjoyment appears as part of God's intention for human living.

Qohelet provides an important theological challenge to the victimization of food outlined previously. We are to eat 'with enjoyment' and drink 'with a merry heart', so presumably not with guilt, fear or anxiety. This is what God intends for us; it is, as Stone puts it, 'the form of life that God has approved for us'.[50] Qohelet's message is that life is fleeting so we must enjoy it while we can. His embrace of pleasure is an embrace of life, an 'opting for life', to cite Stone.[51] Yet Qohelet is not without its problems. Written in a patriarchal context, it not only assumes a male speaker and male audience but also conveys a patriarchal message: 'I found more bitter than death the woman who is a trap, whose heart is snares and nets, whose hands are fetters; one who pleases God escapes her, but the sinner is taken by her' (7.26). This is hardly a life-giving message for women, especially in a context where fears about food and fat repeat the theological assumption that women are closer to sin. Misogynist statements like this can be found in the text (see also 7.27-28), and this potentially renders Qohelet 'unsafe' to consume.[52] But the harmful dimensions of the text need not mitigate the healthful aspects of its teaching. Qohelet still provides a means by which we might rupture theological approaches which would have us be suspicious of pleasure and the enjoyment of food for its own sake.

Returning to a Privatized Selfish Ethic?

At this point some readers may worry that the theology beginning to emerge stands to return to the very neoliberal stance that I have critiqued in earlier chapters, one that defines the highest good as a freedom from need, as limitless possibility unperturbed by anyone or anything and as a type of 'gratuitous desire that answers to no one but ourselves, free-floating, uninformed by any exterior responsibility'.[53] Such a

---

the word wife, 'normalizing sexual assumptions are being imposed' on the text. Ibid., 139.

50. Ibid., 138.
51. Ibid.
52. Ibid., 147.
53. Lilian Calles Barger, *Eve's Revenge: Women and a Spirituality of the Body* (Grand Rapids: Brazos Press, 2003), 28.

prioritization of pleasure may seem to risk a positive endorsement of self-indulgence and over consumption that lacks consideration for others in our global and local food communities. It may also seem to place the burden for sin on the poor given that eating for enjoyment comes at a price and one that only the rich can often afford.[54] The problem becomes even more pronounced if we acknowledge with Korean-Brazilian liberation theologian, Jung Mo Sung, that capitalist societies conflate desire with need in such a way that suggests that people do not really have needs, but just taste.[55] If, as Sung claims, the collapse of need into desire means that there comes to be no limits to what we think we need to fulfil our desire, whether a super-skinny body or a private jet, then desire/taste itself becomes problematic. It is determined by the ambitions of the privileged elite and cemented as need for the masses, despite being only accessible to the few.[56]

Focusing on pleasure also risks overlooking the way good-tasting food is often caught up in distorted capitalist systems that are especially harmful to women of low socio-economic status. In her reflection on obesity, Antronette K. Yancey[57] suggests that feminist work on weight needs to pay much more attention to the socio-economic inequalities that effect access to fresh food and exercise. For Yancey, the increase in attractive, inexpensive, good-tasting, energy-dense nutrient-poor foods over the last thirty years and their promotion by advertising industries has seen the American diet shift in ways that are not conducive to good health.[58] Falling prices in sweeteners and fats has led to an increase in added fats and oils in the US food supply and an increase in fast-food restaurants offering cheap, quick food.[59] Although Yancey restates the sizeist assumption that obesity is 'rooted' in unhealthy eating and a lack of physical activity (laziness),[60] she attentively observes how women's

---

54. Angela West, *Deadly Innocence: Feminist Theology and the Mythology of Sin* (London: Cassell, 1995), 174.

55. Jung Mo Sung, *Desire, Market and Religion: Reclaiming Liberation Theology* (London: SCM, 2007), 32.

56. Ibid., 33-6.

57. Antronette K. Yancey, Joanne Leslie and Emily K. Abel, 'Obesity at the Crossroads: Feminist and Public Health Perspective', *Signs* 31, no. 2 (2006): 425-33.

58. Ibid., 430-1.

59. Ibid., 431.

60. Ibid., 432.

bodies are victims of this poorly nutritious system. Given women still shoulder the responsibility to procure, prepare and serve food and given the demands of work, child care and other caring responsibilities that women are often heavily involved in, fast-food industries especially harm and victimize women's bodies by offering inexpensive options which are nutritionally poor.[61]

The harm here, however, I suggest, is in the restricted access to nutritious food that compromises health and exploits the bodies of working mothers rather than in the so-called fact that fat is an inevitable by-product of unhealthy eating. I want to trouble this assumption, and I will say more about that in Chapter 6. This raises the question, however, of how an emphasis on pleasure ties in with health and justice. If the pursuit of pleasure is the pursuit of life in abundance, then it is also a form of eating that makes for vitality and health. If this is only available to middle-class women like those in the weight loss group who can use their leisure time to cook from scratch, then the pursuit of pleasure is a pursuit of economic privilege that does not attend to inequalities or matters of food justice. We seem to be retreating into the realms of sin once more.

In light of these concerns, I want to challenge us to think about what theological picture might emerge if we take from Jesus's ministry the uniting of joy with the welcome of vulnerable others and from Qohelet the unapologetic endorsement of pleasure. The outcome, I suggest, is a 'sensible' approach to food that understands eating with joy as a relational practice that connects individuals to the lives of others, including the life of God and God's world, and which advocates for the right of all to access nutritious food. Sensible eating does not have to be an expression of class indulgences if we acknowledge it as a practice of self-care that, rather than being a privilege of income, is an aspect of salvation which should be universally available to all.

Salvation and 'Sensible' Eating

Sensible eating is 'sensible', not because it rationalizes food by counting Syn or by making the mind rule over the appetite as in the weight loss group or because it is rooted in 'obvious' knowledge about fat. It is sensible because it invites women who have access to food and who

---

61. Ibid., 433.

nevertheless seek to sterilize their tastes to employ their senses when they eat. For African American feminist writer, Audre Lorde, women 'have been raised to fear the yes within ourselves, our deepest cravings'.[62] Within this passionless patriarchal straight jacket, the spiritual has been reduced to 'a world of flattened affect', she argues, 'a world of the ascetic who aspires to feel nothing'.[63] It is only by embracing sensuality and the capacity for feeling that the politics of self-denial are resisted, she claims, for 'as we begin to recognize our deepest feelings, we begin to give up, of necessity, being satisfied with suffering and self-negation'.[64] Sensible eating is a scandalous means through which women can come into their own 'yes' and experience their own satisfaction. When we eat with sense, we approach our pleasure as good and sacred while maintaining that our sensuality can be trusted.[65] We value our tastes and preferences, and eat in ways that respect and welcome a joyful delight in food rather than approaching food as an instrument that must be used to eradicate fat. In approaching food this way, we refuse to repeat the narrative of self-negation and sacrifice. Instead, we are reminded of our capacity for *feeling*[66] and enact a fearless embrace of joy.[67] We realize that more than simply being thoughtless about food, we often fall into the trap of being senseless about food – eating without feeling, without sense.

In the weight loss group, women are encouraged to take leave of their senses. Food is an object to control and eating, if it is to be 'sensible' or 'intelligent', must be at some point emptied of feeling and emotion. Christian theologies and ascetic practices have highly prized this kind of detachment as we have seen, but sensible eating is a Christian alimentary praxis that radically departs from this. Contrary to the conventional wisdom of Aquinas who considers 'emotional desires' and 'desire for pleasure' dangerous because they threaten to disorder the 'sensory appetite',[68] and distinct from Clement before him, who suggests

---

62. Audre Lorde, *Sister Outsider: Essays and Speeches by Audre Lorde*, New Foreword by Cheryl Clarke (Berkeley: Crossing Press, 2007), 57.

63. Ibid., 56.

64. Ibid., 58.

65. Also see Heyward, *Touching our Strength*, 93.

66. Lorde, *Sister Outsider*, 57.

67. Ibid., 56.

68. Thomas Aquinas, *Summa Theologiæ*, 43 (2a2æ. 141–154), Temperance, trans. Thomas Gilby (Cambridge and New York: Cambridge University Press, 2006), Q148.1.

that the passions should not be captured by the soul's energies because perfection is comprised of a 'passionless state', the call to feel food deeply is an invitation for women to connect with their emotions and tastes, not to abandon them or seek to suppress them. Sensible eating returns value and theological importance to women's sensory experience and to women's sensual pleasure allowing us to be responsible to ourselves. In this way it is a 'per/version'[69] both of dieting logic and of the related vanilla theology that vilifies women's appetites and a re-membering of the practices of self-care women enact in the group. In this sensible economy, oral pleasure is an especial site of women's becoming.

Of course, in Western philosophy and classical theology feeling specifically has been seen as an obstacle to objectivity and to knowing what is good or true.[70] This is mainly because it has been demonized through an association with sex and sexuality, and we have already seen evidence of this. Christianity has placed sex in violent opposition to God in the same way as it has placed pleasure in antagonistic opposition to goodness.[71] Attending to feeling turns this theologically sanctioned vilification of feeling and sensible desire upside down. When we eat with sense, we are 'motivated and empowered from within,'[72] as Lorde puts it, connected to our passions and set against numbness. We recognize that sensation by itself is not enough because as Lorde observes, women need to find themselves in and through their affections. Feeling must accompany sensation as a mode of learning to live from within rather than from without.[73] It drives us to connect with our deepest passions and to return to our sense of self.

Seen in alimentary terms, this calls us to get excited about food: to relish the anticipation of it, savour and delight in the texture of food, the feel of it in our mouths, its taste and smell. It has us salivate at the sizzling pan, value our tastes and preferences and eat in ways that

---

69. Marcella Althaus-Reid, 'Queer I Stand: Lifting the Skirts of God', in *The Sexual Theologian: Essays on Sex, God and Politics*, ed. Marcella Althaus-Reid and Lisa Isherwood (London and New York: T & T Clark, 2004), 107. 'Per/version is a concept that can be theologically related to alternative versions or options which it is our duty to imagine. Per/version (as a different version, or understanding) is the methodological path to take against projects of sameness.'

70. Heyward, *Touching Our Strength*, 6.

71. Ibid., 4.

72. Lorde, *Sister Outsider*, 58.

73. Ibid.

respect the joy of food rather than seeing it as an instrument to be used to aid the project of weight loss. When we eat with sense we take time to feel our food, to savour it and rejoice in it; we are conscious about how our food makes us feel and about other feeling bodies around us. This is the opposite of rushing, hoarding, fuelling, snatching, exploiting, possessing, polluting, starving, purging and renouncing. It calls us to respect the story of food, its history and journey and to let our sensual pleasure feed our aliveness. Sensible eating values food as a site of connection and so encourages more loving and sensual attachments to the things we eat and to other bodies, rather than separation from them. We are called to eat with *jouissance*, which is 'a matter of deep joy, of assured security, of living in the presence of God',[74] and this is very different to the kind of eating that demands that we dispose of the batter from our fish or scoop out the dough from our crusty loaves. Sensible eating rescues the demonization of sensuality and sexuality by patriarchal theology and related philosophical systems and reconnects the body and its passions to God.

This celebration of sensuality begins with a confidence in the body and in women's bodies as created good by God. As such, it 'start[s] from the creation, not from the "fall"'[75] because it deliberately chooses to keep faith with the body in acknowledgement of the Spirit-filled nature of all flesh. To trust our bodies is to honour our bodies as quickened by God whereas to distrust them is to see our bodies as menacing sinful objects that need to be conquered, confessed and tightly managed.[76] Sensible eating allows women to claim back our flesh as a source of power and dignity rather than as a source of poison or deceit. It is, to use Lisa Isherwood's words, 'a proud procession up the vaginal aisle'.[77] Led to enjoy the physical pleasure food brings to our lips, eyes and tastes, we boldly acknowledge the belly as the centre of our bodies, 'sensing it from the inside'[78] rather than being distrustful of the belly as the place 'down there' near the vulva that is a source of shame. To eat with sense ruptures the internalized 'good girl' mentality that demarcates a

---

74. L. Shannon Jung, *Sharing Food: Christian Practices for Enjoyment* (Minneapolis: Fortress Press, 2006), 145.

75. Moltmann-Wendel, *I Am My Body*, 36.

76. Jung, *Sharing Food*, 106–7.

77. Lisa Isherwood, 'Indecent Theology: What F-ing Difference Does It Make?', *Feminist Theology* 11, no. 2 (2003): 145.

78. Roth, *Women, Food and God*, 113.

sanitized and rigorously patrolled space[79] by daring to suggest that it is 'good' for women to acutely feel their bodies for themselves.

This repeats the significance of self-authorization practised by many women in the group, restating its potential to resist compulsory modes of behaviour. In the weight loss community, women become intentional about their eating and consent to caring for themselves, and at points, employ their self-granted permission to refuse the hegemonic expectations of the organization. The principle and practice of sensible eating recovers this emphasis and frames women's prioritization of feeling as a potentially dangerous and transgressive erotic praxis. According to Lorde, the dangerous power of the erotic should not be underestimated. Rather than demarcating the perverse-dirty or being made to constitute 'the confused, the trivial, the psychotic',[80] and instead of being used against women, the erotic is an assertion of the life force of women.[81] It is a self-responsible source of women's power: 'In touch with the erotic, I become less willing to accept powerlessness, or those other supplied states of being that are not native to me, such as resignation, despair, self-effacement, depression, self-denial.'[82] The erotic espouses a responsibility 'not to settle for the convenient, the shoddy, the conventionally expected, nor the merely safe'.[83] Touching the power of the erotic then, for Lorde, has the power to change the world, to turn the patriarchal and capitalist systems upside down. It challenges our ingrained fears and practices of self-denial and is a source of power, creativity and revolution. It also drives us to connect with other bodies and to attend to others' feelings.

Sensible eating is an erotic Christian praxis that can connect women with their feelings and desires and join women's sensual bodies and appetites to the sacred. It is a dangerous activity because it has the power to reshape habituated forms of behaviour and rupture well-established theological norms that sanitize women's tastes and help conform women's eating to fat phobic standards. It directs women beyond the

---

79. For more on the 'good girl' mentality and its association with Christian views about sexuality, see Sonya Sharma, *Good Girls, Good Sex: Women Talk about Church and Sexuality* (Halifax: Fernwood Publishing, 2012).
80. Lorde, *Sister Outsider*, 54.
81. Ibid., 55.
82. Ibid., 58.
83. Ibid., 57.

conventional and beyond the boundaries of 'safe' eating defined by the weight loss organization.

Recovering the principle of permission from the weight loss group and mindful of the ways in which the victimization of food encourages a forgetfulness of others (i.e. of our dependency on the planet, on the workers that produce our food and on other eaters who also must eat to survive), I now suggest that sensible eating is characterized by the two interconnected ethical dynamics and relational practices of 'taste' and 'touch'. As virtues and political postures, these operate to unite food justice with a joyful celebration of pleasure.

Permission to Taste

When we speak of taste in relation to the objects of food and drink we speak about 'gustatory' taste – about our sensory experience of food.[84] Carolyn Korsmeyer explains that gustatory taste has been neglected in philosophical thought through virtue of its association with the feminine and the temporal. Set in opposition to the superior eternal and masculine which has been more readily aligned with the higher sense of sight, taste is more readily associated with the subjectivity of pleasure.[85] Taste concerns our personal dispositions and preferences as they relate to food. It suggests a careful discernment of food for to taste is not simply to eat but to notice and to savour. As such, Korsmeyer argues that taste carries an 'inescapable affective valence [since …] tasting involves registering the sensation as pleasant or unpleasant'.[86] It inevitably has to do with our own judgement about the quality of our sensory experience.[87]

In the group, many are distrustful of taste. Whether the flavour of crisps or the pleasurable consumption of creamy sauces, taste is considered by women to pose a threat to their good intentions and to hinder their weight loss efforts. In this schema women are not meant to be led by taste. As well as repeating the theological tendency and Western philosophical inclination to render the appetite dangerous, the distrust of taste in the group trains women to question their judgement through an association with Syn. Taste, however, need not lend

---

84. Korsmeyer, *Making Sense of Taste*, 38.
85. Ibid., 37–50.
86. Ibid., 41.
87. Ibid.

ideological support to the theological depiction of the bodily senses as 'lower' dimensions of the self. It is not inconsequential that the psalmist impassionedly implores us to 'taste and see that the Lord is good' (Ps. 34.8). Here we are reminded that the pleasurable sensation of food speaks of the manifold splendour and goodness of God in creation and that fullness of life is more than 'God's love made nurture for us',[88] it is God's love made *taste* for us.[89] We know God by eating and tasting God, and this is a sacramental principle communicated by Jesus's food ministry where God's kin-dom is consumed and by the Eucharistic ministry of the church.

The notion of eating God, however, exposes why taste is so dangerous. Unlike sight and sound, taste requires that food enter into the body, blurring the boundaries between the outer and inner, between the object of perception and the perceiver. Eating is 'an experience of extreme nearness, even intimacy', says Angel F. Méndez Montoya, because it transfigures both the food and our bodies.[90] We cannot eat without tasting, and by tasting our food is changed into sensation as well as calories, proteins, vitamins and so on, and our bodies are changed as well. We literally become the food we eat and taste as the borders between our food and our bodies disappear. If we know God by eating and tasting God, then the boundary between God and us breaks down.

The enabling and creative power of taste and its ability to trouble the borders between God and sensual bodies is clearly seen in the Eden narrative. Here desire is not absent. God places in the garden 'every tree that is pleasant to the sight and good for food' (Gen. 2.9) and the attractiveness of the tree and its fruit prompts Eve to eat. She sees that the tree is 'good for food', 'a delight to the eyes' and 'to be desired to make one wise' (Gen. 3.6). God gives food that is attractive. Eve's desire for this food is enabling much like Syn in the group allows women to develop new capacities. It causes her eyes to be opened and to know good and evil – something the serpent accurately predicts (Gen. 3.5), the narrator confirms (Gen. 3.7) and God later acknowledges (Gen. 3.22). Food and pleasure lead to new knowledge and increased (god-like) capabilities exposing the productive and creative power of pleasure. Not only does Eve's eating lead to *'apotheosis'* – 'the possession of knowledge that

---

88. Ibid.
89. Wirzba, *Food & Faith*, xii, xiii.
90. Montoya, *The Theology of Food*, 1–4.

transforms what it means to be human'[91] – this knowledge that troubles the boundary between divinity and humanity[92] is gained through food and by Eve choosing to taste for herself. Thus as French feminist, literary critic and philosopher Hélène Cixous suggests, the story tells us that 'knowledge could begin with the mouth, the discovery of the taste of something … . Knowledge and taste go together.'[93] Eve exposes an economy of pleasure-desire that stands in opposition to the absolute prohibition of God's command.[94] The fruit is 'invested with every kind of power'[95] she says; it symbolizes Eve's 'yes'.

God, then, is not just a word on our tongues but food in our bellies and pleasure between our lips. In the story, God may have banished the primordial pair from the Garden afraid that they may make an already dangerous situation worse by further increasing their God-likeness by eating from the tree of life and living forever, but this punishment speaks more about God's jealousy than anything else.[96] By tasting and choosing to follow her own appetite, Eve becomes the subject of her own destiny and an autonomous person. This reveals taste and self-permission as powerful features of an economy of oral pleasure.

To practise an ethic of taste is to see our own opening to pleasure and the pleasure of others as a dangerous, enabling point of connection with God and as a source of knowledge. As with Eve, taste has the potential to trouble boundaries that lock women out of power. Her eating shows initiative and intentionality and like some women in the slimming group, she chooses for herself and is prepared to risk that there may be more to be had through tasting that which is forbidden than from renouncing. Eve shows that taste is a source of female power,

---

91. Sawyer, 'Hidden Subjects', 313.

92. Ken Stone argues that the Eden story may not be so much about accurately naming the origin of sin and evil in the world as it is about 'working out the distinctions between humankind and the divine'. See Stone, *Practicing Safer Texts*, 38.

93. Hélène Cixous, 'The Author in Truth', in *'Coming to Writing' and Other Essays*, ed. Deborah Jenson, trans. Sarah Cornell, Deborah Jenson, Ann Liddle and Susan Sellers (London and Cambridge: Cambridge University Press, 1991), 151.

94. According to Cixous, desire and prohibition co-exist in Eden as 'opposing currents'. Ibid., 149.

95. Ibid., 151.

96. Ibid., 152.

self-development, knowledge and transformation and that through opening our bodies to pleasure and to one another's pleasure, we hold in our mouths the power to change the world.

Permission to Touch

In Christianity, touch has been approached with a similar degree of fear. Eve symbolizes the danger of touch when she adds the prohibition to not 'touch' the fruit from the Tree of Knowledge (Gen. 3.3) to God's original command to not 'eat' from this forbidden source (Gen. 2.17). It would seem that Eve understands that touch as well as taste is bad for her, so hands off! Of course, traditional Christian thought has considered it rather unwholesome for women to touch themselves sexually. Sex, like food, is not principally for pleasure but for survival (i.e. procreation) so masturbation, much like eating for pleasure, is sin.[97]

We have seen how Jesus displays a healing ministry of touch, astonishing those around him by touching the bodies of people society shuns or views as less worthy, including the bodies of women, children, the sick and the poor.[98] He also makes himself available to be touched and is enriched by tactile friendship with others who become 'food for his own soul'.[99] It is through the courageous touching of Jesus that the woman with the issue with blood is healed (Mk 5.25-34) and that the woman who interrupts Jesus's eating with the Pharisee to bathe, kiss and anoint his body is forgiven.[100] The place of food in his ministry with the poor also foregrounds eating as a practice of touch. When Jesus eats with outcasts, he touches those deemed untouchable and demonstrates a willingness to be touched by them, specifically by the food they prepare and/or share. The touch of Jesus, exercised through food, is a fleshy and loving touch that brings fullness and life. It has an affective quality, appraising bodies as feeling bodies. If the ministry of Jesus shows us anything, it is that touch has the potential to heal distorted

---

97. Julia Collings suggests that in Christianity, 'no sin is greater than the desire to masturbate (masturbation *itself* being completely out of the question)'. Collings cited in Chris Greenough, *Undoing Theology: Life Stories from Non-Normative Christians* (London: SCM, 2018), 133.

98. For more, see Elizabeth Moltmann-Wendel, *I Am My Body*, 63–78.

99. Coleman, 'Sacrifice, Surrogacy and Salvation', 210.

100. For more, see John Hull, *The Tactile Heart: Blindness and Faith* (London: SCM, 2013), 3 and Moltmann-Wendel, *I Am My Body*, 64.

relations. His touch performs a reconciliatory function, returning untouchable bodies to participation in society, healing divisions and splits that victimize and harm.[101]

Sensible eating foregrounds tactility once again reminding us that we feel the world through our skin. However, this is not simply a physical mode of tactility. To practice an ethic of touch in relation to food is not simply to respectfully hold food in our hands, for example, or to avoid rushing to throw it in the bin. It also means to be touched and moved by our encounter with food and so to connect with our emotions.[102] Touch unites the physical, spiritual and emotional. It is what Emily Pennington calls a 'thoroughly embodied language', for through touching we experience the world and one another.[103] When we touch our food, we reach out towards it with thanksgiving and delight, embracing what we eat as created and gifted by God. In allowing our bodies to touch and be changed by food – to be emotionally moved and physically and psychologically transformed by our embodied encounter with it – we receive God's abundant life into our bodies and God's affirmation of our existence. In a world where food is victimized and our bodyselves are divided, this kind of touch can require courage, but the New Testament shows what courageous touch can achieve. In Mk 5.25-34, the woman with the issue of blood dares to touch Jesus's garment and her boldness (like the impertinence of Eve) leads to a share in God's power in defiance of the politics of domination. The unnamed woman in the story immediately feels in her body that she has been healed (5.29). By keeping faith with our food rather than seeking to control and dominate it, we too open ourselves to receive Christ's affirmation that our faith has made us well (5.34).

The practice of touch also determines that eating for pleasure need not mean eating lavishly in ways that fail to acknowledge the impact of privileged foodways on the incomes and livelihoods of the poor or on their capacity to access safe and nutritious food. Touch reminds us that

---

101. For more on this, see Wayne Morris, 'Christian Salvations in a Multi-Faith World: Challenging the Cult of Normalcy', in *Alternative Salvations*, 121-31.

102. Sara Ahmed comments that the word 'emotion' comes from the Latin, *emovere*, meaning 'to move, to move out'. Ahmed, *The Cultural Politics of Emotion*, 11.

103. Emily Pennington, *Feminist Eschatology: Embodied Futures* (Abingdon, Oxon and New York: Routledge, 2017), 173.

our private eating and drinking has global significance and so drives us towards one another. As Carter Heyward reflects,

> *Touching* is a primary relational need. As a sensual, erotic pleasure, it is a life-affirming dimension of human experience. ... We must learn to touch and be touched if we want to respect the needs of our common body. We need to touch and be touched.[104]

According to Heyward, when we reach out and bridge the gaps between ourselves and others, 'God comes to life in the act of reaching, of touching, of bridging'.[105] God is birthed by our right and mutual relating to one another such that 'without our touching, there is no God'.[106] This mode of relating does not simply comprise of reciprocity, for Heyward, but a commitment to share power among ourselves and shape the future together.[107] According to her, our sensory connection with the world is predicated on an innate yearning for connection. This innate desire is the raw power and passion for mutual relation – *dunamis* – that Jesus embodies in his life and ministry.[108] It is a creative, sexual power, a power that 'carries us into lovemaking with our partners, but is moreover present and active in all creative, mutually empowering relations'.[109] This innate erotic passion for connection is a power she identifies as divine: God is erotic power/the power of connection, she claims, and whenever we respect as holy and sacred the power of our embodied yearnings and those of others, we make God present: we 'god'.[110]

This rendering of the divine unites our encounter with one another to our relating to God, but it is weakened by the way it reduces God to the power of right relation. I believe Heyward falls into the trap that Ruether's critics align with her hamartiology, namely, that of removing God's transcendence and difference. Heyward affords no distinction

---

104. Heyward, *Touching Our Strength*, 148–9.

105. Heyward, *Our Passion for Justice*, 140.

106. Carter Heyward, *The Redemption of God: A Theology of Mutual Relation* (Eugene: Wipf & Stock, 2010), 172.

107. Heyward, *Touching Our Strength*, 104 and 34.

108. Heyward, *The Redemption of God*, 36–54.

109. Heyward, *Our Passion for Justice*, 247.

110. Ibid., 140. Heyward maintains that 'to god' is to love God in the act of loving humanity.

between God and the power of right relation, and this leaves it unclear as to how God can touch and be touched by others.[111] Nevertheless, she does show that touch signals a relational kind of pleasure – 'Life cannot be lived in front of a mirror', she rightly warns, 'unless it is to be lived in a distorted, ultimately evil way'.[112] Touch signals exactly this kind of relationality – not just my pleasure but yours as well.

To practise a relation of touch, I propose, means to eat in ways that sustain the environment and other bodies, rather than in ways that impoverish them. 'Only together, in mutual relation, is there any common personal power, any love, any actual God,' says Heyward.[113] This is a thoroughly incarnational principle for it reminds us that God touches and is touched by bodies, that when we respect as sacred our own bodies and those of others, including the body of the world, we celebrate God as flesh and touch the body of Christ. It is also a thoroughly Trinitarian principle because when we relate mutually to one another we live into the Trinitarian image of God. As a community of love where Creator, Redeemer and Sustainer eternally touch one another, and as a community of persons eternally affected by bodies and by the body of the world,[114] God is not equivalent to the sum of our creations, as Heyward infers. Rather, while God is always made flesh through our interdependent mutual touching, God is always more than this as well.

Modelling the Trinity and the inclusive food practices of Jesus, the relational notion of touch is a political virtue and corporate activity.

---

111. If God is equivalent to right relation – or what Heyward terms 'erotic power' – then there is insufficient space between individuals and God for this kind of advance or encounter. My critique here is influenced by Irigaray and her view of 'wonder'. For more of this, see my article, 'What's Right with the Trinity? Thinking the Trinity in Relation to Irigaray's Notions of Self-love and Wonder', *Feminist Theology* 15, no. 2 (2007): 220–35. Also see my book, *What's Right with the Trinity?*, 173–96. Marjorie Suchocki agrees suggesting that 'God appears to be solely the empowering relationality of egalitarian human community'. See her essay, 'God, Sexism and Transformation', in *Reconstructing Christian Theology*, ed. Rebecca S. Chopp and Mark Lewis Taylor (Minneapolis: Fortress, 1994), 40.
112. Heyward, *Touching Our Strength*, 142.
113. Heyward, *Our Passion for Justice*, 167.
114. For more on this, see my book, *What's Right with the Trinity?*, 112–15.

It energizes the hope of transformation and the drive for politics,[115] living out the love of neighbour that Jesus calls those who love God to perform.[116] As a practice underpinned by a view of pleasure as a *shared* encounter, touch is not selfish or bent on possession and consummation of the other. When we touch our food we acknowledge that eating connects us to our friends, families and religious communities who eat with us, to the farmer and food producer, to the distributer, the marketers, to the sea, land and sky, the animals and the Creator who gives food for all. With feminist philosopher, Luce Irigaray, I maintain that touch is not an anaesthetic ethic that divides and separates but one that joins. It does not seize the other's pleasure but suggests an openness to it: 'What affects you, what affects me, as well. I participate in your affections, just as you take pleasure in mine.'[117]

Touch describes an affective relation to food, other bodies and the world whereby we approach our eating as an expansion of ourselves and as an openness to others. It challenges the taken-for-grantedness of food and calls us to see our broken relationship with it as something that does not have to be. It also involves the body in an unfolding towards other bodies that refuses to take others for granted. Understood this way, touch is a value that moves us not only to care about one another's needs but also to respect each other's bodies as passionate, sensual bodies that have the capacity to feel the world deeply. This seems absolutely crucial at a time when around 795 million people are undernourished worldwide, with the majority of these living in developing regions.[118] This amounts to just over one in nine people across the globe.[119] The problem is not simply that there is not enough food to go around but that access to food is uneven. Wide differences between regions around the world mean that some have better access to food than others. An ethic of

---

115. Ibid., 181.

116. Mt. 22.35-40; Mk 12.28-34.

117. Luce Irigaray, *Elemental Passions*, trans. Joanne Collie and Judith Still (New York: Routledge, 1992), 58.

118. Food and Agriculture Organization of the United Nations, 'The State of Food Insecurity in the World. Strengthening the Enabling Environment for Food Security and Nutrition' (2014), http://www.fao.org/3/a-i4030e.pdf (accessed 12 July 2017), 10–12. According to the report, Southern Asia and Sub-Saharan Africa account for substantially larger shares of global undernourishment. In Sub-Saharan Africa, one in four people are estimated to be undernourished.

119. Ibid., 8–9.

touch drives us to care about who has the ability and economic means to get their hands on nutritious food and to quite literally touch it and feel it for themselves.[120] It challenges first-world overconsumption that impacts the ability of others to eat and impoverishes the environment, while demanding better quality food for the poor and more equitable food distribution so that all can eat with passion, joy and pleasure. Touch requires not self-denial but a full-fleshed connection with our food and a passionate desire for food justice.[121]

Food, Feminist Theology and Affect

As a feminist Christian praxis that foregrounds pleasure and joy, sensible eating emphasizes the place of emotion and bodily experience in a feminist theology of food. Reflective of the so-called turn to affect, it extends existing feminist theological emphases on embodiment and emotion[122] to present a distinctive account of how feeling and sense relate to our foodways. In feminist theology, the subject of emotion

---

120. One report claims that even among privileged nations in the West, food insecurity hits minority groups the hardest. See Alisha Coleman-Jensen, Matthew P. Rabbitt, Christian A. Gregory and Anita Singh, 'Household Food Security in the United States in 2015', Economic Research Report no. 215 (2016), https://www.ers.usda.gov/webdocs/publications/79761/err-215.pdf?v=42636 (accessed 5 May 2017). In the United States alone, food insecurity in 2015 was substantially higher than the national average among black non-Hispanic and Hispanic households (15).

121. Also see Lisa Isherwood's description of the 'Fat Jesus' in her book, *The Fat Jesus*, 134.

122. The methodological principle of feminist theologies to value women's experiences as sacred situates embodiment centrally in Christian feminist thought. As such, embodiment has been a key theme in feminist theology from its inception. Of particular influence to me has been the work of Elisabeth Moltmann-Wendel and her view that a theology of embodiment 'seeks to give people once again the courage to use their senses …, to stand by themselves and their experiences and accept themselves with their bodies, to love them, to trust them and their understanding, and to see themselves as children of this earth, indissolubly bound up with it'. See *I Am My Body*, 104. She sees the Jesus of the New Testament relating to bodies in their totality and perceives the healing narratives as testifying to the transformative power of touch.

has been engaged by a number of scholars. As well as challenging the classical tradition of divine *apatheia*,[123] feminist theologians have recovered emotions like anger that have been disparaged and viewed as a threat to God's holy order. For Beverly Harrison, emotions reveal our moral relation to each other; 'The failure to live deeply in "our bodies, ourselves" destroys the possibility for moral relations between us.'[124] She believes that all knowledge is mediated through the body and through our sensuality; hence, we can only know and value the world through the sensible body. Feeling, for Harrison, is 'the basic bodily ingredient which mediates our connectedness to the world'. When we cut ourselves off from feeling, we cut ourselves off from connection with others. 'All power, including intellectual power, is rooted in feeling,' she maintains. 'If we are not perceptive in discerning our feelings, or if we do not know what we feel, we cannot be effective as moral agents.'[125]

The emphasis Harrison, like Lorde, places on feeling as a point of connection is echoed in the account of sensible eating I have proposed, reinforcing emotion and the intellect as important modes of relating to the self, world and one another. However, for Harrison, feelings are never an end in themselves because 'there are no right or wrong feelings'.[126] Morality has to do with acts rather than feelings; hence,

---

123. Elizabeth Johnson, for example, resists the tradition of divine *apatheia* by understanding the suffering of God as an act of love that freely overflows in compassion. For Johnson, God's suffering is active rather than passive; God suffers freely as an act of love that is expressive of God's infinite capacity for solidarity. In a way reminiscent of Jürgen Moltmann, she presents divine suffering as an excellence in God rather than as an imperfection. For more, see Johnson, *She Who Is*, 265–6. Also see Anastasia Philippa Scrutton, *Thinking through Feeling: God, Emotion and Passibility* (London and New York: Bloomsbury, 2011).

124. Beverly Harrison, *Our Right to Choose: Toward a New Ethic of Abortion* (Boston: Beacon Press, 1983), 13.

125. Beverly Harrison, 'The Power of Anger in the Work of Love: Christian Ethics for Women and Other Strangers', in *Making the Connections*, ed. C. S. Robb (Boston: Beacon Press, 1985), 13. Harrison claims that anger is a 'feeling-signal' that our relation with others or the world is not as it should be and is creative in driving us towards action (ibid., 14). For more on feminist theology and anger, see Kathleen Fischer, *Transforming Fire: Women Using Fire Creatively* (New York: Paulist Press, 2000).

126. Harrison, 'The Power of Anger', 14.

the moral question is not 'what do I feel' but 'what do I do with what I feel?'[127] But this may understate the close and complex relationship between feeling and action. Feeling, after all, can unleash destructive forces in women's lives and the lives of others, and this makes it difficult and dangerous to empty feeling of moral content.[128] It is not, as Lorde implies, that everything the body feels is good. Following our deepest cravings has the potential to destroy sources of food, the earth and our friendship with it. Our tastes and pleasures can violate our connectedness by pummelling the earth and by disfiguring our relationships with ourselves and with other bodies. As Kathleen Sands challenges, pleasure can arise even in situations of violence and exploitation.[129] Eating and not eating can harm the body, and the bodies of others, making them sick, hungry and desperate. Rooting sensible eating in an attentiveness to feeling, then, needs to appreciate that although sensuality can be trusted, like any spiritual resource it must be open to scrutiny and critical testing. Feeling is not a neutral or innocent foundation upon which to root a feminist theology of food. It is not a 'basic bodily ingredient', as Harrison claims, nor an innate erotic passion, as Heyward implies, immune from the influence of culture and from the patriarchal codifications of gender and sexuality. What we feel is determined by contact with others and influenced by discourse.

This is one of the difficulties with the so-called turn to affect in recent critical theory. In this literature, the notion of 'affect' has been embraced as a way to rethink the body–mind dualism and to foreground the sensual ways of being in and understanding the world.[130] Among its proponents, affect is usually championed as a challenge to the linguistic turn represented by poststructuralist and deconstructionist thought.

---

127. Ibid.

128. Judith Plaskow makes this point in 'Finding a God I can believe in', in *Goddess and God in the World: Conversations in Embodied Theology*, ed. Carol P. Christ and Judith Plaskow (Minneapolis: Fortress Press, 2016), 107–30. It is a danger Kathleen Sands also debates in her article, 'Uses of the Thea(o)logian: Sex and Theodicy in Religious Feminism', *Journal of Feminist Studies in Religion* 8, no. 1 (1992): 7–33.

129. Sands, 'Uses of the Thea(o)logian', 15.

130. Marianne Liljeström and Susanna Paasonen, 'Introduction: Feeling Differences – Affect and Feminist Reading', in *Working with Affect in Feminist Readings: Disturbing Differences*, ed. Marianne Liljeström and Susanna Paasonen (London and New York: Routledge, 2010), 1.

For Patricia Clough, the affective turn is a movement towards the body that marks a 'substantive shift' in critical theory, returning cultural criticism to bodily matter rather than erasing it through linguistic construction.[131] Affect, she suggests, is an 'imperceptible dynamism' which is immanent to bodily matter.[132] For Brian Massumi, affect is an indeterminate bodily response out of which conscious emotion is subtracted.[133] It has to do with intensity and is not ownable whereas emotion is 'intensity owned and recognized'.[134] For him, affect evades social construction and precedes conscious states of perception.

Understood this way, affect is distinguished from emotion as that which is spontaneous, non-cognitive and bodily physical.[135] As well as repeating the mind–body dualism, this description of affect appears to demarcate a space outside of social signification that is unconditioned by social structures. The image we receive is of an 'untrammelled ontological'[136] out of which our cognitive feelings arise. Cognisant of this difficulty, my understanding of feeling resists a bifurcation between bodily sensation and emotion and between the spontaneous–non-cognitive–physical and the voluntary–intentional–intellectual. It also troubles the related theological split between the sensitive and intellective self upheld by some classical theologies. Sensible eating necessarily attends to bodily sensation and the emotions as integrated features of

---

131. Patricia T. Clough, 'The Affective Turn: Political Economy, Biomedia and Bodies', *Theory, Culture and Society* 25, no. 1 (2008): 1.

132. Ibid., 2.

133. Brian Massumi, *Parables of the Virtual: Movement, Affect, Sensation* (Durham and London: Duke University Press, 2002). Drawing on a neuroscientific experiment that claims to show half a second delay between a body's reaction to stimulus and conscious awareness of the event (195), Massumi suggests that affect is 'never-to-be-conscious' and 'automatic' (25).

134. Ibid., 28.

135. As Clara Fischer argues, by separating the material from the cognitive, and privileging spontaneous impulses over the mind, language and cognition, a wedge is again driven between mind and matter, and a 'reductive physicalist model' produced that tenders 'impoverished metaphysical conceptions of emotion, cognition, and embodiment'. See her article, 'Feminist Philosophy, Pragmatism, and the "Turn to Affect": A Genealogical Critique', *Hypatia* 31, no. 4 (2016): 815.

136. Clare Hemmings, 'Invoking Affect. Cultural Theory and the Ontological Turn', *Cultural Studies* 19, no. 5 (2005): 559.

our embodiment. Feeling has intellectual, emotional, physical, social and discursive components. It can indicate physiological sensation and feelings experienced by the mind, without having to divide the two. Emotion and sense accompany one another.

Sensible eating also resists the distinction Augustine makes between the passive movement of the 'lower' sensory appetite (the *passiones*) and the superior active movement of the rational will (the *affectiones*).[137] Influenced by Paul, Augustine holds that the passions are involuntary movements of the mind that are not subject to reason.[138] Associated with the lusts and desires of the lower self, they are linked with sin and conceived as potential threats to God's harmonious (i.e. rational) order.[139] To follow one's passions is to act in ways that are contrary to reason and to disobey God. I suggest, however, that to eat with feeling and sense involves apprehending our sensory impulses and psychological responses to food and intentionally and rationally choosing to welcome our appetitive desires and passions. Contrary to Augustine, to orient the will towards the sensory appetite and to assent to our passions without apology can mean to orient the will rightly not wrongly, towards God and our God-formed capacity for pleasure. To eat sensibly is a sensitive and intellective performance that places the body and mind, self and sensuality back together.[140]

---

137. See Anastasia Scrutton's discussion of Augustine and his treatment of the passions in *Thinking through Feeling*, esp. 37.

138. Ibid., 15.

139. Ibid., 17.

140. It is worth mentioning Julian of Norwich at this point since she stresses the need for our 'substance' and 'sensuality' to be integrated. Whereas substance designates the essence of the self which is always united with God, sensuality depicts the life of the senses and the mind. Jesus shares not only our substance, being united with God, but also our sensuality. In him, substance and sensuality are harmonized. For Julian, we are only whole when our body and sensuality are integrated into our spirituality. See Grace Jantzen's discussion of Julian in *Power, Gender and Christian Mysticism* (Cambridge and New York and Melbourne: Cambridge University Press, 1995), 146–56. Also see Julian of Norwich, *Revelations of Divine Love: Short Text and Long Text*, trans. Elizabeth Spearing (London: Penguin, 1998). This strikes a very different note to Augustine who considers that the appetitive soul forces the rational soul to exercise mastery over 'the turbulent passions of the lower parts of the soul by directing and controlling them'. Augustine, 'City of God', IX.6.

Feeling and taste are, however, culturally situated, socially and economically positioned and normed by a myriad of intersecting discourses to do with gender, ethnicity, sexuality, class, dis/ability and nation. To attach eating to feeling may, then, appear to overlook the social constructedness of affect and validate feelings shaped by the distorted patterns of relationship previously named as 'sin'. Connecting with our deepest feelings may after all mean welcoming feelings of guilt and shame which are often attached to women's eating. To embrace shame, however, does not have women give up suffering and self-negation and so engage in touching the erotic; rather, it embeds our bodies more deeply within the sacrificial economy that drives us to destroy ourselves. Given this, it is again crucial to remember that feeling must be open to critical examination. Yet, if our emotional responses to food can be informed by fields of meaning that dictate how we ought to eat, then this also suggests that our emotions are not always beyond our control.

Alison Jaggar argues that 'mature human emotions are neither instinctive nor biologically determined. ... Like everything else that is human, emotions in part are socially constructed; like all social constructs, they are historical products, bearing the marks of the society that constructed them.'[141] Emotions are not pre-social even if we experience them as 'gut reactions', she argues. To suggest as such would be to consider that there is no alternative way of living and feeling when we know that it is possible to engage in 'mechanistic behaviour-modification techniques' that sensitize or desensitize our feeling responses and in 'cognitive techniques designed to help us to think differently about situations'.[142] When women in the slimming group feel 'bad' or ashamed when they eat various foods, this is shaped by gendered fields of meaning that dictate how and what 'good' women should eat. Yet, as an example of a 'mechanistic behaviour-modification technique',[143] the slimming process shows that feelings and gut reactions, even physical tastes, can be remodelled and reshaped. Sensible eating parodies this logic but asserts the possibility of being able to live more peacefully and passionately around food without having to apologize.

---

141. Alison M. Jaggar, 'Love and Knowledge: Emotion in Feminist Epistemology', *Inquiry* 32, no. 2 (1989): 179.
142. Ibid., 172.
143. Ibid.

To eat with sense then is not a form of 'intuitive eating'[144] that suggests that our bodies have natural cues that can be followed independent of culture, our own experience, class status and so on. It is not the 'natural knowing' Mary Daly describes in which women know through recalling and rediscovering their 'Original', 'Elemental potency', by reconnecting with their 'instinct, intuition, [and] passion'.[145] It does not hold to such an undifferentiated model of gender essentialism or assume our bodies are passive receptors of knowledge that give us unmediated access to the world around us or to ultimate (or elemental) 'truth'. The body at the centre of sensible eating is not the 'organic body' of Harrison and Daly or the body 'as is'.[146] The body as a feeling body is a 'subversive body'[147] that has the potential to destabilize established orthodoxies by performing counter-cultural behaviours. Feeling and sense are informed by normative injunctions and an atmosphere of evil that trains women to fear their tastes, but the notion of sensible eating recognizes our tastes and bodily desires are not beyond the bounds of change. In the instances where feelings of guilt and shame plague our foodways or where the love and joy of food has left us, we can perform embodied alternatives.

Of course, being able to perceive the senses and consciously observe feeling is a cognitive process. This raises the question of whether sensible eating assumes an able body and homogenizes women's experience of sense. At the start of his book, *The Tactile Heart*, John Hull observes that 'the beauties of touch are, I suppose, largely hidden from many

---

144. The Health at Every Size movement speaks about 'intuitive eating' in this way. See Linda Bacon and Lucy Aphramor, 'Weight Science: Evaluating the Evidence for a Paradigm Shift', *Nutrition Journal* 10, no. 9 (2011): 1–13, https ://www.ncbi.nlm.nih.gov/pmc/articles/PMC3041737/pdf/1475-2891-10-9.pdf (accessed 10 October 2016), and Health at Every Size, http://haescommunity.com/(accessed 10 October 2016).

145. Daly, *Pure Lust*, 7.

146. Marcella Althaus-Reid, '"Pussy, Queen of Pirates": Acker, Isherwood and the Debate on the Body in Feminist Theology', *Feminist Theology* 12, no. 2 (2004): 158.

147. Jane Barter Moulaison presents the 'organic' and 'subversive' body as two types of body which have been theorized within feminist theology. See her article, '"Our bodies, Our Selves?" The Body as Source in Feminist Theology', 342–9.

sighted people'.[148] Recalling his own experience of becoming blind, he explains that those who lose their sight must learn again to *do* with their hands now that the eye has been separated from the hand, to *know* with their fingers rather than through processes of visualization and to discover 'tactile beauty'. He argues that for blind people, beauty is more intimate and concrete – 'we rediscover the loveliness of cups and saucers' and the 'feel of human hair',[149] and a key feature of this tactile beauty is the experience of immediate surprise and the capacity to be surprised by joy. This, he says, is a feature of tactile beauty only accessible to the blind.

The concept of 'sensible eating', similarly, allows that bodies will feel and sense in various ways. In foregrounding the sensible, I do not presume that women who have access to all of their senses are more adept at sensible eating, it simply insists that there is no place outside the eating and drinking body to which we can escape in order to know the world or God. Recalling Gebara's words, we hear again that our bodies provide the first (although not last) word about salvation and hope. Sensible eating expresses that God and the world are known through, in and as bodies, but it does not claim that all bodies know through their flesh and sensuality in the same way. This approach to food is not a universal fix, nor is it appropriate for all women, but it is one redemptive praxis that may resonate with some, who – like women in the weight loss group – find themselves using their intellective capacities to wage war against their appetites.

Conclusion

Eating with sense is an alimentary performance that recovers from the weight loss group the association of eating with the cultivation of self-care. Extending the significance of permission and self-authorization practised by some women in the slimming community, this approach to food invites women to attach their eating to their emotions and sensations and to consume in ways that are attentive to pleasure. Sensible eating is an erotic Christian practice of self-responsibility. It amplifies the transgressive features of slimming glimpsed in the group where women use the permission the organization promotes to transgress the

---

148. Hull, *The Tactile Heart*, 1–2.
149. Ibid., 3.

plan's precepts and eat what is forbidden without apology. To eat with sense means to engage our tastes and refuse to sanitize our appetites. This reveals the dangerous power of women's oral pleasure to transgress gendered codes of decency around food and to shape subjectivities that resist compliance with hegemonic norms. As in the weight loss group and in historic Christian asceticism, food is a way for women to cultivate their own capacities and reorient themselves. Women resist the victimization of food by validating their own sensible bodies as sites of divine revelation, knowledge and insight.

Salvation is a fleshy and 'foody' enterprise. Rather than being confined to another world or imagined as paradise elsewhere, it is the daily 'meaningful work' of eating with feeling, made present through the relational, alimentary and affective practices of 'touch' and 'taste'. Sensible eating calls us to locate our freedom and fullness – our wellness and aliveness – in a hearty full-bodied, sensual appraisal of pleasure. It is a practice of permission that has the potential to help repair the fractures and breaks that characterize distorted modes of relating to food. It is also reconciliatory work, concerned with intentionally joining our eating and feeling back together. In continuity with Jesus's ministry of food, sensible eating refuses to separate relation to others from a joyful encounter with food because the politics of pleasure and justice combine to mutually shape one another. The call to attend to feeling is a call to eat in community and to build communities of inclusion through food.

This makes sensible eating a particular mission for the church as it fulfils its service to God by pursuing the work of reconciliation in the world. The church fulfils a prophetic role of calling the world away from sin towards an unbounded delight in God. The importance of forging communities of solidarity in pursuit of a shared goal is clearly glimpsed in the weight loss group, and I will say more in the next chapter about how this might be recycled to resist the sin of sizeism. We have seen how the slimming community enables women to cultivate genuine friendships and social bonds that encourage them to persist in the face of failure, suffering and frustration. The church as a Eucharistic (foody) community provides a similar revolutionary context for the forging of alternative embodiments and for the particular practice of sensible eating. This is a more rebellious celebration of food than a wafer of bread and a sip of wine. It tasks the church with nurturing the alimentary and relational practices of touch and taste and with providing contexts where women can return to their bodies as sites of joy and divine presence. United in a commitment to celebrate food and the pleasure it brings as a gift from God, Christian communities can be important contexts where the stylized act of sensible eating can be cultivated and where women in particular can make public their pain, worries, joys and frustrations around food without being returned to the cycles of compulsory confession, self-denial and self-sacrifice that harm their flesh. Sensible eating is an intentional and reflective practice of 'micro-salvation' that has the potential to help heal the tears in our relationship with food and to contribute to the larger, political project of building God's future on earth so that all may eat with laughter and delight.

Chapter 6

RETHINKING SALVATION: SABBATH AND FAT PRIDE

Chapter 5 presented food practices as an important site of salvation and as a means through which sin might be resisted. This chapter proposes that a Sabbath sensibility may challenge the relentless work of terrorizing fat, inviting women who habitually strive to escape their size to rest from their labour. Jewish and Christian traditions have long since suggested that wellness, fullness and aliveness are cultivated through the observance of Sabbath. Rest from activity and endless productivity is a divine instruction intended to allow creatures and the land to be rejuvenated. In an extension of this principle, I suggest that repose from the work of frenetically patrolling fat and from the totalitarian project of seeking mastery over it is an opportunity to break with the cycles and systems of sin. By living the Sabbath, salvation again comes to be accessible through life rather than death, in this world rather than in a future perfect world to come. As a performance of salvation and as a pathway to women's flourishing, Sabbath living has the potential to resist the stifling politics of sizeism. Specifically, I suggest that fat pride can be theologically understood as a refusal to keep the body submerged in hiding, being one way for diversely situated women of various sizes to live the Sabbath and bring their bodies and their fat out into the open. Fat pride is a radical Sabbath witness in a fat-hating world.

The Meanings of Sabbath

Sabbath has multiple meanings in the Bible. Genesis tells us that on the seventh day God finished the work of creation by resting (Gen. 2.2). In Exodus, God meets the daily needs of the Israelites in the wilderness, supplying manna from heaven and giving twice as much on the sixth day so that the people can rest on the seventh (Exod. 16.22-30). The Sabbath command to work for six days and rest on the seventh forms part of the Ten Commandments set out in Exodus 20 and 34 and Deuteronomy

5 and corresponds to the concepts of the Sabbath year and the year of Jubilee. According to the Hebrew Bible, every seventh year was to be a Sabbath year when the land was to rest and to allow the poor and wild animals to eat (Exod. 23.10-12; Lev. 25.1-7). All debts were to be forgiven, freeing individuals from crushing cycles of poverty and creating new opportunities in society for the weak (Deut. 15.1-2). After seven Sabbath years (forty-nine years) Israel was to observe a year of Jubilee when slaves would be freed and land returned to its owner (Lev. 25.8-13), thereby making it difficult to retain wealth generation after generation.[1] The Jubilee was to be a time of liberation and rectification of social relations (Lev. 25.8-55). Sabbath thus protected the vulnerable; it spoke of the concreteness of redemption and of God's liberation of the oppressed.

Fundamentally, the concept of Sabbath conveys the importance of rest for the earth and its inhabitants. The instruction in Deuteronomy (5.12-15) and Exodus (20.8-11; 34.21) tells the people of Israel to work for six days and to rest on the seventh. This command addresses the male heads of households and requires them to ensure that no one works.[2] As it says in Deut. 5.14, 'You shall not do any work – you, or your son or your daughter, or your male or female slave, or your ox or your donkey, or any of your livestock, or the resident alien in your towns, so that your male and female slave may rest as well as you.' The mandate is that all should rest – strangers, animals, masters, slaves, women, men and children. The added variant in Deuteronomy that all should rest 'as well as you' simply stresses the equalizing character of this repose.[3]

In Deuteronomy, the motivation for Sabbath is God's liberating activity in Egypt (Deut. 5.15) whereas in the book of Exodus, Israel is commanded to rest because God rested on the seventh day of creation (Exod. 20.11). Despite this difference, reference to the exodus story is not absent from the Exodus account. Here, the liberation of Israel provides the context for the new regime God initiates: 'I am the Lord your God, who brought you out of the land of Egypt, out of the house of

---

1. Randy Woodley, 'An Indigenous Theological Perspective on Sabbath', *Vision: A Journal for Church and Theology* 16, no. 1 (2015): 65; Norman Wirzba, *Living the Sabbath: Discovering the Rhythms of Rest and Delight* (Grand Rapids: Brazos Press, 2006), 40.

2. Kent Blevins, 'Observing Sabbath', *Review and Expositor* 113, no. 4 (2016): 481.

3. Walter Brueggemann, *Sabbath as Resistance: Saying No to the Culture of Now* (Louisville: Westminster John Knox Press, 2014).

slavery' (Exod. 20.2). The appeal to the experience of slavery invites the people of Israel to remember how God saved them from the exploitative economic conditions of Egypt so that they avoid slavish types of working and ensure that everyone has equal opportunity to rest.

According to Walter Brueggemann, the Israelites would have had the memory of Egypt fresh in their minds and so would have found the instruction to remember the Sabbath foreign and frightening. In Egypt, there was no rest for slaves or for Pharaoh. The slaves would be anxious about meeting the brick quotas while Pharaoh would be worried about staying on top of the exploitative system and about the risk of famine and food shortage.[4] Rest was not only unheard of but also dangerous because the Egyptian system made people a threat to one another.[5] He therefore concludes that the call to rest in Exodus signals a break with patterns of anxiety and '*anxious productivity*'.[6] The reference back to creation and God's own rest serves to show that God is not like Pharaoh: God rests, takes delight in what He makes and is confident in creation. God is not anxiously producing.

For Brueggemann this provides an important challenge to modern capitalism. The practice of Sabbath is an act of resistance to the 'anxiety system' that pervades even our world today, he insists, where endless productivity and work fuel a tireless unease about never having done enough. The instruction to the Israelites in Deuteronomy to keep the Sabbath because God rescued them from slavery suggests that observing the Sabbath is an act of resistance to this anxiety system. It also presents the Sabbath repose as a form of resistance to coercion. God led the people of Israel out of Egypt; this means that the challenge of Sabbath is to remember that this pattern of coercion has been broken; it should be no more. A Sabbath sensibility challenges the cycle of coercive competition typical of the Egyptian system and typical also of capitalist economics, he insists, where there are haves and have-nots, insiders and outsiders. The command to remember the Sabbath is to acknowledge 'equal worth, equal value, equal access, equal rest'.[7]

Brueggemann's analysis is helpful because it communicates the significance of Sabbath for practices of justice. Sabbath living is a form of revolutionary living that deliberately seeks to resist patterns of

4. Ibid., 23, 26–7.
5. Ibid., 26.
6. Ibid., 28. Emphasis in original.
7. Ibid., 41.

anxious productivity and systems of coercion. Observing Sabbath, we can say, is a posture of joy and delight that makes us less frantic, less coerced and 'free to be, rather than to do'.[8] The concept of delight is in fact crucial to the principle of Sabbath. Jewish commentators have suggested that on the seventh day of creation God created *měnûhâ*, '*Tranquillity serenity, peace and repose*'.[9] More than a withdrawal from labour or activity, the notion of *měnûhâ* communicates happiness and stillness, peace and harmony.[10] More specifically, it describes the kind of happiness and harmony that come from things being as they ought to be. God's rest on the seventh day is not akin to burn out, but a deep joy that all that has been made is free to be as God intended it. *Měnûhâ* is God's profound and all-encompassing delight in the splendour of creation and a deep expression of joy. When we experience delight and thanksgiving, we live lives of worship and share in the delight of God;[11] we come to see the world as God sees it, with love, care and joy. This is the very reason for why heaven and earth were created – for rest, joy and delight. According to Jürgen Moltmann, God's rest is God's joyful being there with creation – God's resting presence in all that exists – and this is the whole meaning of God's creative work.[12] On the seventh day, God lets creation exist 'before his face', says Moltmann, and allows it to be what it is.[13] This means that when God rests, God is 'wholly present' with creation and in this repose is fully who God is.[14] It also, however, means that we are never more fully ourselves than when we take joy in our existence, than when in our rest, we are also 'wholly present'.[15]

8. Ibid., 42–3.

9. See *Genesis rabba* 10.9, cited in Abraham J. Heschel, 'A Place in Time', in *The Ten Commandments: The Reciprocity of Faithfulness*, ed. William P. Brown (Louisville and London: Westminster John Knox Press, 2004), 221; Dan B. Allender, *Sabbath*, foreword by Phyllis Tickle (Nashville: Thomas Nelson, 2009), 221. Emphasis in original.

10. Heschel, 'A Place in Time', 221.

11. Wirzba, *Living the Sabbath*, 14.

12. Jürgen Moltmann, 'The Sabbath – The Feast of Creation', *Family Ministry* 14, no. 4 (2000): 38.

13. Jürgen Moltmann, *God in Creation: An Ecological Doctrine of Creation* (London: SCM, 1985), 279. Moltmann suggests that God in this way is like an artist who steps back from their painting in order to allow it to have its own life and integrity. Moltmann, 'The Sabbath – The Feast of Creation', 39.

14. Moltmann, *God in Creation*, 279.

15. Ibid., 285.

We can understand the invitation to move into the Sabbath space, then, as an invitation to return to our bodies with delight. Sabbath living deliberately resists the 'anxiety system' that ensures we never feel good enough and is founded on the faith that when we rest in ourselves and in our rest are wholly present, we live into the image of God.[16] Sabbath calls us towards more just communities, to celebrate our life together as creatures who each live and move in the presence of the Living God. When God finishes creation with the Sabbath rest it is because the goal and end of all that God has made is delight, joy and peace. It is also because God's intention is for all to enjoy this sacred repose before God in harmony with all others. The finishing of creation with rest shows that God does not wish to celebrate creation alone.[17] Ultimately, Sabbath is a shared space and corporate duty. All are to rest without exception, which means we embody Sabbath when we resist the will to dominate.[18]

Sabbath and the Meaningful Work of Salvation

Such an understanding of Sabbath locates it squarely within the drama of salvation because every instance of rest and repose is a movement towards fulfilment and life and thus an example of 'mini-salvation'.[19] To cite Moltmann, Sabbath is the 'feast of redemption', offering a way for creatures to participate in God's eternal presence.[20] Rather than being a passive anticipation of a better world, the principle of Sabbath affirms that our mutual and reciprocal relating celebrate and make flesh God's *měnûhâ* in the here and now. When we rest from anxious productivity and coercion, when we touch our bodies with care and affection, we build the repose which is characteristic of the kin-dom of God, a repose where all will exist in the presence of God's uncontainable pleasure, before the face of God, in God's happiness and peace. It is not inconsequential that Deuteronomy cites the exodus as the reason for keeping the Sabbath whereas Exodus cites creation. This simply highlights the interrelatedness of creation and liberation. The

---

16. Ibid.
17. Jürgen Moltmann, 'Sabbath: Finishing and Beginning', *The Living Pulpit* 7, no. 2 (April–June 1998): 4.
  18. Moltmann, *God in Creation*, 285.
  19. See Chapter 5 for more. Also see Gebara, *Out of the Depths*, 125.
  20. Moltmann, *God in Creation*, 277.

replenishing of all persons outside of exploitative systems can never be inseparable from the relinquishment of anxious productivity that comes with resting in God's creative presence. To be wholly present to ourselves and to move into God's rest means to 'comfort all who mourn … to give them a garland instead of ashes, the oil of gladness instead of mourning, the mantle of praise instead of a faint spirit' (Isa. 61.2-3). To embody Sabbath is, therefore, inseparable from the meaningful work of salvation understood as the struggle for fullness of life for all of God's creatures.[21] It is the hope of creation, a taste of God's redemptive future, the materialization of God's delight.

To relate Sabbath to 'work', however, seems somewhat contradictory given the Sabbath command invites us to cease from our labours. Embracing Sabbath, however, is not equivalent to inactivity. Sabbath does not call us to do nothing. It invites us to rest from our ordinary work and from modes of doing that are exploitative, fraught and harried so that our repose becomes a site of resistance to these exhausting patterns of behaviour. When we enter the Sabbath space, we have room to do and think differently. Sabbath is not empty time but holy time filled with a different kind of work.[22] It is the invitation to engage in '"out of ordinary" activities'[23] that replenish our bodies and cause us to move and breathe more freely. When we embody the Sabbath we inhabit an extraordinary space that resists the distorted relations of domination and participate in God's work of love for creation, cherishing the integrity of all creatures and performing God's generosity and care.[24]

In the Sabbath economy, rest and work feed and nourish one another.[25] The rest we are called to enjoy galvanizes social action and fuels a commitment to work for justice. If all should rest because God is the God of the exodus who freed the people of Israel from exploitation, then the command to remember and sanctify the Sabbath is a call to join with God in the redemptive work of reconciliation and to challenge the coercive politics of domination that encourages restlessness in our bodies. The Sabbath repose energizes meaningful work that contributes

---

21. See Ross Kinsler and Gloria Kinsler, *The Biblical Jubilee and the Struggle for Life: An Invitation to Personal, Ecclesial, and Social Transformation* (Maryknoll: Orbis, 1999).
22. See Blevins, 'Observing Sabbath', 487.
23. Ibid.
24. Wirzba, *Living the Sabbath*, 100.
25. Ibid., 14.

to the quality of life and care of the self, and which is invested in the replenishing of all persons. It is also, however, enabled in the first place by activities and alternative rituals that move us to slow down. Such rituals are practices of delight – Sabbath practices – through which we participate in God's rest and break with patterns of anxiety and slavish productivity. Salvation then is tightly bound to Sabbath as the meaningful work that makes for the Sabbath repose and as the working out of this repose in concrete, everyday life.

At its best, Sabbath is *lived* so that all our activities fall within its own orbit.[26] This denies any straightforward and absolute distinction between rest and the work and activity related to it. Caught up in the drama of salvation where God's love is enjoyed by all and all are free to be, the observance of Sabbath has the potential to transform the world; it depicts a journey towards change. As a productive and generative space characterized by creativity and fecundity, Sabbath is a space of release as opposed to loss or lack. Rather than offering a temporary reprieve from overdoing or burn out which is followed by an inevitable return to the same old anxiety systems and exploitative patterns of labour, it is a space to inhabit which has the potential to enrich the everyday away from frenzied activity. Taking time away from harried patterns of productivity may cause us to notice, sense and feel more deeply and may therefore contribute to the project of sensible living that I began to sketch in the previous chapter. It has the power to transform the mundane and ordinary, to reorient our priorities and integrate all aspects of our embodiment. Sabbath, as a practice of salvation, opens our bodies to feel and sense our worlds more intensely and invites us to celebrate existence 'because existence itself is glorious'.[27]

The living of Sabbath is not another form of frenetic work resourced by an obsession with completion. Wendell Berry is right that the aspiration to 'get away' in order to be at rest can often turn out to fuel another form of anxiety involving us in 'the haste, speed, and noise, the auxiliary pandemonium, of escape'.[28] Sabbath, as I envisage it, however, is not a call to inhabit guilt or repeat the sentiment of the weight loss group that has women only focus on endings (i.e. 'getting there'). It is a movement towards fulfilment and rest where each step is acknowledged and celebrated. Rather than a call to escape into a perfect paradise, it

---

26. Ibid.
27. Moltmann, *God in Creation*, 286.
28. Wendell Berry, 'Foreword', in Norman Wirzba, *Living the Sabbath*, 11.

describes a peaceful but gutsy return to our bodies, without overlooking or glamorizing the multiple struggles women experience in daily life. Sabbath is a 'gentle, compassionate discipline',[29] as Nicola Slee argues, a way of living at peace with ourselves, the world and God in a harried world.

Slimming and Sabbath?

Slimming does not inherently flout a Sabbath sensibility. In fact, weight loss communities can provide women especially with access to rest and recuperation amidst the frenzy of trying to balance the competing demands of work, home and family life. In my group, attending the weekly meeting provides Tracy with a break from her son's bath routine and gives her time away from her domestic role. As we have already seen, for many the enterprise of slimming opens up opportunities to pursue their own projects, goals and ambitions in a break from servicing the needs of husbands, children and others. Time together in the meeting is sacred time where women break with habituated attitudes and behaviours, do and think differently in relation to food and observe their eating in new ways.

The pursuit of weight loss is itself a quest for rest. The redemptive motif of 'getting there' narrated by women like Hevala, Helen, Joy and Lucy casts slimming as the search for completion. Reminiscent of the way God rests on the seventh day in celebration of the work God has concluded, Helen desires nothing more than to look at her recreated body and ecstatically exclaim that it is good. If Sabbath is the finishing of creation, then slimming grants opportunities for women to complete their bodies and to rest in the knowledge that they are finally as they ought to be. The completed body of course, though, is the body liberated from fat and assumed to be healthier and more attractive.

Slimming meetings, as Sabbath-like spaces, are also liminal spaces. In my group, this interval exists between seven o'clock and half-past eight, between the frenzy of family routines at night and the pressures of work the next day, between the body before joining the group and the body after finishing the work and obtaining a target weight. As an 'in between' space, time in the group allows members the freedom

---

29. Nicola Slee, 'Into the Woods – and Out Again: Reflecting on Sabbath and Sabbatical Time' (unpublished), 2.

to think about different possibilities whether other possible selves, new recipe ideas or other ways of combining foods together. Like the Sabbath space, it is generative and productive, not simply a time to stop, withdraw and close down but a time to think again, reassess and dream. Since the pursuit of weight loss gives many women the room they need to make changes to their lives and to shape them for themselves, it offers a similar type of 'breathing space'[30] to that which Nicola Slee identifies with Sabbath. Like silences in a piece of music or a clearing in the woods through which the light comes, the spacious living of Sabbath, she argues, brings colour, soul and life to work.[31] For many women in the group, the process of slimming gives purpose to life and makes way for the expansion of their selves moving them to become more vibrant and more alive. That this takes place within the context of community and in the company of other women parallels the corporate emphasis of Sabbath, for just as the whole of creation shares in God's delight in all that has been made, so the sabbatical space of the meeting provides a context for women to celebrate in front of one another.

Of course, in other important ways, slimming frustrates a Sabbath sensibility. Although there is celebrating in the weight loss group, whether or not a member is applauded by others and Louise is dependent on how well they have done on the scale. Joy in thinness rather than joy in existence is lauded, and this is extolled as women's ultimate purpose. Delight is not found in just being; in fact, the willingness to feel content with the way one is without striving to produce a thinner self stands to locate women in a 'danger zone', close to Syn and duty-bound to confess. As such, slimming does not condone the type of rest where women can be wholly present to themselves because it inevitably entails a rush to get somewhere else and to become some-body else. In the group, the desire to be at ease makes some women frantic and fearful about staying still. Even in the case where women achieve their target weight, they strive to protect and maintain the bodies they have shaped. As we have seen, this means there can be no rest from the work of frenetic and anxious production. Salvation is not for the idle. In this version of the Protestant ethic, members come to define themselves on the basis of their weight loss achievements, and this not only encourages women to see themselves as the sum of their accomplishments but also urges

30. Slee, 'Into the Woods', 6.
31. Ibid.

them to perceive the undoing of their bodies as an instance of personal success. Nothing could be further from a Sabbath sensibility.

Sabbath also speaks of the cancellation of debt. The Jubilee mandates the remission of debt and freeing of those who have fallen into slavery, requiring families to return to their land and houses. In the New Testament, Jesus continues this message, proclaiming the cancellation of debts and release from slavery. Debt and sacrifice, however, are crucial features of slimming logic. In this respect, slimming flouts a Sabbath sensibility, validating coercive and exploitative relations to fatness and bolstering oppressive sizeist systems that victimize fatter bodies. Since the debt narrative supports a hatred of fat and services the notion that it is morally wrong to live in peace with fat and with people who refuse to 'get rid' of it, the reconciliatory, liberative character of Sabbath is frustrated.

Living and Sanctifying the Sabbath: Resisting Sizeism

In his discussion of Sabbath, Kent Blevins reminds us that the Sabbath command is general rather than specific: 'It points in a particular direction, but leaves us to sort out what heading in that direction might mean in our own specific circumstances.'[32] The command informs us that we should do no ordinary work, but it fails to answer the question of 'how' we should rest. I want to suggest that the religious and moral duty to remember and honour the Sabbath can take material form in a number of 'embodied alternatives'[33] women perform in protest against the exploitative system of sizeism. The principal invitation of Sabbath is to stop, and this provides a radical but simple challenge to the frenzy of sizeism, encouraging those who frantically pursue thinness to cease from this work and from the striving it entails. This does not deny the enabling dimensions of slimming previously observed or neglect the ways in which Syn-watching allows women to take their lives into their own hands. It does, however, present the observance of Sabbath as an alternative performance of self-care through which women can cultivate creativity and perform their own agency without repeating the logic of sacrifice. Sabbath opens up a space away from the body-policing

---

32. Blevins, 'Observing Sabbath', 485.

33. I use this phrase in Chapter 5 also. It is borrowed from Isherwood, 'Sex and Body Politics', 33.

techniques of slimming where women can flourish and be wholly present to themselves without having to erase their flesh.

At its simplest, women can observe the Sabbath by taking a day or period of respite from weight loss activity. Amidst the daily work of patrolling the body, calories, Syn and stepping on and off the scale, the invitation to remember the Sabbath invites women who habitually police their weight to stop, question and slow down. According to Norman Wirzba, the Sabbath 'compels us to reconsider and question with depth and seriousness what all our striving is ultimately for'.[34] As an act of resistance against the anxiety system and coercive politics of sizeism, Sabbath challenges women to consider whether the exertion of patrolling and despising fat grants our bodies enough space to breathe and live as creatures made by God, intended for aliveness. It encourages reflection on whether this kind of labour and restless striving makes for a joyful delight in existence.

As a yearly Sabbath, we may be drawn to observe International No Diet Day[35] which takes place on 6 May in defiance of unrealistic body norms and the pleasure-diminishing expectation that women must relentlessly patrol their eating. On No Diet Day, people are encouraged to cease from dieting and weight obsessions and bring public awareness to size-based prejudice.[36] Observing the Sabbath may also consist of a period of committed respite from shaming and insulting fat – our own fat and the fat of others. By ceasing from what Mimi Nichter calls 'fat-talk' and 'diet-talk', we deliberately refuse to participate in modes of complaining about fat and speaking about dieting and resist the system of fat shame. According to Nichter, these speech performances establish women's and girls' bodies as credible because they signal to others around them that they are appropriately concerned about their appearance.[37] Refraining from them as one performance of the Sabbath repose will, therefore, be costly. Like other Sabbath postures that break with habitual patterns of work and frenzy, they involve risk. Where women's status and identity are built around patrolling weight and

---

34. Wirzba, *Living the Sabbath*, 38.

35. International No Diet Day was created by Mary Evans Young, a non-diet activist, and was first celebrated on 5 May 1992 by Young with a group of friends and relatives. See Cooper, *Fat and Proud*, 154–7.

36. Ibid., 156.

37. Mimi Nichter, *Fat Talk: What Girls and Their Parents Say about Dieting* (Cambridge and London: Harvard University Press, 2000), 73.

appearance, Sabbath presents the terrifying prospect of giving up what is familiar and venturing into the unknown. It calls us to face who we are without these things and without this work. It also, however, offers itself as a gift, inviting us to let go and to be refreshed. Before us in the Sabbath space is the chance to be still, to be wholly present in the place of our *now* bodies and to be, feel, see and think at a distance from the usual habits of despising fat and striving to 'get rid' of it. In this space our first response to fatness can be silence rather than slander, a finger on lips rather than attack.

If God rests on the seventh day because there is no other place God would rather be,[38] then Sabbath is the invitation to live at home in the dwelling place of the body. 'Sabbath teaches us to *savor* the places we are in as God's delight made delectable,'[39] says Wirzba. To savour the place of our present bodies means to celebrate all bodies in all their magnificent diversity as equally loved by God and to 'see in each other the trace of God'.[40] The uniform goal of thinness conforms a multiplicity of bodies to one body standard, defying the wonderful variety that characterizes God's creation and refuses to permit every-body to be. The movement into the Sabbath space, on the other hand, directs us to honour everybody as good. When we do this we enter more deeply into God's rest and unbounded delight and are free to be the glorious bodyselves that God has made. In this way we participate in God's pleasure in creation and celebrate God's presence in all things.

As an invitation to relinquish control and to wander into the unknown, the call to remember the Sabbath also encourages us to suspend what we think we know about fat and all that we usually do to defend against it. According to Slee, Sabbath is the invitation to 'explore off the beaten path, enter the unbounded space of our hearts and imagination' and step into 'the freefall where the normal rules fall away'.[41] Like venturing into the woods, Sabbath depicts an entry into a wild, free, magical place, she suggests; it is the opportunity to 'think outside the box' and to do and think in unforeseen ways.[42] Of course, in the weight loss group, slimming provides some women with similar

---

38. Norman Wirzba, *Food & Faith: A Theology of Eating* (New York: Cambridge University Press, 2011), 46.
39. Ibid.
40. Wirzba, *Living the Sabbath*, 53.
41. Slee, 'Into the Woods', 3.
42. Ibid.

opportunities, but in the Sabbath space I envisage, women venture outside the permitted boundaries of fat hatred in search of other words about fat. Here the journey into the wild is a dangerous rebellious journey into forbidden territories, into words, thoughts and actions that shock and defy convention. If the invitation of Sabbath is to play and explore, then it is an invitation to be daring. The Sabbath space is a transgressive space occupied by women who choose to think for themselves and permit their bodyselves to play and produce new truths. When we release our minds and bodies to imagine and creatively wander rather than be confined to the predictable and tiresome 'obvious truths' about fat, we cross the boundary into this liberating space.

As an interval, Sabbath is a period of time we can define to playfully craft these types of repose and engage in other modes of doing that resist the compulsion to shame fat. Rendered this way, Sabbath emerges once more as a site of resistance to systems of anxiety and coercion that cause us to hate our fat and attack it.

Facing Fat and Restoring Face to Fat

Moltmann describes the Sabbath day as a time when God rests '*in face* of his works'.[43] The world is not only made *by* God, he argues, but exists *before* God and lives *with* God.[44] When God rests, creation is free to be in all of its splendour and glory; hence, God's repose allows each created thing to unfold in their own way before God and in God's presence. For Moltmann, this means that human beings sanctify the Sabbath by recognizing that everything that is is made by God and exists before the face of God. To enter the Sabbath rest is to cease from frenetic activity and simply be, in celebration of existence and life, with joy and thanksgiving.

If this is so, then Sabbath is an invitation to notice the presence of God in all bodies, in fatness and fat bodies and to rest in the face of fat with peace and joy. It offers a challenge to sizeism because it encourages us towards thankfulness rather than hatred or regret for our now bodies and to face fat rather than rush to destroy it. Sabbath calls us into a space where we allow our fat to be, to exist before our eyes and in God's face. This kind of repose, this letting be of fat, does not depict a toleration of fat because we are too shattered to keep trying to 'beat it' – it is not

---

43. Moltmann, *God in Creation*, 279. Emphasis in original.
44. Ibid.

equivalent to burnout. Nor does it invite us to take joy in our existence *in spite* of fatness. Rather, we are encouraged towards a full-fleshed delight in the bodies we are, as fat and as bodies that display fatness.

This presentation of Sabbath as bound up with the politics of fat acceptance rejects an 'assimilationist' approach to fat liberation that tries to make fat existence more bearable or suggest that fat people are valuable *even though* they are fat. Kathleen LeBesco describes this political approach to fat as one that seeks greater toleration of fat, the securing of fat rights and greater awareness of fat oppression but which may also continue to conceive of fat as a problem.[45] To embody and live the Sabbath is to embody a 'liberationist' position which aligns with a confident and gutsy delight in fat existence and an acceptance that fat can stay, to believe that one can indeed *be* fat and live and that fat need not be burnt or beaten.

For fat activist Nomy Lamm, facing fat squarely in the mirror with elation is an important practice of resistance to the dominant hegemony of fat phobia. Speaking about the movement of fat acceptance and fat positivity, she reflects, 'My body is fucking beautiful, and every time I look in the mirror and acknowledge that, I am contributing to the revolution.'[46] One way to let our bodies be in front of our faces and before God's face is to look at them without apology and to joyously affirm our fat as wonderful and good. This could involve us taking time in our weeks or days to stop and practise the art of beholding our bodies as beautiful, glorious, sensual, feeling bodies.

This strategy, detectable in fat activism, resists sizeist regulatory norms by claiming fat as sexually attractive. It has, however, been criticized for assimilating with a thin-centric symbolic system. Samantha Murray, for example, claims that by announcing fat as beautiful, fat activist campaigners simply swap the fat-phobic politics of sizeism for the 'celebratory politics' of size acceptance,[47] repeating rather than resisting the heteropatriarchal 'visual regime' that assesses the female body on the basis of appearance. Given that concentration on beauty and appearance are pivotal features of thin-centric culture,

---

45. LeBesco, *Revolting Bodies?*, 42.

46. Nomy Lamm, 'It's a Big Fat Revolution', http://www.tehomet.net/nomy.html (accessed 23 June 2018).

47. Samantha Murray, *The 'Fat' Female Body* (Basingstoke and New York: Palgrave Macmillan, 2008), 133–4.

assimilating with them stands to further inculcate thin privilege.[48] Although it is fat now which is to be gazed at and adored, this still relies on the 'objectification of women as beautiful bodies', Murray suggests.[49] Seen in these terms, living the Sabbath by living at home in the place of fat may simply validate the heteronormative neoliberal assumption that women must be judged according to how they look.

One theological response to this is to argue that beauty is an inherent quality of creation which does not depend on normative frameworks. This position would claim that in Genesis, beauty and goodness are intrinsic to God's world. God's delight in creation does not derive from creation's compliance with external regulatory norms. Everything is good without qualification. In this sense, the performance of Sabbath begins with the acknowledgement that all bodies are good, not the so-called 'real' person beneath the layers of fat but the enfleshed person, the fat person, the person as fat. At the same time, however, Genesis does little to displace the male gaze since created things are good because the male God 'sees' that what 'he' has made is good. Beauty also does not exist in a vacuum. Even if the principle of Sabbath teaches us that corporeal things are inherently valuable, this does not change the fact that 'beauty' as a concept is wedded to time and place and to body norms. The claim that fatness should be included into this category then stands to further entrench the assumption that beauty is timeless (eternal) and constant, exposing what LeBesco names as 'beauty's clever trick of making *itself* not seem [like] a social construction'.[50]

Notwithstanding these difficulties, we should not rush to abandon all reference to the fat female body as sexy or beautiful. Murray may be right that emphasizing beauty in fat politics is unrealistic and problematic because to live a beautiful life means to comply with the normative ascetic of slenderness, but given that fatness is constructed in the weight loss setting as antithetical to beauty and in ways that discredit and erase women's sexualities and given Christian traditions have lent support to this symbolic system, restoring face to fat by affirming fat as beautiful and sexy remains important, albeit contentious. 'Just being fat and positively sexual is radical in a culture thoroughly inculcated with

---

48. Ibid., 117.
49. Ibid., 119.
50. LeBesco, *Revolting Bodies?*, 51. Emphasis in original.

sexism and anti-fat prejudice,'[51] argues fat activist Heather McAllister.[52] Kimberly Dark similarly observes that her fat must be made to disappear if she is to be thought beautiful and sexy. Like McAllister she tells her readers that 'nothing cancels out female beauty as quickly as being fat'[53] and that sexy fat women demonstrate another way of living and loving the body that troubles the normative model.[54]

Facing fat positively then – as good, glorious and beautiful – can be an important act of resistance against fat phobia if beauty is pulled down from its pedestal and redefined 'in its own very intimidating and self-proclaimedly inert face'.[55] Rather than assimilating with thin heteronormative culture by suggesting that fat women can wear bikinis or miniskirts, as is sometimes the suggestions in fat politics, this rethinks what counts as attractive in the first place. Beauty is a social construct so Sabbath living allows us to be inventive, to conjure up multiple images and multiple namings so that women like those in the weight loss group whose bellies and breasts protrude across tables and whose baby-weight still shows can rejoice in their heft rather than see their bodies as vile and disgusting.

Facing fat in the mirror may be one radical outworking of a Sabbath sensibility through which women can rewrite the script of beauty and give themselves permission to be and delight in their flesh. This seems especially important in light of the way fat bodies are frequently defaced and beheaded in the public media. According to fat activist Charlotte Cooper, the image of the 'Headless Fatty' is commonplace in news reporting on obesity. The image carries powerful symbolism, she suggests, communicating that fat people loom large but have nothing of value to say:

> As Headless Fatties, the body becomes symbolic: we are there but we have no voice, not even a mouth in a head, no brain, no thoughts or opinions. Instead we are reduced and dehumanised as symbols of cultural fear: the body, the belly, the arse, food. There's a symbolism,

---

51. Heather McAllister, 'Embodying Fat Liberation', in *The Fat Studies Reader*, 305.
52. Ibid., 306. McAllister founded the world's first all-fat burlesque troupe and deliberately sought to challenge anti-fat hatred through fat performance.
53. Kimberly Dark, 'Coming Out Fat', in *Fat Sex*, 216.
54. Ibid., 218.
55. LeBesco, *Revolting Bodies?*, 51.

too, in the way that the people in these photographs have been beheaded. It's as though we have been punished for existing, our right to speak has been removed by a prurient gaze, our headless images accompany articles that assume a world without people like us would be a better world altogether.

By facing fat in the mirror and using our mouths to celebrate our flesh, we return our faces to our fat and give ourselves back our mouths, our voices and the right to say our bodies for ourselves. In so doing, we join our bodies back together and challenge the assumption of the slimming organization that fat is a 'thing' extraneous to the self that confesses a discredited identity without women even saying a word. As a Sabbath practice of delight, facing fat rejects the conventional wisdom that fat should cause individuals, especially women, to lose face (respect) and instead restores face to our fat, moving us to face our bodies with pride.

A Return to the Voluntarist Liberal Humanist Project?

Aligning the practice of a fat-positive stance with a Sabbath sensibility presents our bodies once more as testimonies. But rather than 'confessing' our guilt or outing Syn as in the slimming group, by allowing our fat to be without apology, before our faces and before the face of God, our flesh announces that fat bodies are loveable, beautiful and valuable. By breaking with compulsive anti-fat attitudes and languages, by ceasing from the work of shaming fat and from the frantic pursuit of its obliteration, our bodies witness to the boundless joy and abundant love of God in a bounded fat-hating world. Such embodied performances are 'Sabbath signs' that point towards God's 'yes' in relation to all flesh, incarnating and corporealizing a different message about fat.

This, however, may appear to suggest that women can only embody the Sabbath space if they step outside of fat-hating culture into a parallel universe of fat acceptance and if they somehow cut themselves off from their fat-hating selves. Such a vision of flight obviously repeats the damaging logic already observed in the group and also shown to parallel Western Christian soteriology, endorsing the need for detachment and evacuation. It also assumes that such a retreat from sizeism is possible in the first place. According to Samantha Murray, this is a further related weakness with fat politics since fat activism assumes that people can change the way they feel about their fat simply by deciding to. For Murray, this only repeats the mind-over-matter motif forwarded by the voluntarist liberal humanist project and so once again falls into the trap of assuming the primacy of the individual and the supremacy of reason and the will.[56]

I would argue, conversely, that a fat-positive stance does not have to assume an escape from fat-phobic discourse or repeat the mind-over-matter mantra that dominates weight loss culture. A Sabbath sensibility has us be realistic at the same time as practice a measure of hope because Sabbath is a liminal space. As an interlude, it does not depict a place outside of fat-hating/thin-adoring culture or a shiny new paradise where the evils of sizeism are abolished in the twinkling of an eye. Rather, it is a break in the midst of fat-hating culture, a clearing in the woods, a breathing space. Embodying fatness without regret or apology is not equivalent to the '"liberatory" moment' Murray identifies with the utopic vision of fat politics, when we suddenly opt to see the world and fat differently and never look back. She is right that we cannot simply remove ourselves from the embedded knowledges that have shaped our seeing, thinking and feelings about fat, simply by choosing to.[57] Observing Sabbath, however, is not this kind of intellectual 'heady' enterprise, reminiscent of the 'click in the mind' or dramatic moment of conversion narrated by some women in the group in relation to their thinning projects. It invites us to cross a border, to dare to rest from the usual habits of slandering fat and anxiously working to produce a thinner 'me'. But for many, it will be a temporary repose because it is difficult to sustain. However, the Sabbath call is an invitation to inhabit hope and rest time and again. Sabbath is a place of *return*, a rhythm that embraces replenishment in the midst of travail and one that welcomes us back often, without fear or reproach.

By repeating and returning to more fat-positive body performances we gradually reorient our bodyselves away from fat-phobic performances and equip ourselves to carry the Sabbath stance through into the rest of our lives. In this sense, although Sabbath is an interlude rather than an escape from sizeist culture, it does nevertheless mark the opening of a new horizon because it has the power to transform our bodywork rather than fuel a more determined return to fighting fat. Sabbath is redemptive and recreative.[58] Repeated repose from the

56. Murray, *The 'Fat' Female Body*, 108.

57. Samantha Murray, '(Un/Be)Coming Out? Rethinking Fat Politics', *Social Semiotics* 15, no. 2 (2005): 161.

58. Barbara Reid, 'Sabbath: Recreation and Liberation', *The Living Pulpit* 7, no. 2 (April–June 1998): 42.

anxious work of trying to produce or protect a thinner self can awaken our senses and our minds. It may draw us to return to the ordinariness of daily life more able to perceive the gloriousness of our bodies/fat and the bodies/fat of others and more attentive to instances of fat phobia and fat shaming in our everyday worlds. Through entering the Sabbath space, we will build resilience and become more adamant in our refusal to comply with such normative conventions and more committed to protesting against them. Resting from what sizeist culture expects us to think, say and do about fat has the potential to reshape our mundane habits. As well as restructuring our fat-phobic attitudes and behaviours, it has the power to open up time for other things, for noticing a sunset, a flower opening, a lover's eyes[59] and for reconnecting with hobbies or parts of ourselves we have neglected.

Of course, our best intentions may end in failure for Sabbath as an outworking of salvation, may be practised only then to be lost. But unlike the pattern of slimming, the failure to rest fully from fat shaming and from rigorously patrolling the appetite does not demand guilt or confession. The Sabbath space is forever a place of welcome and refreshing and never insists that we crucify the body for its failure to comply. To move into the Sabbath rest and repose is to understand that structural forces intervene to make women fraught. Hence, although Sabbath could be another motivation for frenetic activity as the desire to abstain from slandering fat manifests as an additional form of anxious striving, the call to rest is an invitation to practise peace with our bodyselves, not war. Sabbath is the gentle whisper that says 'the cross is not our goal'.[60]

Beyond the Private: Sabbath as a Corporate and Political Practice

So far, I have considered how Sabbath as a practice of delight may be observed by women in ways that resist the sin of sizeism. Murray's charge above would suggest that Sabbath and the performance of fat positivity are individualist projects that lack a concern for politics. However, the account of sin I have already forwarded makes clear that even personal acts are not empty of politics because all of our individual doings are necessarily located in networks of relationships and in social

---

59. See also Moltmann, 'The Sabbath – The Feast of Creation', 41.
60. Ruether, *Introducing Redemption*, 79.

worlds. Given that private actions are always embedded in societies and communities, no clear distinction can be made between the private and political. Change at an individual level can be conceived as an instance of 'micro' activism, defined by Charlotte Cooper as a form of activism that 'takes place in everyday spaces, is generally performed by one person, sometimes two, but rarely more, and happens in small, understated moments'.[61] This kind of revolt against fat hatred, she argues, is crucial because it builds esteem and encourages alternative ways of being.[62] When we live the Sabbath by resisting the need to shame, remove or police fat, our rest actually becomes a form of micro-activism and an instance of 'mini-salvation'. Such micro-politics need not be understood as 'solipsistic individualism'[63] not only because they are embedded in social networks but also because they are opinion changing. They are valid in their own right for producing embodied esteem and for supporting women in 'creating liveable lives for themselves and others'.[64]

Sabbath keeping is, however, also a call for the people of God. The sanctification of Sabbath is never a purely solitary or private affair because it is a duty for the worshipping community as it seeks to serve the world and love God. It is a communal practice that energizes the Christian churches to unite in praise of God and to resist exploitative systems of relationship that hinder the Sabbath repose. Liturgy and ritual provide important Sabbath spaces outside of the daily humdrum of life for harried believers to come together before God, to break slavish patterns of labour and to name the forces of evil and frustration that deprive their bodies of God's peace. Marjorie Procter-Smith reminds us that liturgy is our common work before God on behalf of the world. It is a work and common life founded upon reconciliation with God and one another.[65] Seen in these terms, liturgy draws the people of God towards out of ordinary activities. Rather than assisting in the customary reproduction of exploitative patterns of relationship marked by frantic activity, liturgy has the potential to open up a space for women to practise rest and perform the salvific task of healing wounds, building justice and restoring peace.

61. Ibid.
62. Charlotte Cooper, *Fat Activism: A Radical Social Movement* (Bristol: HammerOn Press, 2016), 81.
63. Ibid.
64. Ibid., 82.
65. Marjorie Procter-Smith, 'Reconciliation: Hope and Risk', *Liturgy* 23, no. 4 (2008): 1.

I thus want to suggest now that liturgical settings can be important Sabbath spaces for resisting sizeism and for cultivating the Sabbath sensibility of delight. If the sin of sizeism vilifies fat and separates women from enjoying their bodies and food, dividing their bodies against themselves, then liturgical environments may provide communal contexts where Christian women can join together to cease from the work of policing and shaming fat in renunciation of the evils of fat phobia. I imagine these grassroots groups as providing contexts where praise of God unites with a different kind of doing, where women can hold their fat before God and one another, let go of the cultural obsession with weight and venture into the unknown. Liturgy as work, of course, returns us to the close association between Sabbath and work and between salvation and Sabbath. The rituals and alternative practices women perform in these groups are, however, distinct from the frenetic work of anxious productivity and from slavish labour. This work is directed and performed by women to encourage a rest from the exploitative patterns of fat phobia and to cultivate delight in the body as a practice of self-care and self-responsibility. Through ritual and sharing, women enact their communal resolve to resist the sin of sizeism that robs so many of their rest time. Such ritual performances, I suggest, are ways of living a Sabbath sensibility, of connecting with joy and affirming the glorious creation of women's flesh.

Women's Liturgies and Meaning-making

The significance of ritual for the formation of knowledge and meaning-making is plain to see in the weight loss meetings. Here, the rites women perform (such as confession, passing around lumps of lard and standing on the scale) together with the symbols and languages they adopt and adapt (including the nomenclature and symbolism of Syn) help conform their bodies to fat-phobic body standards. Women use their hands to celebrate one another's weight loss, and although there are no set words members must speak or actions they must perform, each meeting has women obey tacit scripts that assume fat must be confessed and abandoned. Speech and movement are mostly repetitive and predictable and constitute 'stylized'[66] acts that perform fat-phobic norms. As a corporate entity, women act and speak their bodies in ways

---

66. Judith Butler, *Gender Trouble: Feminism and the Subversion of Identity* (New York and London: Routledge, 2007), 191.

that produce the cultural truth that fat is a virtual confession of moral failure. At the same time, the meetings provide contexts for women to produce their own bodies and tell their own stories. Interweaving their narratives with the narratives of others, women get to value their own bodies and hear to speech their experiences and the lives of other women. They celebrate one another's achievements, build confidence and form social bonds. Together they encourage one another to shape their own worlds and become intentional human agents.

Suggesting that the Sabbath repose can be embodied in corporate liturgical settings and in women's ritual making acknowledges that ritual has the power to shape new worlds. It echoes the way the embodied actions of women in the slimming community construct new realities and fashion new habits and behaviours. Christian feminist grass-roots women's groups, however, will radically differ to slimming clubs because they will be committed to resisting the toxic distortions of sizeism and be intentionally motivated by a communal resolve to rest from the frantic work of upholding the thin ideal. Populated by women who are 'weary and are carrying heavy burdens' (Mt. 11.28), by those who wish to be at peace with their flesh but whose attempts to do so are thwarted by the pervasiveness of fat phobia, and by women who are furious with the demands of a fat-hating world, these communities will provide liminal spaces away from the daily 'noise' of anti-fat discourse for women to embrace one another and let one another's bodies be. They may encourage a reorientation of our bodies to time, allowing women to become more conscious of time, of the people, places and things that matter most. Such ritual contexts will be purposefully intended to liberate fatness from the theological and cultural web of 'obvious' truths that encourage women to experience their bodies as uninhabitable. As Sabbath spaces, they will offer opportunities for women to break with patterns of fat shame and diet-talk and will enable women to build community with other women. Groups will meet at regular intervals to observe the Sabbath repose: in women's homes, outside or in a diversity of other places.

Since thinner women are attacked in their skin by the same fat-phobic attitudes that make fat embodiment so obscene and given that the evils of sizeism influence patterns of relating to food, fat and the bodyself for women of various shapes and sizes, such liturgical groups will welcome differently sized women and not just women who identify as fat. This, though, does not mean that women's bodies and experiences are homogenized. Because the politics of size inevitably benefit skinnier women, the journey from fat shame towards body positivity will not be the same for fatter women as for thinner women. Other sites of difference intersect with women's experience of size making every woman's journey unique. However, because the corporate liturgical settings imagined are communities of diverse women united by a shared commitment to resist sizeism, they will be enriched by the varieties of embodied experience women bring. Such liturgical communities will provide alternative material contexts to weight loss organizations where women can cultivate equivalent capacities of self-care, creativity and agency. Facilitated by rites and rituals that stubbornly refuse to repeat fat hatred, these material contexts have the capacity to motivate women to take the rest and repose from fat hatred into their everyday lives.

Of course, the concept of women's groups raises important questions about exclusion given that men are also affected by weight-related bias and are increasingly expected to aspire to a thin ideal. Mixed groups will be important, as will men-only groups perhaps, but in a culture where slimming still continues to be a predominantly female affair and in response to the dynamics observed in the weight loss group attended almost exclusively by women, there is a need, I believe, for liturgical groups generated and populated by women. Feminist practical theologian Jan Berry observes that many women's liturgies are not open to outsiders which has the effect of including some while simultaneously excluding others. She compellingly argues that this is justified on the basis that some kind of boundary must be drawn in order to provide participants with a sense of safe and sacred space.[67] In the same way, the social pressures on women to be skinny and to adhere to normative feminine aesthetics may mean that in many cases, women will feel more comfortable in the company of other women and benefit from having their own space and time.

Women's worship groups and communities have emerged in multiple contexts as alternatives to the clerical domination of the liturgy and as ways of acknowledging women's experiences. Such groups have provided women with the opportunity to own their worship and to come together to share the events of their lives.[68] Women's groups have challenged the way women's voices and bodies have been excluded in

---

67. Jan Berry, *Ritual Making Women: Shaping Rites for Changing Lives* (London and Oakville: Equinox, 2009), 19.

68. Susan A. Ross, *Extravagant Affections: A Feminist Sacramental Theology* (New York: Continuum, 1998), 220–1.

official liturgical settings,[69] recovering forgotten texts and traditions and providing contexts for a reimagining of faith. Elisabeth Schüssler Fiorenza's notion of the *ekklēsia gynaikon* – the '*ekklēsia* of wo/men' or simply 'women-church' – has taken concrete shape in a number of women's groups. Conceived by Fiorenza as a 'political site of debate, persuasion, and opposition within the framework of Christian community',[70] women-church is a democratic assembly of free citizens who gather to decide their own affairs in challenge of 'hegemonic "common sense" theological discourses'.[71] It offers itself as a challenge to the institutional church and to other institutions and organizations that assist with the propagation of kyriarchy and so is both 'ideal vision and ... historical reality'.[72]

The feminist worship and liturgical groups I imagine constitute examples of women-church. They prioritize women's experiences of fat shame, exclusion and weight-based prejudice and seek to use words, imagery, symbols, sights and sounds, gestures and movements to both build a Sabbath delight in all flesh and orientate women towards extended forms of committed action against sizeism. Such groups will take account of the multiple layers of oppression that structure women's lives – and so of how race, class, culture, age, ability, religion and gender intersect with fat and body size. They will also be politically and religiously motivated towards transformation. In this sense, they offer instances of liturgical spaces where ritualizing has the power to change reality, helping to elevate the position of women of a variety of sizes in

69. See, for example, Janet R. Walton, *Feminist Liturgy: A Matter of Justice* (Collegeville: The Liturgical Press, 2000), 12.

70. Elizabeth A. Castelli, 'The Ekklesia of Women and/as Utopian Space: Locating the Work of Elisabeth Schüssler Fiorenza in Feminist Utopian Thought', in *On the Cutting Edge: The Study of Women in Biblical Worlds*, ed. Jane Schaberg, Alice Bach and Esther Fuchs (New York and London: Continuum, 2004), 43.

71. Elisabeth Schüssler Fiorenza, *Jesus: Miriam's Child, Sophia's Prophet: Critical Issues in Feminist Christology* (London and New York: Continuum, 1994), 17.

72. Elisabeth Schüssler Fiorenza, *Discipleship of Equals: A Critical Feminist Ekklēsia-logy of Liberation* (New York: Crossroad Publishing Company, 1998), 344. For Fiorenza, the term 'wo/men' points away from essentialism to signal the ways in which 'women' are fragmented and fractured by the complex structures of race, class, religion, heterosexuality, colonialism, age and health.

defiance of fat phobia.[73] As 'feminist' groups they embody what Majorie Procter-Smith sees as the crucial feature of Fiorenza's vision of women-church, forging a democratic assembly of equals who are committed to political and religious change and where diverse women can come together to share experience without this being reduced to sameness or assimilated into another normative hegemony.[74] As 'Christian' groups they constitute Sabbath communities, places of rest for those who are tired and furious with the coercive system of sizeism that separates women from their bodies, others and God. They allow women to enter a slowed down existence, to replenish their energies and to laugh, speak, eat and sing together. These Christian communities use the Sabbath space to trouble hegemonic 'common sense' theological discourses that feed the impersonal system of sizeism and which train women to see the war on fat as a holy war concerned with overcoming sin and achieving salvation. As Sabbath spaces motivated by the principle of equal worth, equal value and equal rest, these communities are rooted in faith and in an alternative vision of society and church, one that 'has as its goal to make experientially available here and now the well-being and inclusivity … of God's intended world'. Those who gather to rest and who use their repose to energize projects that challenge sizeism form a pilgrimage community who journey together in the power of the Spirit that gives life. They are 'inside-outsiders'[75] or 'resident-aliens',[76] to use Fiorenza's description, fully aware that there can be no exodus from the structures of sizeism but prepared to cross the boundary into a counter-cultural space that allows their bodies to breathe and which helps make present God's eschatological repose.

In these contexts, liturgies refuse to position fatness in opposition to God and remember with praise and thanksgiving that God calls all bodies into being. Scriptures may be read as well as a myriad of other texts but always to build faith in our flesh and confirm fat people as 'equivalent human persons'.[77] In feminist liturgical groups, women who

---

73. See Lesley A. Northup, *Ritualising Women* (Cleveland: The Pilgrim Press, 1997), 103.

74. Marjorie Procter-Smith, 'Feminist Ritual Strategies', in *Toward a New Heaven and a New Earth: Essays in Honour of Elisabeth Schüssler Fiorenza*, ed. Fernando F. Segovia (Maryknoll: Orbis, 2003), 505.

75. Fiorenza, *Discipleship of Equals*, 328.

76. Ibid., 326.

77. Ruether, *Sexism and God-Talk*, 173.

experience the violence of sizeism and who hope for change are free to inhabit the Christian story of liberation for themselves and to narrate their own bodies within its drama. By 'staring down' the pervasive evil of sizeism,[78] such communities of women-church join with God in moving creation towards the Sabbath delight and rest for which it groans (Rom. 8.22).

Feminist Women's Liturgical Groups as Instances of Fat Activism

I have already argued that the line between the Sabbath repose and work is rightly blurred. At its best, Sabbath is a way of living that cannot be straightjacketed into a tidy pocket of time distinct from the everyday. When the Sabbath sensibility of thankfulness and delight heightens our attentiveness to the beauty of God's world, driving us to face our own fat and the fat of others with joy, then we allow the Sabbath principle to shape our everyday worlds. I have also suggested that liturgy and ritual are activities through which women can challenge 'obvious' truths about fat. As out of the ordinary work that encourages rest from the ordinary work of shaming and patrolling fat and as activity that is motivated by a radical faith commitment to make flesh God's repose in the here and now, liturgy and ritual are also sites of activism. Arguing this does not suggest that liturgy is a way for women to anxiously and slavishly labour to combat sin and remake the world. The kind of activism that women perform through liturgy is one stimulated by rest and directed towards the Sabbath principle that all should rest and experience the delight of God. As an opening where women generate their own words about their fat and narrate their own bodies, liturgy forwards the meaningful work of salvation, helping women rest from their sacrificial projects while fuelling the political commitment to change.

As religious instances of activism, these liturgical groups mirror feminist fat activist groups in using community as a tool for rescuing fat from a spoiled identity. Charlotte Cooper describes community building as a political process that helps fat people form networks of support that can influence change. 'Building community', she says, 'simply getting together, is a project of generating social capital, developing connections

---

78. Emilie Townes suggests that when we reject suffering and injustice as inevitable and to dare to imagine an alternative reality, we 'stare down suffering with an apocalyptic vision'. Emilie M. Townes, *In a Blaze of Glory: Womanist Spirituality as Social Witness* (Nashville: Abingdon Press, 1995), 122–3.

that enable people to exercise power, become agentic and visible, and be legitimised'.[79] It can comprise the 'cultural work' of creating texts, images, art, poetry, photographs, digital artefacts, moving images and so on that make fat bodies visible and which offer new possibilities for imaging fat.

A number of fat feminist groups have emerged since the formation of the Fat Underground in the early 1970s – the founding organization of the feminist fat liberation movement.[80] Grass-roots groups have developed resources engaging with health, fitness, self-esteem, fashion and defending against discrimination.[81] Many are online communities, and personal blogs and social media sites have become increasingly common.[82] In the United States, the feminist punk movement, Riot Grrrl, and feminist music and arts festival, Lady Fest, have been important sites of transmission for fat activism. Online platforms are also providing digital spaces for fat Christians to come together to affirm their bodies. Social media pages such as *Fat and Faithful*,[83] *All Bodies Are Good Bodies*[84] and *Fat, Catholic and Loved*[85] offer fat Christians – often women in particular – opportunities to debate faith and fat politics,

---

79. Cooper, *Fat Activism*, 60–1.

80. NAAFA was founded in 1969 as the National Association to Aid Fat Americans but now goes by the name of the National Association to Advance Fat Acceptance. The Fat Underground emerged as a critique of NAAFA and in particular objection to the way it marginalized women and failed to properly confront the injustices of sexism, homophobia and women's sexual exploitation. For more, see Zora Simic, 'Fat as a Feminist Issue: A History', in *Fat Sex*; and Cooper, *Fat Activism*, 115–29.

81. Marilyn Wann, 'Foreword: Fat Studies: An Invitation to Revolution', in *The Fat Studies Reader*, x.

82. Helen Hester and Caroline Walters, 'Riots Not Diets!: Sex, Fat Studies and DIY Activism', in *Fat Sex*, 4.

83. 'Fat and Faithful', https://www.facebook.com/FatAndFaithful/ (accessed 23 June 2018).

84. Amanda Martinez Beck, 'All Bodies Are Good Bodies', https://www.facebook.com/groups/allbodiesaregoodbodies/ (accessed 15 June 2018). This group states that it exists 'to create a digital space for people to learn that it is okay to take up as much space as they need – physically, emotionally, spiritually, and mentally'.

85. Amanda Martinez Beck, 'Fat, Catholic and Loved', https://www.facebook.com/fatcatholicandloved/ (accessed 15 June 2018).

promoting fat acceptance as a faithful practice of Christian self-care and stewardship.[86] This form of Christian activism conducts the important work of making fat bodies visible in online faith spaces and in ways that build networks of solidarity among fat people.

The liturgical groups I imagine, however, differ in that they are premised on the notion of shared physical space, and actual face-to-face/body-to-body encounter, not unlike the commercial slimming group in this study. As a form of fat activism, feminist worship and liturgical groups committed to resisting sizeism will engage in the cultural work of artistic, literary and symbolic representation and so follow feminist fat activism in employing cultural devices to challenge social norms of appropriateness. In Christian feminism, the charge has been that women's bodies have been feared and invalidated in ecclesial contexts and that the language and imagery of liturgy has promoted women's submission rather than encouraging women to seek their own liberation.[87] Fatness, however, has also failed to find positive expression in official Christian liturgies. Verbal languages may reference the 'weight' of sin and its 'heavy' burden; visual languages may depict girls and women as skinny and Jesus as toned and 'buff'; worship spaces may assume worshippers are thin and may compel restricted movement; worship leaders and those involved in other forms of leadership may be banned from performing ministerial roles on the basis of their size[88] and food and drink may be 'celebrated' as redemptive through the sharing of miniscule pieces of bread and a sip of wine. In worship contexts where 'fat' is a word that is seldom spoken and thinness is assumed as normative, liturgy fails to be the work of the people.[89] Instead,

---

86. Nicole Morgan and Amanda Martinez Beck are among the Christian fat activist women whose blogs, podcasts and personal websites seek to fulfil this vision. See, for example, Nicole Morgan's blog, 'J. Nicole Morgan', https://jnicolemorgan.com/ (accessed 23 June 2018).

87. Berry, *Ritual Making Women*, 11.

88. See, for example, Leonardo Blair, 'Church Bans Fat People from Worship Team Because They Would Interrupt Flow of Anointing', *Christian Post Reporter*, https://www.christianpost.com/news/church-bans-fat-people-from-worship-team-because-they-would-interrupt-flow-of-anointing-170814/#eyCubqUEYsORSjxD.99 (accessed 4 May 2018).

89. Marjorie Procter-Smith argues this point in relation to the androcentric nature of liturgical language. See *In Her Own Rite: Constructing Feminist Liturgical Tradition* (CreateSpace Independent Publishing Platform, 2013), 50.

women who identify as fat or who are terrified by fat and subsequently diminished by the politics of sizeism are silenced and rendered invisible and so not encouraged to seek social change. Furthermore, in a cultural frame where anti-fat sentiment is premised on the assumption that fat is the result of unruly eating, the reluctance to celebrate appetite in worship buttresses sizeism. These kinds of liturgical expression reinforce rather than dismantle distorted structures of oppression and so violate the social vision of Sabbath. They also fail to adequately witness to the abundance of God.

Feminist women's groups committed to the political struggle against sizeism will attend to movement, to visual imagery, to the use of space and time and to what is seen, touched and sensed. As Sabbath spaces which galvanize women to work against sizeism, women's liturgical groups will provide contexts for breaking the rules, for the performance of 'sensible eating' where women can connect with their bodies and desires and where food and drink can be touched and tasted with riotous laughter and with attention to justice, passion and feeling. 'Fat art'[90] and images of differently sized women and representations of God may be employed and used for meditation, in lament of the politics of sizeism that cause so many women to hate their flesh. Space and movement will be used to liberate women so that all are free to stand, leap, dance, roll, sit and bend without being forced to squeeze into tight, unforgiving and painful places. In these Sabbath spaces, women will be encouraged to touch their fat, not as extraneous lumps of lard as in the weight loss meeting but as an integral feature of their bodies that is loved by others and cherished by God. If a central feature of shame is the incentive to '*hide, disappear or flee*' as Stephen Pattison argues,[91] then women's grass-roots groups offer worshipping environments where women do not have to keep their fat at arm's length (like Jane does when she stands inside her skirt), fear the judgement of others and God or feel the need to reprimand their fat as some 'thing' defective. In these spaces, fat is not untouchable.

---

90. Stefanie Snider defines fat art as 'art with a fat-positive viewpoint'. See her article 'Fatness and Visual Culture: A Brief Look at Some Contemporary Projects', *Fat Studies* 1, no. 1 (2012): 13. Fat-positive art, she argues, laughs at fatness, defies fatness as problematic and rejects the cultural truth that says that fat bodies are ugly 'wretched cultural artefacts' (14).

91. I discuss this further in Chapter 1. Also see Pattison, *Shame: Theory, Therapy, Theology*, 75. Emphasis in original.

Writing may figure as a tool of resistance in feminist liturgical contexts as it does in the weight loss group and in fat activism, allowing women opportunities to practise creativity and take charge of their own lives. Women may come together to craft liturgies and rites that enable fat bodies to enter discourse proudly and to give voice to body-positive and fat-accepting words, songs, prayers and chants. Feminist theologians have drawn attention to the predominance of male language used for God in the spoken and written words of liturgies. Concerned that women have been prevented from saying their own words about themselves and their lives, feminist liturgies have sought to return the power of naming to women. In Christian feminist communities of women committed to resisting sizeism, the spoken and written words of women become tools through which the scripts of compulsory thinness can be troubled and rewritten. For fat activist Kimberley Dark, 'coming out' as fat comprises the refusal to erase fat from conversation. It requires that fat people talk about and discuss their fat bodies rather than talk around them to protect others. By voicing fat experience she believes fat people open fat-hating culture to a level of critique that could cause reality itself to crumble.[92] In feminist Christian liturgies, women bring their fat to speech and allow their fat to be. The need to say 'fat' – to use the 'f' word without reproach – is something feminist liturgies will embrace, but its descriptive meaning will be determined by those who speak it. The word will be uttered with confidence in full knowledge that fat bodies are invested with the fullness of God and God's image. If fat bodies are loved by God and are fully in the image of God, then faithful speech about God expresses that *God is fat*. In praise of a God who is Trinity and who is, therefore, vast, expansive and uncontainable, we proclaim that God is not a God of thinness.[93]

Yet, saying the 'f' word is not all that is needed. Feminist liturgical contexts will also provide important Sabbath spaces for variously sized women to come together to name for themselves in their own words the many complex ways in which their bodies are harmed by sizeism. The gathering of women-church will be formed of women who

---

92. Dark, 'Coming Out Fat', 219.

93. I develop this argument in 'Expanding Bodies, Expanding God: Feminist Theology in Search of a "Fatter" Future', *Feminist Theology* 21, no. 3 (2013): 309–26.

are committed to hearing to speech the ambiguities and tensions that women often experience around fat. For women opposed to fat phobia but who nevertheless struggle to shake off the irrepressible urge for thin, liturgy may give expression to their pain and frustration, to how sizeism curtails their freedom, and provide an opportunity for them to hold their bodies with honesty before God and other women. In this sense, liturgy enables women to engage in acts of 'truth-telling'.[94] In such feminist networks, women use their bodies to expose the pain of self-hatred and fat shame and the community serves as an important resource for challenging this. Like in weight loss groups, women develop various forms of capital, harnessing their corporate vision to drive a determined commitment to change. Here, however, women join with one another to resist the coercive system of confession that denies women the chance to think for themselves. They no longer accept words that shame their bodies and passions and use their social bonds to support their communal resolve. If Sabbath is an invitation to wander into the unknown and to stray from the usual paths so that we can be replenished, then feminist liturgies may provide important Sabbath spaces where women of all sizes can carve out room for their bodies and ignite their imaginations.[95]

Reflecting on her own sense of what it means to pray as a woman, Nicola Slee suggests that 'we must question, hypothesize, challenge, reconceptualise. We must ask the unaskable, speak the unsayable, chart the unnavigable.'[96] In providing contexts where women can bring their bodies and fat to speech, feminist liturgical groups involve women in giving themselves permission to transgress all boundaries of reverent speech by describing their unruly bulges, bumps, lines, curves, dimples and folds in rebellious ways. They present an opportunity for women to develop new languages about fat in the context of faith, to 'play as we pray'[97] and to unite worship with the pursuit of justice. With no blueprint, this, for some, will be a journey into new knowledge and insight which only comes from going where we are told not to go and from journeying into the wild. It is a Sabbath course that Eve shows us,

94. Walton, *Feminist Liturgy*, 12.
95. Ibid., 31.
96. Nicola Slee, *Praying Like a Woman* (London: Society for Promoting Christian Knowledge, 2004), 2.
97. Walton, *Feminist Liturgy*, 31.

and it is a venture feminist women embark on with others in order to 'push against the blockages [and] help each other move the stones'.[98]

Living the Sabbath, Embodying Pride

To end this chapter I want to argue more explicitly a point that should already be starting to emerge – that fat pride is a crucial Sabbath sensibility and practice of salvation that resists the sin of sizeism. When Jane wins the Woman of the Year award and stands in her skirt pulling out the edges, we not only see how the generation of pride cleverly functions to validate sizeism but also how greater levels of body positivity enable her to flourish and expand. Fat pride recovers this latter feature of slimming but makes fatness a source of positivity.

Following the pattern of other pride movements such as gay pride, the civil rights and women's rights movement, the feminist fat liberation and fat acceptance movement invokes fat pride as a political stand against prejudice, discrimination and oppression. Originating in the United States in the 1960s but now evident throughout the West, the movement advocates for fat people and includes a collective of various organizations.[99] Notwithstanding the eclectic mix of commitments,

---

98. Slee, *Praying Like a Woman*, 2–3.

99. Sobal, 'The Size Acceptance Movement and the Social Construction of Body Weight', 237. For an excellent discussion of how fat acceptance groups use social media and other online platforms, see A. A. Afful and R. Ricciardelli, 'Shaping the Online Fat Acceptance Movement: Talking about Body Image and Beauty Standards, *Journal of Gender Studies* 24, no. 4 (2015): 453–72. NAAFA was founded by William Fabre, a self-identified fat admirer (ibid., 454). It is the dominant fat acceptance organization, but numerous groups have emerged within the fat acceptance network including The Fat Underground, The London Fat Women's Group and, more recently, The Chubsters, Health at Every Size and Pretty Porky and Pissed Off. The Fat Underground sought to bring feminism together with fat politics and began with Aldebaran and Judy Freespirit. (For more on the Fat Underground, see Cooper, *Fat and Proud*, 133–7 and Cooper, *Fat Activism*, 116–29.) Together they wrote the Fat Liberation Manifesto which aligned fat oppression with the stigmatization of other oppressed groups. The London Fat Women's Group began in 1987 but experienced infighting around issues of class, race and sexuality that were splitting the feminist movement at the time and so eventually disbanded. (See Cooper, *Fat and Proud*, 141.) The

views and political goals represented within the fat acceptance movement by a diversity of networks and groups, the notion of 'fat pride' is a defining feature. The principle emerged in the United States and the United Kingdom in response to the negative ways in which fatness was being portrayed in public discourse[100] and has been adopted by fat activists as a revolutionary political stance that replaces fat hatred with the principles of self-acceptance, body positivity and celebration.[101] Fat pride takes from LGBTQI politics the significance of 'coming out' as a radical act of confronting and dismantling social prejudice. For fat activist Charlotte Cooper, for example, being 'out and open' means having the courage as a fat woman to no longer live in fear or in camouflage.[102] Echoing the mantra of ACT-Up and Queer Nation, 'We're here, we're queer! Get used to it!,' Marilyn Wann captures the meaning of coming out as fat in the parallel refrain, 'We're here, we're spheres! Get used to it!'[103] According to Wann, the closet is just as dangerous for fat people as for LGBTQI persons, holding 'the dangers of unlived life, self-hatred, teen suicide, and brutalizing, futile "cures"'.[104] Fat people lack a language to celebrate fatness, she argues, because the only acceptable way to speak about fat is to speak about the need to do something about it. To reject shame and self-hatred as a fat person, she claims, is nothing short of revolutionary.

Feminist Christian women's liturgical groups provide a setting for developing new languages about fat from the contexts of women's bodies and so offer important faith spaces for the cultivation of fat pride. However, if fat pride is to be understood as a Sabbath sensibility

---

UK-based fat activist group, The Chubsters, was formed by Charlotte Cooper in 2003 as a queer feminist girl gang. (See Cooper, *Fat Activism*, 201–5.) The Health at Every Size movement stresses the importance of health over body size and contends that no conclusions can be made about a person's health on the basis of their weight. (For more, see Deb Burgard, 'What is "Health At Every Size?"', in *The Fat Studies Reader*, 42–53.) Pretty Porky and Pissed Off is a Toronto performance art and fat acceptance group founded by Allyson Mitchell and Ruby Rowan in 1996. (See Lupton, *Fat*, 81 and Afful and Ricciardelli, 'Shaping the Online Fat Acceptance Movement', 455.)

    100. Murray, *The 'Fat' Female Body*, 8.
    101. Ibid., 6.
    102. Cooper, *Fat and Proud*, 144.
    103. Wann cited in LeBesco, *Revolting Bodies?*, 95.
    104. Wann, *FAT!SO?*, 122.

and if it is to be promoted as an embodied response to the compulsory pursuit of thinness, it will need to take account of the bodies of women who slim. The concept, therefore, requires much broader definition and needs to attend to the way fat is constructed through discourse and confession and closely tied to individual and social perception. In distinction from the dominant narrative of fat acceptance, I suggest that fatness is not a brute fact. Fat 'materializes' through the performance of regulatory norms. As Judith Butler argues, social norms produce through force bodies that give the impression of fixity and surface that we call 'matter'. According to Butler, matter always materializes because the impression of 'naturalness' and the body as a fixed surface is only maintained by these norms being repeatedly performed in time, through the body.[105] We have seen already in this book that fat bodies are produced by sizeist norms. This means fat can never be simply viewed as a neutral description of unmediated reality. Fat is not just a 'hypervisible'[106] stigma or 'discredited identity' that shames women's bodies; it is produced by the power play of confession. In the group, fat is also a matter of perception, only outed on the scale and by Louise who exposes it. Fat pride as an expression of self-appreciation will, therefore, be an important practice of self-care that stands to assist women of a variety of sizes to resist the normative requirement to 'get rid'. Contrary to what Marilyn Wann suggests, it is not exclusive to fat people and is not only for the 'flabulous fatso'.[107]

Of course, appreciating that sizeist norms must be reiterated in order to materialize fat exposes that the process of materialization is never complete and that re-materialization is possible.[108] One way to re-materialize fatness is through individual and communal 'reiterative and ritual practices'[109] that 'flout' fat – that is, by repeatedly performing generosity and acceptance towards fat without apology. Liturgical settings allow women to develop and engage in rites that cultivate this affective posture, as do women's various forms of micro-activism. Both are expressive of the kind of Sabbath living that has the potential to transform the harried pursuit of thinness.

105. Butler, *Bodies That Matter*, 9–10.
106. Saguy and Ward, 'Coming Out as Fat', 54.
107. This is one of Marilyn Wann's famous descriptors. See her 'Fat! So? manifesto' in *FAT!SO?*, 28.
108. Butler, *Bodies That Matter*, 2.
109. Ibid., 10.

A Challenge to Theological 'Knowingness' about Pride

As a living out of Sabbath, fat pride is a religious as well as political performance that sees loving fat as inseparable from observing the Sabbath command to rest in God's uncontainable pleasure. This not only violates conventional theological approaches to fatness but also flouts normative theological understandings of, and Christian 'knowingness' about pride. According to mainstream theological tradition, pride is a heinous sin – a 'deadly' sin – that upsets a proper orientation towards God. For the fourth-century desert-dwelling monk Evagrius Ponticus, pride accompanies gluttony, impurity, avarice, sadness, anger, acedia and vainglory as a category of (evil) thought or 'logismoi', preventing a person from engaging in true knowledge of God.[110] 'Pride is a tumour of the soul filled with pus,' he teaches; 'When it has ripened, it will rupture and create a great disgusting mess.'[111] John Cassian takes Evagrius's ideas and develops them into 'eight principal vices that attack humankind', naming pride as one of these.[112] Pope Gregory the Great then identifies pride as the root sin and as the source of other so-called deadly sins.[113] According to Gregory, pride is a sin that swells the mind.[114]

For these early Christians, pride means hubris, an overestimation of the self. Although contemporary meanings may describe pride more positively as 'self-respect' or 'self-assurance', the term continues to carry negative association with arrogance and conceit. Proud people think they are bigger than others; they are full of themselves and inflated with

---

110. Scott Sullender, 'The Seven Deadly Sins as a Pastoral Diagnostic System', *Pastoral Psychology* 64 (2015): 218.

111. Evagrius Ponticus cited in George Tsakiridis, *Evagrius Ponticus and Cognitive Science: A Look at Moral Evil and the Thoughts* (Eugene: Pickwick, 2010), 31. According to Evagrius, pride is the failure to acknowledge God as the source of all virtue.

112. John Cassian, *The Conferences*, trans. Boniface Ramsey (New York and Mahwah: The Newman Press, 1997), 183.

113. Gregory identified the seven deadly sins as pride, lust, anger, envy, sloth, gluttony and avarice. For more on this, see Hoverd, 'Deadly Sin: Gluttony, Obesity and Health Policy', 215 and 218.

114. Gregory the Great, *The Book of Pastoral Rule*, trans. and intro. by George E. Demacopoulos (New York: St Vladimir's Seminary Press, 2007), 141. The seven deadly sins inspired medieval and renaissance writers like Dante whose *Inferno* interwove the deadly sins with the nine circles of hell. See Sullender, 'The Seven Deadly Sins as a Pastoral Diagnostic System', 219.

a sense of self. These popular descriptions resonate with theological accounts of pride and expose the sizeist connotations of the concept. Whether a 'swollen' mind as with Gregory, a boasting self who puffs up like leavened bread, as Paul suggests to the Corinthians (1 Cor. 5.6-8), hearts that are arrogant, 'fat and gross' as in Ps. 119.70, or an 'inflated' self, the tacit message is that it is morally wrong to be big, to grow and expand.

Appended to this is the assumption that virtue is found away from a fully centred-self. Pride is about being self-serving and self-centred, and this view has been rightly challenged by feminist theologians on the grounds that it discourages women from pursuing selfhood. Famous critiques forwarded by the likes of Valarie Saiving, Judith Plaskow and Susan Nelson have made clear that the conflation of sin with pride fails to take sufficient account of women's experiences of sin. If women's sin is found in the temptation to think too little of themselves, to depend on others for self-definition, in self-negation[115] and in refusing the freedom to name themselves,[116] then pride, for women, is more expressive of salvation than sin.

Although such feminist positions have raised legitimate concerns about gender essentialism,[117] tending to accuse all women of the sin

115. Valerie Saiving, 'The Human Situation: A Feminine View', *The Journal of Religion* 40, no. 2 (1960): 109. Plaskow describes women's sin as 'drifting' through life, a scenario that occurs when without even realizing, women look to others for self-definition and fail to take responsibility for their own lives. 'The language of self-sacrifice conflicts with personhood and becomes destructive when it depicts that the struggle to become a centred self, to achieve full independent selfhood, is sinful.' Judith Plaskow, *Sex, Sin and Grace: Women's Experience and the Theologies of Reinhold Niebuhr and Paul Tillich* (Lanham and London: University Press of America, 1980), 87.

116. Susan Nelson Dunfee, 'The Sin of Hiding: A Feminist Critique of Reinhold Niebuhr's Account of the Sin of Pride', *Soundings: An Interdisciplinary Journal* 65, no. 3 (1982): 316–27.

117. Susan Thistlethwaite, for example, has levelled this critique at Saiving: 'Without a historically accurate definition of what it means to be female in different racial, class, and sexual role definitions, Saiving's contribution to understanding "sin for women" is misleading.' See Susan Brooks Thistlethwaite, *Sex, Race, and God: Christian Feminism in Black and White* (Eugene: Wipf & Stock, 1989), 78–9. Also see Jacquelyn Grant, *White Women's Christ, Black*

of self-negation and all men of the opposite sin of pride,[118] they have provided a crucial challenge to mainline Protestant theology by identifying pride as an avenue to salvation. As a Christian outworking of Sabbath, the practice of fat pride continues in this pattern and confidently confesses that women can be fat, big, powerful and full of self without having to apologize. Fat pride expresses confidence in women's created goodness and prophetically witnesses to the fact that fat bodies are valuable, loveable and revelatory of God. Pride is not an emotion that tears the self from God nor is it a barrier to salvation; it attaches women to their bodies and feelings and enables them to come into their 'yes' and participate in the delight of God. In cultural contexts where women's fat is especially vilified, women's performance of fat pride contributes to the meaningful work of self-care and salvation. Such a posture refuses to repeat the regulatory norm that says women must keep their fat under cover. When women hide their bodies because they are ashamed of their size, they become buried beneath shame and guilt. Fat pride on the other hand signals a 'coming out' from the closet of fat shame into 'a *life* to be lived'.[119] 'Coming out' is a coming out against sizeism and a coming out against body shame, a coming out in support of fatness. All are theo-political acts of 'holding our bodies together', to cite disability theologian Nancy Eiesland, because they have us 'affirm … our bodies as whole, good and beautiful' rather than as incomplete or disgusting.[120]

Fat Pride Overlooks the Fact that Fat is Unhealthy?

Of course, whether performed through micro-activism or in liturgical groups, fat pride is controversial. Some will worry that presenting it as salvific and as one Sabbath practice of delight glamorizes obesity and fails to acknowledge the real threat that fat poses to health. Elspeth Probyn sees this tendency in fat activism. For her, fat pride is an ineffectual political strategy because it keeps people fat and fails to challenge the

---

Women's Jesus: Feminist Christology and Womanist Response (New York: Oxford University Press, 1989), 14.

118. See, for example, Angela West, *Deadly Innocence: Feminist Theology and the Mythology of Sin* (London: Cassell, 1995).

119. Dunfee, 'The Sin of Hiding', 325. Emphasis in original.

120. Nancy L. Eiesland, *The Disabled God: Toward a Liberatory Theology of Disability* (Nashville: Abingdon Press, 1994), 95–6.

socio-economic structures that produce larger bodies.[121] Antronette Yancey, Joanne Leslie and Emily Abel make a similar point when they suggest that by overlooking the 'accumulating data' on the health risks of being fat, feminists ignore the socio-economic inequalities that place women at higher risk of obesity.[122] They argue that feminists should care more about the vested interests of corporations profiting from fast-food industries, about access to physical activity and healthy food because women are usually at the centre of these inequalities.

It is certainly the case that feminists and feminist theologians should care about women's health and about women's access to nutritious food and exercise, but lurking behind both of these arguments is the assumption that fatness is caused by unhealthy eating[123] and results in a greater risk of death. In Yancey, Leslie and Abel's piece, statistics about obesity are presented in support of their overarching view that fat is a 'serious health problem',[124] and it is this generalization that the political posture of fat pride appropriately challenges. What constitutes health is by no means obvious. Health is not a fixed or self-evident reality but a discursive construct produced through relations of power/knowledge that serve to stigmatize certain groups. In the case of fat, mainline health discourses confirm fat as a disease and moral impediment that must be corrected and such narratives systematically function to build a climate of fear about weight.

Often there are sinister financial interests being served through the transmission of anti-obesity discourses. A 2008 White Paper published by the Obesity Society defending the notion of 'obesity' as disease, for example, discloses at the end that its authors 'have accepted funds from multiple food, pharmaceutical, and other companies with interests in

---

121. Elspeth Probyn, 'Silences Behind the Mantra: Critiquing Feminist Fat', *Feminism & Psychology* 18, no. 3 (2008): 402.

122. Antronette K. Yancey, Joanne Leslie and Emily K. Abel, 'Obesity at the Crossroads: Feminist and Public Health Perspective', *Signs* 31, no. 2 (2006): 425.

123. Feminist writers challenging size discrimination have sometimes failed to question this assumption. Susie Orbach and Kim Chernin, for example, both reinforce the view that fat results from compulsive overeating and is an expression of mental or physical ill health. For a discussion of this feature of early feminist engagements with weight, see Tina Jenkins and Barbara Smith, 'Fat Liberation', *Spare Rib: A Women's Liberation Magazine* 182 (1987): 14–18.

124. Yancey, Leslie and Abel, 'Obesity at the Crossroads', 427.

obesity'.[125] In the UK, the general public are told that lifestyle choices now cause 37 per cent of cancers, with obesity and overweight being substantial factors,[126] but Cancer Research UK is funded by the weight loss organization I joined, and generously so. Both examples reveal how health organizations and weight loss industries are financially invested in transmitting anti-fat messages.[127] The fact is that public health officials who wage war against fat are often paid consultants for weight loss and drug companies. Many who run weight loss clinics are often on the staff of medical institutions or serve on health panels which define health priorities and that obtain research grants.[128] This again suggests that anti-obesity health-talk is in no way neutral or objective.

Furthermore, not all health experts agree on the physical dangers of fatness.[129] Some argue that fat cannot be established unambiguously as the cause of high-risk diseases like cardiovascular disease, hypertension and diabetes.[130] For health professionals researching in the Health at

---

125. TOS Obesity as a Disease Writing Group, 'Obesity as a Disease: A White Paper on Evidence and Arguments Commissioned by the Council of the Obesity Society', *Obesity* 16 (2008): 1177.

126. Alex Therrien, 'Rise in Cancers "Caused by Weight"', *BBC News*, http://www.bbc.co.uk/news/health-43502144 (accessed 4 May 2018).

127. Eric Oliver suggests that the source of America's obesity 'epidemic' is not Burger King or McDonald's but the country's health establishment that has set low and arbitrary definitions of ideal weight rendering most Americans 'overweight' or 'obese'. As well as exaggerating the dangers of fat, the construction of obesity as a 'disease' in the 1990s, he argues, served the financial interests of government health agencies, scientists and pharmaceutical companies, extending the size of their budgets and enabling new drugs to be developed that would inflate stock prices. He notes how most reports identifying obesity as a 'disease' have been written by those standing to benefit from this pathological framing of fat. See J. Eric Oliver, *Fat Politics: The Real Story behind America's Obesity Epidemic* (Oxford and New York: Oxford University Press, 2006), 5–6.

128. Pat Lyons, 'Prescription for Harm', in *The Fat Studies Reader*, 79–80.

129. See Maria Grazia Franzosi, 'Should We Continue to Use BMI as a Cardiovascular Risk Factor?', *The Lancet* 368 (2006): 624–5 which shows how typical associations between obesity and increased risk of mortality and 'cardiovascular events' are being questioned; Ernsberger, 'Obesity is an Early Symptom of Diabetes', 67–9; Fontaine et al., 'Body Mass Index and Mortality Rate among Hispanic Adults'.

130. Bacon and Aphramor, 'Weight Science', 4.

Every Size (HAES) movement, where evidence suggests a link between high BMI and such diseases, it does not prove that fatness produces them. Not only are these diseases present in thinner people, access to good quality food, medical care, weight-based stigma and weight cycling are among the other possible explanations for the connection.[131] Co-founder of the organization, Deb Burgard, argues that for every weight there are people who are healthy and unhealthy, making the distinction between 'acceptable' and 'unacceptable' weight contentious. High BMI becomes a protective factor after the age of seventy, she finds, with some health conditions being less prevalent in people with higher BMIs.[132] She also notes that weight loss can cause physiological and psychological harm when it is followed by patterns of weight cycling, such patterns having been correlated with hypertension and adverse body fat distribution.[133]

What all this means is that the conflation of health with thinness is far too simplistic. Although measures of ideal weight like the BMI make it extremely hard to acknowledge, thin people can be unhealthy and fat people can be healthy.[134] Assuming fat is synonymous with unhealthiness also often assumes that fatness results from eating too much and/or from poor diet, but fat cannot be straightforwardly associated with volition in this way. While some data shows that weight loss can be sustained after leaving a commercial dieting setting,[135] a number of other studies show that slimming people's best efforts fail to produce permanent and safe weight loss.[136] Most women in my group had experimented with multiple diets before joining the group and though some had been successful, where weight had been lost, it had inevitably been regained, provoking their renewed attempts to 'get rid'.

---

131. Burgard, 'What is "Health at Every Size?"', 46.

132. Ibid., 44.

133. Ibid., 47.

134. See Bacon and Aphramor, 'Weight Science', 6.

135. See, for example, Michael R. Lowe, Tanja V. E. Kral and Karen Miller-Kovach, 'Weight-Loss Maintenance 1, 2 and 5 Years after Successful Completion of a Weight-Loss Programme', *The British Journal of Nutrition* 99, no. 4 (2008): 925–30.

136. See, for example, F. Grodstein, R. Levine, L. Troy, T. Spencer, G. A. Colditz and M. J. Stampfer, 'Three-Year Follow-Up of Participants in a Commercial Weight Loss Program: Can You Keep It Off?', *Archives of Internal Medicine* 156, no. 12 (June 1996): 1302–6.

It is also important to recognize that genetic and physiological factors potentially impact body size. Robinson, Hunger and Daly suggest that low resting metabolic rate and high respiratory quotient may influence weight gain;[137] for Jeffrey Friedman, genetics may account for as much as 70 per cent of factors contributing to weight. For him, the pursuit of weight loss is a fight we are bound to lose because in the end, it is a 'battle against biology'.[138]

These alternative accounts of fat will make some feel uncomfortable, but they suggest that the foundational claims of anti-obesity discourse are contentious. People in the United Kingdom and the United States are getting fatter, but that does not mean that the public's health is in decline.[139] Health problems in these countries are considerable, but few of these can be causally linked with the population's increasing weight.[140] All this suggests that fatness cannot be unambiguously associated with unhealthiness. It also indicates that slimming should not be endorsed as an 'obvious' good. Sustained weight loss or weight fluctuation can pose worse risks to health than remaining overweight[141] and the mental

137. In their study of perceived weight status and the risk of weight gain across life in US and UK adults, Robinson, Hunger and Daly also found that perceiving oneself as overweight actually increased the likelihood of weight gain since individuals were more likely to overeat as a result and in response to being part of a stigmatized group. See E. Robinson, J. M. Hunger and M. D, 'Perceived Weight Status and Risk of Weight Gain across Life in US and UK Adults', *International Journal of Obesity* 38, no. 12 (2015): 1725.

138. Jeffrey Friedman, 'A War on Obesity, Not the Obese', *Science* 299 (2003): 858. His position is echoed by fat activist writers like Wann and Pat Lyons who see fat more as a brute fact that is biologically determined. Marilyn Wann argues that 'anatomy is destiny. ... Some people are left-handed, just like some people are fat. In both cases, it's pretty much something you're born with' (Wann, *FAT!SO?*, 47). Pat Lyons refers to fat people as 'those of us whose genetically determined bodies refuse to conform to "ideal" weight charts'. See Pat Lyons, 'Fitness, Feminism and the Health of Fat Women', in *Overcoming Fear of Fat*, ed. Laura S. Brown and Esther D. Rothblum (London and New York: Routledge, 1989), 65–6.

139. Lyons, 'Prescription for Harm', 77.

140. Oliver, *Fat Politics*, 2.

141. See, for example, K. D. Brownell and J. Rodin, 'Medical, Metabolic, and Psychological Effects of Weight Cycling', *Archives of Internal Medicine* 154, no. 12 (June 1994): 1325–30.

anguish many women experience as they slim (observed in my group where fear of fat keeps some locked in cycles of anxiety) diminishes their well-being and frustrates a Sabbath sensibility. Ultimately, weight can never be a stand-alone measure for health, nor can it be simplistically tied to volition. Other factors also contribute to health such as psychological well-being, self-esteem, enjoying what we eat and having access to reliable health care, nutritious food and physical exercise.[142]

On this reading, practising the Sabbath repose by refusing to relentlessly patrol our size may have health benefits, contributing to women's wellness and wholeness, and so to our projects of salvation. A focus on health over weight has, indeed, been shown to improve blood pressure, blood lipids, mood, self-esteem and body image.[143] Yet, some may question whether the concept of 'fat pride' returns ultimate significance to size and poundage celebrating fat as unequivocally good and so as indisputably healthy. The account of fat pride I am proposing presents the embodiment of pride by women as a practice of self-care. This resists myopic discourses about fatness and health and embraces a body-positive posture that has the power to improve the physical and psychological well-being of women. When we embody fat pride we affirm our bodies as good: our bodies that are fat and that display fatness, all without exception. Taking pride in fat is to embrace fat and fat bodies as valid and as expressive of God. This does not announce that all fat bodies are healthy or that all thin bodies are either, but it does proclaim that all fat bodies are valuable. Fat pride refuses to repeat the assumption that fat is synonymous with disease and ill health, while conversely acknowledging that fat acceptance and body positivity have the potential to enrich women's health and help heal the fractured relationship with fat that many women experience. Weight can never tell us anything 'obvious' about a person's health. In the end Marilyn

---

142. Bacon and Aphramor suggest that people with strong self-esteem are more likely to demonstrate positive health behaviour, engaging in regular exercise and connecting their eating to how their bodies feel. Bacon and Aphramor, 'Weight Science', 7.

143. Bacon and Aphramor claim that while evidence does not support the view that weight loss is synonymous with health, findings from a number of randomized controlled trials show that shifting emphasis away from weight and the pursuit of weight loss can improve health. Bacon and Aphramor, 'Weight Science', 2.

Wann is right that 'the only thing anyone can diagnose by looking at a fat person is their own level of prejudice toward fat people'.[144]

Fat Pride Overlooks the Pain and Discomfort of Fatness?

Aligning salvation with the Sabbath sensibility of fat pride may also appear to overlook the negative ways in which fatness is experienced by some women. Suggesting women should be euphoric about their size may seem to ignore the ambiguities of fat embodiment. Samantha Murray criticizes the notion of 'fat pride' on these grounds. She suggests that the principle is flawed because it assumes one is '"fat and proud", with no grey areas, no contradictions'.[145] She recounts her own experience as a fat woman of feeling 'strong, powerful, [and] swollen with my fat identity' as she wore a sleeveless top with her dimpled arms proudly visible, only to, moments later, squirm at her own reflection in a shop window.[146] She describes too an instance when she followed her mother's advice and tried on a pair of 'Control Top' underpants designed to keep her fat in, only to, moments later, feel horrified by her actions and the way the undergarment hurt and branded her body, preventing her from moving and breathing freely.[147] The red marks left imprinted on her skin served to remind her that her fat body was a transient body, always on its way to becoming and, more specifically, to becoming thin.[148] Fat pride is problematic, she argues, because it assumes a unitary subject, and this fails to bear witness to the divided embodiment fat women often experience.

At the centre of this worry is that a fat-positive stance encourages the kind of escape from the body already addressed in this chapter and consistently challenged in this book. In the case where fat existence is characterized by messy contradictions, the solution appears to be one of flight.[149] Yet as an outworking of Sabbath, fat pride does not call women

---

144. Marilyn Wann, 'Fat & Choice: A Personal Essay', *MP: An Online Feminist Journal*, http://academinist.org/wp-content/uploads/2005/09/010308Wann_Fat.pdf, 62 (accessed 5 May 2018).
145. Murray, '(Un/Be)Coming Out?', 160.
146. Ibid., 153.
147. Ibid., 154–6.
148. Ibid., 155.
149. Similar concerns have been raised by disability scholars in response to the so-called 'social' model of disability. For theologian Nancy Eiesland,

to crucify their bodies and tear their selves apart for being unable to unambiguously celebrate fat. As I have already argued, the Sabbath space is a place of return that invites compassion and kindness towards our bodyselves rather than harshness and judgement. Liturgical settings provide women with contexts for sharing honestly and openly and so are environments where women can narrate the contradictions they embody. This may involve bringing to speech 'the jumbled pleasure-pain that is our bodies'.[150] Fat pride, as a practice of salvation, is an enactment of self-care that we will need to begin again and again.

Accepting fat with delight is grounded in respect for the body and for the complexity of being bodies. Physical discomfort and pain do cause some women to opt for surgical intervention, and there is no shame in this because physical distress can be 'persistent and real', as Murray herself experiences.[151] What I am arguing, however, is that weight loss need not be the 'obvious' solution to health issues it is said to be. Given health complaints are often not caused by fat, a myriad of other health options or social and economic changes may be more appropriate. If socio-economic conditions are impacting a woman's ability to access nutritious food and are producing ill health; if the material environments of church, office, home, hospital, pub, restaurant and plane cause physical pain; if the stress of being fat in a fat-hating world produces high blood pressure and makes women less likely to visit the doctor, then this signals the need for other types of change in order to facilitate women's Sabbath repose. To have pride in fat is to protest against the way sizeist society forces fat women in particular to see fat embodiment as uninhabitable and to reject the conventional wisdom that says weight loss is the only way to live a liveable life.

---

coming to terms with the body for disabled people can mean facing the reality of bodies that twitch or fall over, that feel uncomfortable and that are sources of distress. 'Embodiment is not a purely agreeable reality,' she reflects; 'It incorporates profound ambiguity – sometimes downright distress. There is simply no denying it.' Eiesland, *The Disabled God*, 95.

150. Ibid., 96.

151. Samantha Murray, 'Women Under/In Control? Embodying Eating After Gastric Banding', in *Whose Weight Is It Anyway?: Essays on Ethics and Eating*, ed. Sofie Vandamme, Suzanne van de Vathorst and Inez de Beaufort (Leuven: Acco Academic, 2010), 43–4. Murray explains how she had a laparoscopic gastric band fitted due to the continuous pain and lethargy she experienced as a fat woman.

Conclusion: Salvation, Sabbath and Fat Pride

Salvation is whatever helps individuals and communities to thrive. It is not only the work of God but also the work of human creatures who are called by God to build God's future of peace in the here and now. This chapter has argued that to practise the Sabbath repose by ceasing from slavishly patrolling fat and appetite is to prophetically embody this future and to resist sin. In a world dominated by fears about food and fat and in response to the anxiety system of slimming that punishes women for feeling content with their bodies, the call to observe Sabbath energizes women towards counter-cultural practices of delight that can help heal distorted relationships with food, fat and the bodyself.

The Sabbath space is a hush in the busyness of our thinning projects. It is an invitation to reappraise our bodies and their relationship with time, to journey into unknown territories, to play and experiment with 'obvious' knowledge about fat and to delight in existence for its own sake. The call to rest encourages us to break from the usual work of patrolling fat and to engage in the extraordinary work of savouring and delighting in the place of our present bodies. As a repose that is lived and worked out in everyday life, Sabbath is cultivated through deliberate and purposeful action. By ourselves, we may engage in forms of micro-activism where we intentionally cease from fat shaming and take a deliberate break from slimming and from slavishly patrolling our bodies, but if Sabbath is a calling for the people of God it will need to be a communal repose also, motivated by the social and political vision of equal rest and equal worth. Feminist liturgical women's groups ('women-church') are politically motivated towards the transformation of society and towards the Christian vision of remembering God's call away from slavish productivity and making God's eschatological repose present in the here and now. They provide important Sabbath spaces where women can come together in search of rest from body hatred, from fat shame and to break with the systems of anxiety and coercion that alienate us from our bodies. As an outworking of a Sabbath sensibility, fat pride may be cultivated as women share and meet together, pray, dance, eat, sing, speak, think and move in ways that challenge fat phobia and in ways that allow their fat to venture out of the closet into the open. Here, ritual becomes a religious and political activity that helps reshape the world, opening up spaces for women to caress their fat with kindness and to face their size with celebration. Women bring their fat to speech and celebrate the value of their bodies together. Rites and liturgies rupture assumptions about appropriate thought, speech, behaviour and religious observance, providing creative spaces where women can celebrate their bumps, bulges, folds and curves and form communities of solidarity committed to resisting sin. Through a hearty embrace of fat, women engage in the Sabbath practice of delight which has the potential to challenge cultural scripts and 're-materialize' fatness.

Such an account of Sabbath takes from the slimming group the importance of community for forming social bonds and for challenging normative expectations. It also extends the principle of permission that galvanizes women's transgressive actions by aligning the Sabbath repose with a practice of agency that has the potential to subvert and resist sin. Living the Sabbath through individual and communal activities that break with the ordinary work of shaming fat calls women towards the cultivation of similar capacities as those observed in the group but without re-placing women into a sacrificial economy. Self-authorization, self-determinism, creativity, self-reflection, valuing other women's experiences, self-esteem, narrating one's own life and body, building solidarity with other women through fellowship and food – through the sharing of stories and experience – and practising a new cultural habit are all capacities that can be developed by the kind of Sabbath living outlined in this chapter.

Fat pride is a Christian act of 'coming out' of the closet of fat shame. It recovers the emotion of pride from the theological waste bin of sin, presenting it instead as a site of wellness and salvation. This performance of a Sabbath sensibility is a form of resurrection, but one that bids us rise just as we are. It does not encourage a soteriological flight from the present, from time, age and all things corporeal. Nor does it require that we be 'born again' into a different body or that we crucify our fat so that a thinner body can emerge victorious. Fat pride renounces the claim that God is elated by the odour of burning fat. As a mode of practical living that arises from our thankful disposition, fat pride has us join with the Psalmist in exclaiming, 'For you, O Lord, have made me glad by your work; at the works of your hands I sing for joy' (Ps. 92.4). In praise of God's goodness in creation and in celebration of each person's embodied uniqueness, it is a journey into aliveness. When we allow our fat to be without apology, we live into God's tactile and intimate embrace and into a future where seemingly untouchable bodies are lovingly touched by God. This may be one of the most 'sensible' futures we can imagine.

CONCLUSION: FOR THE LOVE OF FOOD, FOR THE LOVE OF FAT

My weight loss book looks pretty haggard. The spine is practically broken because of the amount of times it has been opened and closed by the volunteer on the scale, by me in the meeting and at home and through the course of me doing this research. It feels nice in my hands. It bulges with slips of paper that have been handed out in meetings, with recipes, pages of my food diary, certificates I have been awarded. When I look at my 'personal progress record' that is contained in the book and which appears directly after the seventeen-page list of Syns, I see how my weight changed, incrementally reducing almost weekly. I lost 9.5 kilograms in total while in the group. I was what might be called a 'successful' slimmer. Like so many other women who slim, I have regained most of the weight I lost, and even though I am absolutely convinced that it is better to learn to love my body rather than punish it, I still miss feeling thinner. Such is the struggle for life and salvation. The ambiguity of these feelings does not worry me though, exactly because I recognize that I am a woman who cannot escape the hegemony of the thin ideal. I think it is better to be honest about my ambivalence, because then I stand a better chance of touching my body with kindness and permitting myself to enjoy my food. But there are no quick-fix solutions to the self-division many women experience or to the multiple ways in which food and fat are victimized in our culture. The work of reconciliation requires not only stamina but also kindness and grace, for as we imagine and attempt to live into a different future in our now bodies, we will inevitably stumble and so must learn to practise forgiveness with ourselves and with one another.

In her reflections on reconciliation, Ada María Isasi-Díaz suggests that three requisites need to be met before we can really know the reality of brokenness. First, one has to be in the midst of it and one's body touched by it; second, one has to accept and understand one's role in it and third, one has to do something to heal it.[1] Through the

---

1. Isasi-Díaz, *La Lucha Continues*, 226.

course of writing this book, I have lived all three of these features. Through participation in the weight loss group, my body has known and experienced what it means to patrol food and my desire for it and has experienced the shame and disappointment of fat. I have come to observe how my worrying about food and weight diminishes my aliveness before God and how even nodding at others who joke about being 'good' in the face of food or who poke fun at fat makes me complicit in the sins that I profoundly wish to challenge. This book is one form of action I take to heal the divisions I have observed and felt, but it is a journey about doing rather than writing. The challenge is not to replace food with words (as in the weight loss group) by substituting better foodways with an academic book on weight but to commit with my mouth, gut, mind and hands to a better future by intentionally trying to change the present.

Part of this healing comes from observing and respecting the enabling aspects of slimming culture. Although I do not wish to endorse the pursuit of thinness, there are nevertheless things feminist theologians can glean from weight loss communities, and a central ambition of this book has been to identify some of those features and to put them to work in alternative ways. The emphasis women place on pride, community and social bonds, on valuing and summoning the power they hold in their bodies and mouths to shape and reform their lives, on food as a locus of salvation, on the importance of writing and speaking their bodies into being, on self-permission and its capacity to be performed in ways that transgress hegemonic norms – these are all enabling and worthwhile dimensions of slimming that can be uncoupled from the sacrificial project of burning fat and channelled into activities that resist it. If feminist theologians are to respect as 'holy ground' the lives and bodies of women who slim, then we need to take seriously the ways in which slimming increases women's capacities, at the same time as appreciating how the possibilities for flourishing operate in tandem with the intensification of power relations.

In plotting the resonances with ancient Christian thought, I have shown that the secular rhetoric and discourses that the organization and its members develop and transmit have theological vestiges. These alliances allow the company to profit from the historic efficacy of theological idioms to discipline women's appetites. Christian notions of 'sin' and 'salvation' surface as theological residues that feed the tensions of modernity and consumer anxieties of advanced capitalism. As well as exposing the ongoing purchase of sin and salvation in Western culture, the cultural borrowing from Christianity moves beyond a mere general appropriation. By plotting the particulars of women's weight loss narratives against multiple layers of theological meaning, we have seen the intricate and multifaceted ways in which theological ideas surface in, and resonate with, patriarchal weight loss ideologies.

We have seen too that slimming does not simply continue the worst aspects of Christian religion. While this book has argued that that women in the group follow well-established Christian discourse in aligning food with sin, in lauding self-abnegation and techniques of detachment from pleasure and emotion as virtuous and by deferring ultimate fulfilment to a life-after-fat, they also repeat healthful aspects of ancient theological tradition, foregrounding food and body in their salvation projects and acknowledging the power of eating to reorient the self, produce insight and shape intentional attitudes and actions. By amplifying the aspects of women's Syn and salvation narratives together with related theological traditions shown to be healthful and by modifying or rejecting those aspects which engender harm, I have developed feminist theological accounts of sin and salvation that speak back to theological tradition and the culture of slimming. Sin is a relational tear. The term provides a distinctly Christian way of describing exploitative and domineering ways of relating to food, fatness and our bodyselves. This adds thin privilege and weight-related fears about food to the intersecting politics of domination named by Ruether and other Christian feminists. Sin describes the way we use our freedom to create and assent to exploitative patterns of relationship that diminish the self and others, violating the aliveness which is God's intention. The life-diminishing realities of sin are, however, located within the hopeful grasp of God's grace. Knowledge of sin drives us towards redemptive action. Salvation is the meaningful work of reconciliation, a praxis that emerges from a refusal to let the sins of sizeism, the victimization of food and the divided self have the last word. It is imagined in this book as the alimentary and erotic practices of 'sensible eating' – a mode of eating that reconnects food with feeling, pleasure, sensuality and passion, and as a living out of the Sabbath repose – an individual and communal practice of rest from the frenetic sacrificial work of burning fat. Theology has important work to do in restoring face to fat people so that fatness is not maligned through the resources of faith. The principles of Sabbath and fat pride assist with this.

This book responds to the call marshalled by some working in Fat Studies for the discipline to attend more closely to religion.[2] By plotting the various ways in which theologies intersect with the commercial enterprise of slimming and by showing how theologies might resource more healthful discourses and practices around food and fat, I have sought to contribute a distinctly religious perspective to current debates surrounding fat politics. This book also enriches and extends current feminist theological discussion on weight and fat by studying the micro-practices of ordinary women who slim and by delving into the layers of theological meaning that are recycled in the context of a commercial weight loss setting. Ultimately, I present size-acceptance as a thoroughly Christian political stance that calls for faith-based action in our world.

According to Mary McClintock Fulkerson, 'Theologies that matter, arise out of dilemmas – out of situations that matter'. The contemporary marketization of women's fears about food and fat and the multiple ways in which Christian discourse assists the war on fat is a situation that matters. It is a dilemma observed within the particular situation of the group I attended and one that is replicated in various ways and to various degrees in cultural discourses about fat. As such, it demands our time and attention. It is too straightforward to say that women are tricked by the 'false' promises of weight loss culture or duped into believing that self-abnegation is good for them. However, if the enabling dimensions of slimming are cleverly recycled back into the lucrative business of burning fat, then Christian theology has an important role to play in resourcing a faith-based call away from this sacrificial economy. The challenge for Christian communities of faith is to provide prophetic and nourishing contexts where the compulsion to 'get rid' is met by real opportunities for women to embrace their bodies with delight and their fat with pride.

---

2. This invitation is extended by Lynne Gerber, Susan Hill and LeRhonda Manigault-Bryant in their introduction to the special issue of the journal, *Fat Studies*, designed to engage with the intersection between religion and fat in light of this deficit. See 'Religion and Fat = Protestant Christianity and Weight Loss? On the Intersections of Fat Studies and Religious Studies'.

Bibliography

Afful, Adwoa A. and Ricciardelli, Rose. 'Shaping the Online Fat Acceptance Movement: Talking about Body Image and Beauty Standards'. *Journal of Gender Studies* 24, no. 4 (2015): 453–72.

Ahmed, Sara. *The Cultural Politics of Emotion*, 2nd edition. Edinburgh: Edinburgh University Press, 2014.

Alcoff, Linda. 'Feminism and Foucault: The Limits to a Collaboration'. In *Crises in Continental Philosophy*, edited by Arlene B. Dallery, Charles E. Scott with P. Holley Roberts, 69–87. New York: State University of New York Press, 1990.

Alexander, Saffron. 'Is a Glass of Wine a Night Healthy?'. *The Telegraph*, 3 March 2016. Accessed 8 September 2016. http://www.telegraph.co.uk/food-and-drink/wine/is-red-wine-really-healthy/

Allender, Dan B. *Sabbath*, foreword by Phyllis Tickle. Nashville: Thomas Nelson, 2009.

Althaus-Reid, Marcella Maria. '"Pussy, Queen of Pirates": Acker, Isherwood and the Debate on the Body in Feminist Theology'. *Feminist Theology* 12, no. 2 (2004): 157–67.

Althaus-Reid, Marcella Maria. 'Queering the Cross: The Politics of Redemption and the External Debt'. *Feminist Theology* 15, no. 3 (2007): 289–301.

Althaus-Reid, Marcella Maria and Isherwood, Lisa. 'Introduction. Slicing Women's Bodies: Christianity and the Cut, Mutilated and Cosmetically Altered Believers'. In *Controversies in Body Theology*, edited by Marcella Althaus-Reid and Lisa Isherwood, 1–6. London: SCM, 2008.

Aquinas, Thomas. *Summa Theologiæ*, 16 (Ia2æ.1-5), Purpose and Happiness, translated by Thomas Gilby. Cambridge, New York: Cambridge University Press, 2006.

Aquinas, Thomas. *Summa Theologiæ*, 25 (Ia2æ. 71-80), Sin, translated by John Fearon. Cambridge, New York: Cambridge University Press, 2006.

Aquinas, Thomas. *Summa Theologiæ*, 26 (Ia2æ. 81-85), Original Sin, translated by T. C. O'Brien. Cambridge, New York: Cambridge University Press, 2006.

Aquinas, Thomas. *Summa Theologiæ*, 43 (2a2æ. 141-154), Temperance, translated by Thomas Gilby. Cambridge, New York: Cambridge University Press, 2006.

Athanasius. 'Life of Anthony'. In *A Select Library of Nicene and Post-Nicene Fathers of the Christian Church*, translated by Rev. A. Robertson, edited by Philip Schaff and Henry Wace, Second Series, vol. IV. Grand Rapids: William B. Eerdmans Publishing Company, 1978.

Augustine. *Answer to the Pelagians*, introduction, translation, and notes Roland J. Teske, edited by John E. Rotelle. New York: New City Press, 1997.

Augustine. *Answer to the Pelagians, II*, introduction, translation and notes Roland J. Teske, edited by John E. Rotelle. New York: New City Press, 1998.

Augustine. 'City of God'. In *A Select Library of the Nicene and Post-Nicene Fathers of the Christian Church*, vol. 11, edited by Philip Schaff, 1–511. Grand Rapids: William B. Eerdmans Publishing Company, 1979.

Augustine. 'On Christian Doctrine'. In *A Select Library of the Nicene and Post-Nicene Fathers of the Christian Church*, vol. 11, edited by Philip Schaff, 516–97. Grand Rapids: William B. Eerdmans Publishing Company, 1979.

Augustine. *On the Trinity*, Books 8–15, edited by Gareth B. Matthews, translated by Stephen McKenna. Cambridge, New York: Cambridge University Press, 2002.

Augustine. *Sermons*, III/3 (51–94). 'On The New Testament', translated by E. Hill, edited by J. E. Rotelle. New York: New City Press, 1991.

Augustine. *Sermons*, III/7 (230–272B). 'On the Liturgical Seasons', translated and notes by E. Hill, edited by J. Rotelle. New York: New City Press, 1993.

Augustine. *Sermons* III/10 (341–400). 'On Various Subjects', translated by E. Hill, edited by J. Rotelle. New York: New City Press, 1995.

Augustine. *The Confessions*, introduction, translation and notes Maria Boulding, edited by John E. Rotelle. New York: New City Press, 1997.

Augustine. *The Enchiridion on Faith, Hope and Charity*, translated by Bruce Harbert, edited by Boniface Ramsey. New York: New City Press, 1999.

Australian Institute of Health and Welfare. 'Overweight and Obesity'. Accessed 10 November 2016. http://www.aihw.gov.au/risk-factors-overweight-obesity/

Authaus-Reid, Marcella. 'Queer I Stand: Lifting the Skirts of God'. In *The Sexual Theologian: Essays on Sex, God and Politics*, edited by Marcella Althaus-Reid and Lisa Isherwood, 99–109. London and New York: T & T Clark, 2004.

Bacon, Hannah. 'Dieting for Salvation: Becoming God by Weighing Less'. In *Alternative Salvations: Engaging the Sacred and the Secular*, edited by Hannah Bacon, Wendy Dossett and Steve Knowles, 41–51. London and New York: Bloomsbury Academic, 2015.

Bacon, Hannah. 'Expanding Bodies, Expanding God: Feminist Theology in Search of a "Fatter" Future'. *Feminist Theology* 21, no. 3 (2013): 309–26.

Bacon, Hannah. 'Fat, Syn, and Disordered Eating: The Dangers and Powers of Excess'. *Fat Studies* 4 (2015): 92–111.

Bacon, Hannah. 'Sin or Slim? Christian Morality and the Politics of Personal Choice in a Secular Commercial Weight Loss Setting'. *Fieldwork in Religion* 8, no. 1 (2013): 92–109.

Bacon, Hannah. *What's Right with the Trinity? Conversations in Feminist Theology*. Farnham and Burlington: Ashgate, 2009.

Bacon, Hannah. 'What's Right with the Trinity? Thinking the Trinity in Relation to Irigaray's Notions of Self-love and Wonder'. *Feminist Theology* 15, no. 2 (2007): 220–35.

Bacon, Linda and Aphramor, Lucy. 'Weight Science: Evaluating the Evidence for a Paradigm Shift'. *Nutrition Journal* 10, no. 9 (2011): 1–13.
Bailey, Edward. '"Implicit Religion"? What Might That Be?'. *Implicit Religion* 15, no. 2 (2012): 195–207.
Bailey, Edward. *Implicit Religion in Contemporary Society*. Kampen: Kok Pharos, 1997.
Barger, Lilian Calles. *Eve's Revenge: Women and a Spirituality of the Body*. Grand Rapids: Brazos Press, 2003.
Barter Moulaison, Jane. '"Our Bodies, Our Selves?" The Body as Source in Feminist Theology'. *Scottish Journal of Theology* 60, no. 3 (2007): 341–59.
Bartky, Sandra Lee. *Femininity and Domination. Studies in the Phenomenology of Oppression*. New York and London: Routledge, 1990.
Basil the Great. 'On Fasting'. Accessed 10 July 2018. https://www.crkvenikalendar.com/post/post-svetivasilije_en.php.
Basil the Great. 'The Hexaemeron'. In *The Nicene and Post-Nicene Fathers*, vol. VIII, translated with notes by Rev. Blomfield Jackson, edited by Philip Schaff and Henry Wace. Grand Rapids: William B. Eerdmans Publishing, 1978.
Basil the Great. 'The Letters'. In *The Nicene and Post-Nicene Fathers*, vol. VIII, translated with notes by Rev. Blomfield Jackson, edited by Philip Schaff and Henry Wace. Grand Rapids: William B. Eerdmans Publishing, 1978.
BEAT, 'The Costs of Eating Disorders. Social, Health and Economic Impacts'. Accessed 2 May 2018. https://www.beateatingdisorders.org.uk/uploads/documents/2017/10/the-costs-of-eating-disorders-final-original.pdf
Beckford, James. 'SSSR Presidential Address: Public Religions and the Postsecular: Critical Reflections'. *Journal for the Scientific Study of Religion* 51, no. 1 (2012): 1–19.
Bell, Kristen and McNaughton, Darlene. 'Feminism and the Invisible Fat Man'. *Body & Society* 13, no. 1 (2007): 107–31.
Bell, Rudolf. *Holy Anorexia*. Chicago and London: The University of Chicago Press, 1985.
Bergman, S. Bear, 'Part-Time Fatso'. In *The Fat Studies Reader*, edited by Esther Rothblum and Sondra Solovay, 139–42. New York and London: New York University Press, 2009.
Berry, Jan. *Ritual Making Women: Shaping Rites for Changing Lives*. London and Oakville: Equinox, 2009.
Berry, Wendell. 'Foreword'. In *Living the Sabbath: Discovering the Rhythms of Rest and Delight*, 11–12. Grand Rapids: Brazos Press, 2006.
Bible Hub. 'Strong's Exhaustive Concordance of the Bible'. Accessed 18 August 2017. http://biblehub.com/greek/264.htm
Bieler, Andrea and Schottroff, Luise. *The Eucharist: Bodies, Bread, Resurrection*. Minneapolis: Fortress, 2007.
Biltekoff, Charlotte. 'The Terror Within: Obesity in Post 9/11 U.S. Life'. *American Studies* 48, no. 3 (2007): 29–48.

Blair, Leonardo. 'Church Bans Fat People from Worship Team because they Would Interrupt Flow of Anointing'. *Christian Post Reporter*. Accessed 4 May 2018. https://www.christianpost.com/news/church-bans-fat-people-from-worship-team-because-they-would-interrupt-flow-of-anointing-170814/#eyCubqUEYsORSjxD.99

Blevins, Kent. 'Observing Sabbath'. *Review and Expositor* 113, no. 4 (2016): 478–87.

Boeve, Lieven, Geybels, Hans and Van den Bossche, Stijn. *Encountering Transcendence: Contributions to a Theology of Christian Religious Experience*. Leuven: Peeters Publishers, 2005.

Boff, Leonardo. *Trinity and Society*, translated by Paul Burns. Eugene: Wipf & Stock, 1988.

Bordo, Susan. *Unbearable Weight: Feminism, Western Culture, and the Body*. Berkeley, Los Angeles and London: University of California Press, 1993.

Bourdieu, Pierre. *Distinction: A Social Critique of the Judgement of Taste*, translated by Richard Nice. London and New York: Routledge, 2010.

Bovey, Shelley. *The Forbidden Body: Why Fat is not a Sin*. London: Pandora, 1989.

Boyce, James. *Born Bad: Original Sin and the Making of the Western Mind*. London: SPCK, 2014.

Boyce, James. 'How Original Sin Led to a Western Obsession with Self-Help'. *The Guardian*. Accessed 7 March 2017. https://www.theguardian.com/culture/australia-culture-blog/2014/jul/23/how-original-sin-led-to-a-western-obsession-with-self-help

Braziel, Jana Evans. 'Sex and Fat Chics: Deterritorializing the Fat Female Body'. In *Bodies Out of Bounds: Fatness and Transgression*, edited by Jana Evans Braziel and Kathleen LeBesco, 231–54. Berkeley, Los Angeles and London: University of California Press, 2001.

Braziel, Jana Evans and LeBesco, K., eds. *Bodies Out of Bounds: Fatness and Transgression*. Berkeley, Los Angeles, London: University of California Press, 2001.

Bringle, Mary Louise. *The God of Thinness: Gluttony and Other Weighty Matters*. Nashville: Abingdon Press, 1992.

Brock, Rita Nakashima. *Journeys by Heart: A Christology of Erotic Power*. Eugene: Wipf & Stock, 1988.

Brock, Rita Nakashima and Parker, Ann. *Saving Paradise: How Christianity Traded Love of this World for Crucifixion and Empire*. Boston: Beacon Press, 2008.

Brown, Catrina and Jasper, Karin. 'Why Weight? Why Women? Why Now?'. In *Consuming Passions. Feminist Approaches to Weight Preoccupation and Eating Disorders*, edited by Catrina Brown and Karin Jasper, 16–35. Toronto: Second Story Press, 1993.

Brown, Joanna Carlson and Parker, Rebecca. 'For God so Loved the World'. In *Christianity, Patriarchy and Abuse. A Feminist Critique*, edited by Joanna Carlson Brown and Carole R. Bohn, 1–30. Cleveland: Pilgrim Press, 1989.

Brown, Laura and Rothblum, Esther D. 'Editorial Statement'. In *Overcoming Fear of Fat*, edited by Laura Brown and Esther D. Rothblum. New York: Routledge, 2015.

Brown, Wendy. 'American Nightmare: Neoliberalism, Neoconservatism, and De-Democratization'. *Political Theory* 34, no. 6 (2006): 690–714.

Brownell, K. D. and Rodin, J. 'Medical, Metabolic, and Psychological Effects of Weight Cycling'. *Archives of Internal Medicine* 154, no. 12 (1994): 1325–30.

Brueggemann, Walter. *Sabbath as Resistance: Saying No to the Culture of Now*. Louisville: Westminster John Knox Press, 2014.

Butler, Judith. *Bodies that Matter: On the Discursive Limits of 'Sex'*. New York: Routledge, 1993.

Butler, Judith. *Gender Trouble: Feminism and the Subversion of Identity*. New York and London: Routledge, 2007.

Bulter, Judith. *Undoing Gender*. New York: Routledge, 2004.

Burgard, Deb. 'What is "Health at Every Size?"'. In *The Fat Studies Reader*, edited by Esther Rothblum and Sondra Solovay, 42–53. New York and London: New York University Press, 2009.

Bynum, Caroline Walker. *Holy Feast and Holy Fast: The Religious Significance of Food to Medieval Women*. Berkeley, Los Angeles and London: University of California Press, 1987.

Cable News Network. 'Surgeon General to Cops: Put Down the Donuts'. *CNN.com/Health*. Accessed 16 April 2013. http://edition.cnn.com/2003/HEALTH/02/28/obesity.police/

Cairus, Kate and Johnston, Josée. 'Choosing Health: Embodied Neoliberalism, Postfeminism, and the "Do-diet"'. *Theory and Society* 44, no. 2 (2015): 153–75.

Calvin, John. *Institutes of the Christian Religion*, translated by Ford Lewis Battles, edited by John T. McNeill. Louisville and London: Westminster John Knox Press, 2006.

Campbell, Dennis. 'Eating Disorder Patients' Lives at Risk due to Long Waits for NHS Treatment'. *The Guardian*, 14 June 2015. https://www.theguardian.com/society/2015/jun/14/eating-disorders-long-waits-nhs-treatment-lives-risk

Caspary, Almut. 'The Patristic Era: Early Christian Attitudes toward the Disfigured Outcast'. In *Disability in the Christian Tradition: A Reader*, edited by Brian Brock and John Swinton, 24–64. Grand Rapids and Cambridge: William B. Eerdmans Publishing Co., 2012.

Cassian, John. 'Conferences'. In *Nicene and Post-Nicene Fathers*, Second Series, vol. 11, edited by Philip Schaff and Henry Wace, translated by C. S. Gibson. Buffalo: Christian Literature Publishing Co., 1894. Revised and edited for New Advent by Kevin Knight. Accessed 27 May 2018. http://www.newadvent.org/fathers/350801.htm

Cassian, John. 'Institutes'. In *Nicene and Post-Nicene Fathers*, Second Series, vol. 11, edited by Philip Schaff and Henry Wace, translated by C. S. Gibson. Buffalo: Christian Literature Publishing Co., 1894. Revised and edited for

New Advent by Kevin Knight. Accessed 27 May 2018. http://www.newadvent.org/fathers/350705.htm

Cassian, John. *The Conferences*, translated by Boniface Ramsey. New York and Mahwah: The Newman Press, 1997.

Castelli, Elizabeth A. 'The Ekklesia of Women and/as Utopian Space: Locating the Work of Elisabeth Schüssler Fiorenza in Feminist Utopian Thought'. In *On the Cutting Edge: The Study of Women in Biblical Worlds*, edited by Jane Schaberg, Alice Bach and Esther Fuchs, 36–52. New York and London: Continuum, 2004.

Centers for Disease Control and Prevention (CDC). 'Adult Obesity Causes & Consequences'. Accessed 10 November 2016. http://www.cdc.gov/obesity/adult/causes.html

Centers for Disease Control and Prevention (CDC). 'Adult Overweight and Obesity'. Accessed 10 November 2016. https://www.cdc.gov/obesity/adult/

Chen, Eva. 'Neoliberalism and Popular Women's Culture'. *European Journal of Cultural Studies* 16, no. 4 (2013): 440–52.

Chernin, Kim, *The Obsession: Reflections on the Tyranny of Slenderness*. New York: HarperCollins Publishers, 1981.

Christ, Carol P. *Diving Deep and Surfacing: Women Writers on Spiritual Quest*, 3rd edition. Boston: Beacon Press, 1995.

Chrysostom, John. 'Homily XXXV on the Acts of the Apostles'. In *Nicene and Post-Nicene Fathers*. First Series, vol. XI, edited by Philip Schaff. Edinburgh: T & T Clark, 1889. Accessed 5 February 2018. https://www.ccel.org/ccel/schaff/npnf111.vi.xxxv.html.

Cipriani, Roberto. '"Diffused religion" and New Values in Italy'. In *The Changing Face of Religion*, edited by J. A. Beckford and T. Luckmann, 24–48. London: Sage, 1989.

Cixous, Hélène. 'The Author in Truth'. In *"Coming to Writing" and Other Essays*, edited by Deborah Jenson, translated by Sarah Cornell, Deborah Jenson, Ann Liddle and Susan Sellers, 136–82. London and Cambridge: Cambridge University Press, 1991.

Cixous, Hélène, Cohen, Keith and Cohen, Paula. 'The Laugh of the Medusa'. *Signs* 1, no. 4 (1976): 875–93.

Clement of Alexandria. 'The Instructor'. In *Ante-Nicene Fathers: Translations of the Writings of the Fathers Down to AD 325*, vol. II, edited by Rev. Alexander Roberts and James Donaldson. Grand Rapids: William B. Eerdmans Publishing Company, 1977.

Clement of Alexandria. 'The Stromata, or Miscellaneous'. In *Ante-Nicene Fathers: Translations of the Writings of the Fathers Down to AD 325*, vol. II, edited by Rev. Alexander Roberts and James Donaldson. Grand Rapids: William B. Eerdmans Publishing Company, 1977.

Clough, Patricia T. 'The Affective Turn: Political Economy, Biomedia and Bodies'. *Theory, Culture and Society* 25, no. 1 (2008): 1–22.

Coakley, Sarah. *Religion and the Body*. Cambridge: Cambridge University Press, 2000.

Colbert, Don. *What Would Jesus Eat? The Ultimate Program for Eating Well, Feeling Great and Living Longer*. Nashville: Thomas Nelson, 2002.

Coleman, Monica A. 'Sacrifice, Surrogacy and Salvation'. *Black Theology: An International Journal* 12, no. 3 (2014): 200-12.

Coleman-Jensen, Alisha, Rabbitt, Matthew P., Gregory, Christian A. and Singh, Anita. 'Household Food Security in the United States in 2015'. Economic Research Report no. 215 (2016). Accessed 5 May 2017. https://www.ers.usda.gov/webdocs/publications/79761/err-215.pdf?v=42636

Colls, R. 'Review of Bodies out of Bounds: Fatness and Transgression'. *Gender, Place and Culture: A Journal of Feminist Geography* 9, no. 2 (2002): 218-20.

Coogan, Michael D. 'Salvation'. In *The Oxford Companion to the Bible*, edited by Bruce Metzger and Michael D. Coogan, 670. New York and Oxford: Oxford University Press, 1993.

Cooper, Charlotte. *Fat Activism: A Radical Social Movement*. Bristol: HammerOn Press, 2016.

Cooper, Charlotte. *Fat and Proud: The Politics of Size*. London: The Women's Press, 1998.

Cooper, Charlotte. 'Headless Fatties'. *Obesity Epidemic*, January 2007. Accessed 10 February 2016. http://charlottecooper.net/publishing/digital/headless-fatties-01-07

Dallam, Marie W. 'Introduction: Religion, Food and Eating'. In *Religion, Food, & Eating in North America*', edited by Benjamin Zeller, Marie W. Dallam, Reid L. Neilson and Nora L. Rubel, XVII–XXXII. New York: Columbia University Press, 2014.

Daly, Mary. *Beyond God the Father: Towards a Philosophy of Women's Liberation*. London: The Women's Press, 1986.

Daly, Mary. *Pure Lust: Elemental Feminist Philosophy*. London: The Women's Press, 1998.

Dark, Kimberly. 'Coming Out Fat'. In *Fat Sex: New Directions in Theory and Activism*, edited by Helen Hester and Caroline Walters. Farnham and Burlington: Ashgate, 2015.

Davaney, Sheila Greeve. 'Continuing the Story but Departing the Text: A Historicist Interpretations of Feminist Norms in Theology'. In *Horizons in Feminist Theology: Identity, Tradition and Norms*, edited by Rebecca S. Chopp and Sheila Greeve Davaney, 198-214. Minneapolis: Fortress Press, 1997.

Davaney, Sheila Greeve. 'The Limits of the Appeal to Women's Experience'. In *Shaping New Vision. Gender and Values in American Culture*, edited by Clarissa W. Atkinson, Constance H. Buchanan and Margaret R. Miles, 31-50. London: UMI Research Press, 1987.

Davis, Angela. *Women, Race and Class*. New York: Random House, 1981.

Dennett, Andrea Stulman. 'The Dime Museum Freak Show Reconfigured as Talk Show'. In *Freakery: Cultural Spectacles of the Extraordinary Body*, edited by Rosemary Garland Thomson, 315-26. New York and London: New York University Press, 1996.

Department of Health. 'Annual Report of the Chief Medical Officer 2002: Health Check, on the State of the Public Health'. Accessed 16 April 2014. http://webarchive.nationalarchives.gov.uk/+/www.dh.gov.uk/en/PublicationsAndStatistics/Publications/AnnualReports/DH_4006432

Department of Health. 'Healthy Lives, Healthy People: A Call to Action on Obesity in England'. Accessed December 2013. https://www.gov.uk/government/uploads/system/uploads/attachment_data/file/213720/dh_130487.pdf

Department of Health. 'Policy Paper. 2010 to 2015 Government Policy: Obesity and Healthy Eating'. Accessed 10 November 2016. https://www.gov.uk/government/publications/2010-to-2015-government-policy-obesity-and-healthy-eating/2010-to-2015-government-policy-obesity-and-healthy-eating

Davis, Sally. *Annual Report of the Chief Medical Officer, 2014: The Health of the 51%: Women.* London: Department of Health, 2015.

Desjardins, Michel. 'Clement's Bound Body'. In *Mapping Gender in Ancient Religious Discourses*, edited by Todd Penner and Caroline Vander Stichele, 411–30. Leiden, Boston: Brill, 2007.

DeVault, Marjorie L. *Feeding the Family: The Social Organization of Caring as Gendered Work.* Chicago and London: The University of Chicago Press, 1991.

DeVault, Marjorie L. and Gross, Glenda. 'Feminist Qualitative Interviewing. Experience, Talk, and Knowledge'. In *The Handbook of Feminist Research. Theory and Praxis*, 2nd edition, edited by Sharlene Nagy Hesse-Biber, 206–36. Los Angeles, London, New Delhi, Singapore and Washington: Sage, 2012.

Donne, John. *The Works of John Donne*, vol. I, edited by Henry Alford. London: John W. Parker, 1839.

Douglas, Mary. *Purity and Danger: An Analysis of Concept of Pollution and Taboo.* London and New York: Routledge, 2002.

Dunfee, Susan Nelson. 'The Sin of Hiding: A Feminist Critique of Reinhold Niebuhr's Account of the Sin of Pride'. *Soundings, The Interdisciplinary Journal* 65, no. 3 (1982): 316–27.

Edwards, Katie. *Admen and Eve: The Bible in Contemporary Advertising.* Sheffield: Sheffield Phoenix Press, 2012.

Eiesland, Nancy L. *The Disabled God: Toward a Liberatory Theology of Disability.* Nashville: Abingdon Press, 1994.

Ellmann, Maud. *The Hunger Artists. Starving, Writing & Imprisonment.* London: Virago Press, 1993.

Engel, Mary Potter. 'Evil, Sin, and Violation of the Vulnerable'. In *Lift Every Voice: Constructing Christian Theologies from the Underside*, edited by Susan Brooks Thistlethwaite and Mary Potter Engel, 152–64. San Francisco: Harper and Row, 1990.

Ernsberger, P. 'Obesity is an Early Symptom of Diabetes, Not Its Cause'. *Health at Every Size Journal*, no. 18 (2004): 67–9.

Evagrius Ponticus. 'To Eulogios. On the Confession of Thoughts and Counsel in their Regard'. In *Evagrius of Pontus: The Greek Ascetic Corpus*, edited and translated, introduction and commentary by Robert E. Sinkewicz, 12–59. Oxford: Oxford University Press, 2003.

Evans, Bethan. 'Anticipating Fatness: Childhood, Affect and the Pre-emptive "War On Obesity"'. *Transactions of the Institute of British Geographers* 35, no. 1 (2010): 21–38.

Evans, Bethan. '"Gluttony or Sloth": Critical Geographies of Bodies in (Anti) Obesity Policy', *Area* 38, no. 3 (2006): 259–67.

Faludi, Susan. *Backlash: The Undeclared War against Women*. London: Vintage, 1993.

Fat and Faithful. 'Fat and Faithful'. Accessed 23 June 2018. https://www.facebook.com/FatAndFaithful/

Feldman, M. and Meyer, I. 'Eating Disorders in Diverse, Lesbian, Gay, and Bisexual Populations'. *International Journal of Eating Disorders* 40, no. 3 (2007): 218–26.

Fiddes, Paul. *Past Event and Present Salvation: The Christian Idea of Atonement*. Louisville: Westminster/John Knox Press, 1989.

Finlan, Stephen. *Problems with Atonement: The Origins of, and Controversy about, the Atonement Doctrine*. Collegeville: The Liturgical Press, 2005.

Fiorenza, Elisabeth Schüssler. *Bread not Stone: The Challenge of Feminist Biblical Interpretation*. Boston: Beacon Press, 1984.

Fiorenza, Elisabeth Schüssler. *But She Said: Feminist Practices of Biblical Interpretation*. Boston: Beacon Press, 1992.

Fiorenza, Elisabeth Schüssler. *Discipleship of Equals: A Critical Feminist Ekklēsia-logy of Liberation*. New York: Crossroad Publishing Company, 1998.

Fiorenza, Elisabeth Schüssler. 'Feminist Theology as a Critical Theology of Liberation'. *Theological Studies* 36, no. 4 (1975): 605–26.

Fiorenza, Elisabeth Schüssler. *Jesus: Miriam's Child, Sophia's Prophet: Critical Issues in Feminist Christology*. London and New York: Continuum, 1994.

Fischer, Clara. 'Feminist Philosophy, Pragmatism, and the "Turn to Affect": A Genealogical Critique'. *Hypatia* 31, no. 4 (2016): 810–26.

Fischer, Kathleen. *Transforming Fire: Women Using Fire Creatively*. New York: Paulist Press, 2000.

Fisk, Anna. *Sex, Sin, and Our Selves: Encounters in Feminist Theology and Contemporary Women's Literature*. Eugene: Pickwick Publications, 2014.

Flood, Gavin. *The Ascetic Self: Subjectivity, Memory, and Tradition*. Cambridge: Cambridge University Press, 2004.

Fontaine, K. R., McCubrey, R., Mehta, T., Pajewski, N. M., Keith, S. W., Bangalore, S. S., Crespo, C. J. and Allison, D. B. 'Body Mass Index and Mortality Rate among Hispanic Adults: A Pooled Analysis of Multiple Epidemiologic Data Sets'. *International Journal of Obesity* 36, no. 8 (2012): 1121–6.

Food and Agriculture Organization of the United Nations. 'The State of Food Insecurity in the World: Strengthening the Enabling Environment for Food Security and Nutrition' (2014). Accessed 12 July 2017. http://www.fao.org/3/a-i4030e.pdf

Foucault, Michel. *Discipline and Punish: The Birth of the Prison*. London: Penguin Books, 1977.

Foucault, Michel. *Power/Knowledge. Selected Interviews and Other Writings 1972-1977*, edited by Colin Gordon. New York: Pantheon, 1980.

Foucault, Michel. 'Self Writing'. In *Ethics. Essential Works of Foucault 1954-1984*, vol. 1, edited by Paul Rainbow, translated by Robert Hurley, 207-22. London: Penguin Books, 1994.

Foucault, Michel. 'Technologies of the Self'. In *Ethics. Essential Works of Foucault 1954-1984*, vol. 1, translated by Robert Hurley, edited by Paul Rainbow, 223-51. London: Penguin Books, 1994.

Foucault, Michel. 'The Ethics of the Concern for Self as a Practice of Freedom'. In *Ethics: Essential Works of Foucault 1954-1984*, vol. 1, translated by Robert Hurley, edited by Paul Rainbow, 281-301. London: Penguin Books, 1994.

Foucault, Michel. *The History of Sexuality, Vol. 1, The Will to Knowledge*, translated by Robert Hurley. London: Penguin Books, 1976.

Foucault, Michel. *The History of Sexuality, Vol. 2, The Use of Pleasure*, translated by Robert Hurley. London: Penguin Books, 1985.

Foucault, Michel. *The History of Sexuality, Vol. 3, The Care of the Self*, translated by Robert Hurley. London: Penguin Books, 1986.

Franzosi, Maria Grazia. 'Should We Continue to Use BMI as a Cardiovascular Risk Factor?'. *The Lancet*, no. 368 (2006): 624-5.

Friedan, Betty. *The Feminine Mystique*. London: Penguin, 1963.

Friedman, Jeffrey. 'A War on Obesity, Not the Obese'. *Science* 299 (2003): 856-8.

Fulkerson, Mary McClintock. *Changing the Subject. Women's Discourses and Feminist Theology*. Minneapolis: Fortress Press, 1994.

Fulkerson, Mary McClintock. 'Interpreting a Situation: When is "Empirical" also "Theological"?'. In *Perspectives on Ecclesiology and Ethnography*, edited by Pete Ward, 124-44. Grand Rapids and Cambridge: William B. Eerdmans Publishing Company, 2012.

Fulkerson, Mary McClintock. *Places of Redemption: Theology for a Worldly Church*. Oxford: Oxford University Press, 2007.

Fulkerson, Mary McClintock. 'Sexism as Original Sin: Developing a Theacentric Discourse'. *Journal of the American Academy of Religion* 59, no. 4 (1991): 653-75.

Gaesser, Glenn. 'Is "Permanent Weight Loss" and Oxymoron? The Statistics on Weight Loss and the National Weight Control Registry'. In *The Fat Studies Reader*, edited by Esther Rothblum and Sondra Solovay, 37-40. New York and London: New York University Press, 2009.

Gaspar, Prata and Clara de Moraes, Maria. 'Control of Eating Behaviour and Eating Pleasure among French Female College Students'. *Menu: Journal of Food and Hospitality Research* 1, no. 1 (2012): 92–6.

Gebara, Ivone. *Out of the Depths: Women's Experience of Evil and Salvation*. Minneapolis: Fortress, 2002.

Gerber, Lynne. 'My Body is a Testimony: Appearance, Health and Sin in an Evangelical Weight-loss Program'. *Social Compass* 56, no. 3 (2009): 405–18.

Gerber, Lynne. *Seeking the Straight and Narrow: Weight Loss and Sexual Reorientation in Evangelical America*. Chicago and London: University of California Press, 2011.

Gerber, Lynne, Hill, Susan and Manigault-Bryant, LeRhonda. 'Religion and Fat = Protestant Christianity and Weight Loss? On the Intersections of Fat Studies and Religious Studies'. *Fat Studies* 4, no. 2 (2015): 82–91.

Gill, Rosalind. *Gender and the Media*. Cambridge and Malden: Polity Press, 2007.

Gill, Rosalind. 'Postfeminist Media Culture: Elements of a Sensibility', *European Journal of Cultural Studies* 10, no. 2 (2007): 147–66.

Gill, Rosalind and Arthurs, Jane. 'Editors' Introduction. New Femininities?'. *Feminist Media Studies* 6, no. 4 (2006): 443–51.

Gill, Rosalind and Scharff, Christina. 'Introduction'. In *New Femininities. Postfeminism, Neoliberalism and Subjectivity*, edited by Rosalind Gill and Christina Scharff, 1–20. New York: Palgrave Macmillan, 2011.

Goffman, Erving. *Stigma: Notes on the Management of a Spoiled Identity*. New York: Prentice Hall, 1963.

Gortmaker, Steven L., Must, Aviva, Perrin, James M., Sobol, Arthur M. and Dietz, William H. 'Social and Economic Consequences of Overweight in Adolescence and Young Adulthood'. *The New England Journal of Medicine* 329 (1993): 1008–12. Accessed 1 May 2017. http://www.nejm.org/doi/full/10.1056/NEJM199309303291406

Graham, Elaine. *Apologetics without Apology: Speaking of God in a World Troubled by Religion*. Eugene: Cascade Books, 2017.

Graham, Elaine. *Between a Rock and a Hard Place: Public Theology in a Post-Secular Age*. London: SCM Press, 2013.

Granberg, Ellen. '"Is That All There Is?" Possible Selves, Self-Change, and Weight Loss'. *Social Psychology Quarterly* 69, no. 2 (2006): 109–26.

Grant, Jacquelyn. *White Women's Christ, Black Women's Jesus: Feminist Christology and Womanist Response*. New York: Oxford University Press, 1989.

Greene-McCreight, Kathryn. *Feminist Reconstructions of Christian Doctrine. Narrative Analysis and Appraisal*. New York and Oxford: Oxford University Press, 2000.

Greenough, Chris. *Undoing Theology: Life Stories from Non-Normative Christians*. London: SCM, 2018.

Gregory of Nyssa. 'On the Making of Man'. In *A Select Library of Nicene and Post-Nicene Fathers of the Christian Church*, Second Series, vol. 5, edited by Philip Schaff and Henry Wallace, XVII.2. Grand Rapids: William B. Eerdmans Publishing Company, 1979.

Gregory the Great. *The Book of Pastoral Rule*, translated and introduction by George E. Demacopoulos. New York: St. Vladimir's Seminary Press, 2007.

Grey, Mary. *Redeeming the Dream: Feminism, Redemption and Christian Tradition*. London: SPCK, 1989.

Grey, Mary. *The Outrageous Pursuit of Hope, Prophetic Dreams for the Twenty-First Century*. London: Dart Longman & Todd, 2000.

Griffith, R. Marie. *Born Again Bodies: Flesh and Spirit in American Christianity*. Berkeley, Los Angeles and London: University of California Press, 2004.

Griffith, R. Marie. *God's Daughters: Evangelical Women and the Power of Submission*. Berkeley, Los Angeles and London: University of California Press, 2000.

Griffith, R. Marie. 'The Promised Land of Weight Loss: Law and Gospel in Christian Dieting'. *The Christian Century* 114, no. 15 (1997): 448–54. Accessed 10 November 2016. http://www.religion-online.org/showartic le.asp?title=249

Grimshaw, Jean. 'Practices of Freedom'. In *Up against Foucault. Explorations of Some Tensions between Foucault and Feminism*, edited by Caroline Ramazanoğlu, 51–71. London and New York: Routledge, 1993.

Grodstein, F., Levine, R., Troy, L., Spencer, T., Colditz, G. A. and Stampfer, M. J. 'Three-year Follow-up of Participants in a Commercial Weight Loss Program: Can You Keep It Off?'. *Archives of Internal Medicine* 156, no. 12 (1996): 1302–6.

Grosz, Elizabeth. *Space, Time and Perversion: Essays on the Politics of Bodies*. New York and Abingdon: Routledge, 1995.

Grosz, Elizabeth. *Volatile Bodies: Toward a Corporeal Feminism*. Bloomington: Indiana University Press, 1994.

Guthman, Julie and DuPuis, Melanie. 'Embodying Neoliberalism: Economy, Culture and the Politics of Fat'. *Environment and Planning D: Society and Space* 24, no. 3 (2006): 427–48.

Guthman, Julie. 'Neoliberalism and the Constitution of Contemporary Bodies'. In *The Fat Studies Reader*, edited by Esther Rothblum and Sondra Solovay, 187–98. New York and London: New York University Press, 2009.

Habermas, Jürgen. 'Secularism's Crisis of Faith: Notes on Post-Secular Society'. *New Perspectives Quarterly* 25 (2008): 17–29.

Hampson, Daphne. *Swallowing a Fishbone? Feminist Theologians Debate Christianity*. London: SPCK, 1996.

Harmless, William. 'Christ the Paediatrician: Augustine on the Diagnosis and Treatment of the Injured Vocation of the Child'. In *The Vocation of the Child*, edited by Patrick McKinley Brennan, 127–53. Cambridge and Grand Rapids: William B. Eerdmans Publishing Company, 2008.

Harrison, Beverly. *Our Right to Choose: Toward A New Ethic of Abortion.* Boston: Beacon Press, 1983.

Harrison, Beverly. 'The Power of Anger in the Work of Love: Christian Ethics for Women and Other Strangers'. In *Making the Connections: Essays in Feminist Social Ethics*, edited by Carol S. Robb, 3–21. Boston: Beacon Press, 1985.

Hartley, Cecilia. 'Letting Ourselves Go: Making Room for the Fat Body in Feminist Scholarship'. In *Bodies out of Bounds: Fatness and Transgression*, edited by J. E. Braziel and K. LeBesco, 60–73. Berkeley, Los Angeles and London: University of California Press, 2001.

Health at Every Size, 'Health at Every Size'. Accessed 10 October 2016. http://haescommunity.com/

Hemmings, Clare. 'Invoking Affect: Cultural Theory and the Ontological Turn'. *Cultural Studies* 19, no. 5 (2005): 548–67.

Herndon, April. 'Disparate but Disabled: Fat Embodiment and Disability Studies'. *National Women's Studies Journal* 14, no. 3 (2002): 120–37.

Heschel, Abraham J. 'A Place in Time'. In *The Ten Commandments: The Reciprocity of Faithfulness*, edited by William P. Brown, 214–22. Louisville, London: Westminster John Knox Press, 2004.

Hesse-Biber, Sharlene. *The Cult of Thinness.* New York and Oxford: Oxford University Press, 2007.

Hester, Helen and Walters, Caroline. 'Riots Not Diets!: Sex, Fat Studies and DIY Activism'. In *Fat Sex: New Directions in Theory and Activism*, edited by Helen Hester and Caroline Walters, 1–14. Farnham and Burlington: Ashgate, 2015.

Heyes, Cressida J. 'Foucault Goes to Weight Watchers'. *Hyatia* 21, no. 2 (2006): 126–49.

Heyes, Cressida J. *Self-Transformations. Foucault, Ethics, and Normalized Bodies.* Oxford and New York: Oxford University Press, 2007.

Heyward, Carter. 'Heterosexist Theology: Being above It All'. In *Feminist Theological Ethics: A Reader*, edited by Lois K. Daly, Robin W. Lovin and Douglas F. Ottata, 172–82. Louisville: Westminster John Knox Press, 1994.

Heyward, Carter. *Our Passion for Justice: Images of Power, Sexuality, and Liberation.* New York: The Pilgrim Press, 1984.

Heyward, Carter. *The Redemption of God: A Theology of Mutual Relation.* Eugene: Wipf & Stock, 2010.

Heyward, Carter. *Touching our Strength: The Erotic as Power and the Love of God.* New York: Harper San Francisco, 1989.

Hill, Susan E. *Eating to Excess: The Meaning of Gluttony and the Fat Body in the Ancient World.* California: Praeger, 2011.

Hogan, Linda. *From Women's Experience to Feminist Theology.* Sheffield: Sheffield Academic Press, 1995.

Hollows, Joanne. *Feminism, Femininity and Popular Culture.* Manchester: Manchester University Press, 2000.

Hollywood, Amy. *Sensible Ecstasy: Mysticism, Sexual Difference, and the Demands of History*. Chicago, London: University of Chicago Press, 2002.

hooks, bell. *Ain't I a Woman? Black Women and Feminism*. Boston: Pluto Press, 1981.

House of Commons. 'Obesity: Third Report of Session 2003-04', vol. 1. London: The Stationery Office Limited.

Hoverd, William James. 'Deadly Sin: Gluttony, Obesity and Health Policy'. In *Medicine, Religion and the Body*, edited by Elizabeth Burns Coleman and Kevin White, 205–30. Leiden: Brill, 2010.

Hull, John. *The Tactile Heart: Blindness and Faith*. London: SCM, 2013.

Irenaeus. 'Against Heresies'. In *The Ante-Nicene Fathers: Translations of the Writings of the Fathers Down to AD 325*, vol. I, edited by Rev. Alexander Roberts and James Donaldson. Grand Rapids: William B. Eerdmans Publishing Company, 1981.

Irigaray, Luce. *An Ethics of Sexual Difference*, translated by Carolyn Burke and Gillian C. Gill. Ithaca: Cornell University Press, 1993.

Irigaray, Luce. *Elemental Passions*, translated by Joanne Collie & Judith Still. New York: Routledge, 1992.

Irigaray, Luce. *Speculum of the Other Woman*. New York: Cornell University Press, 1985.

Irigaray, Luce. *This Sex Which Is Not One*, translated by Catherine Porter with Carolyn Burke. Ithaca: Cornell University Press, 1985.

Irigaray, Luce. 'Women-Mothers, the Silent Substratum of the Social Order'. In *The Irigaray Reader*, edited by Margaret Whitford, 47–52. Oxford: Blackwell Publishers Ltd., 1991.

Isasi-Díaz, Ada María. *La Lucha Continues. Mujerista Theology*. New York: Orbis, 2004.

Isherwood, Lisa. 'Indecent Theology: What F-ing Difference Does it Make?'. *Feminist Theology* 11, no. 2 (2003): 141–7.

Isherwood, Lisa. 'Sex and Body Politics: Issues for Feminist Theology'. In *The Good News of the Body: Sexual Theology and Feminism*, edited by Lisa Isherwood, 20–34. New York: Sheffield Academic Press, 2000.

Isherwood, Lisa. *The Fat Jesus. Feminist Explorations in Boundaries and Transgressions*. London: Darton, Longman and Todd, 2007.

Isherwood, Lisa and Stuart, Elizabeth. *Introducing Body Theology*. Sheffield: Sheffield Academic Press, 1998.

Isono, Maho, Watkins, Patti Lou and Ee Lian, Lee. 'Bon Bon Fatty Girl: A Qualitative Exploration of Weight Bias in Singapore'. In *The Fat Studies Reader*, edited by Esther Rothblum and Sondra Solovay, 127–38. New York and London: New York University Press, 2009.

Jaggar, Alison M. 'Love and Knowledge: Emotion in Feminist Epistemology'. *Inquiry* 32, no. 2 (1989): 151–76.

Jamie Oliver Enterprises Limited. 'Jamie's Ministry of Food'. Accessed 5 May 2017. http://www.jamieoliver.com/jamies-ministry-of-food/

Jantzen, Grace M. *Becoming Divine: Toward a Feminist Philosophy of Religion.* Manchester: Manchester University Press, 1998.

Jantzen, Grace M. 'Feminism and Flourishing: Gender and Metaphor in Feminist Theology'. *Feminist Theology* 4, no. 10 (1995): 81–101.

Jantzen, Grace M. *Power, Gender and Christian Mysticism.* Cambridge: Cambridge University Press, 1995.

Jenkins, Tina and Smith, Barbara. 'Fat Liberation'. *Spare Rib: A Women's Liberation Magazine* 182 (1987): 14–18.

Johnson, Elizabeth. *Quest for the Living God: Mapping Frontiers in the Theology of God.* London: Continuum, 2007.

Johnson, Elizabeth A. *She Who Is: The Mystery of God in Feminist Theological Discourse.* New York: The Crossroad Publishing Company, 1992.

Jones, Serene. *Feminist Theory and Christian Theology: Cartographies of Grace.* Minneapolis: Fortress, 2000.

Julian of Norwich. *Revelations of Divine Love: Short Text and Long Text,* translated by Elizabeth Spearing. London: Penguin, 1998.

Jung, L. Shannon. *Sharing Food: Christian Practices for Enjoyment.* Minneapolis: Fortress Press, 2006.

Justin Martyr. 'Fragments of the Lost Work of Justin On the Resurrection'. In *The Ante-Nicene Fathers. Translations of the Writings of the Fathers Down to AD 325,* vol. I, edited by Rev. Alexander Roberts and James Donaldson, translated by Rev. M. Dods. Grand Rapids: William B. Eerdmans Publishing Company, 1981.

Kenardy, Justin, Brown, Wendy J. and Yogt, Emma. 'Dieting and Health in Young Australian Women'. *European Eating Disorders Review* 9, no. 4 (2001): 242–54.

Kent, Le'a. 'Fighting Abjection: Representing Fat Women'. In *Bodies out of Bounds: Fatness and Transgression,* edited by J. E. Braziel and K. LeBesco, 130–52. Berkeley, Los Angeles and London: University of California Press, 2001.

Kinsler, Ross and Kinsler, Gloria. *The Biblical Jubilee and the Struggle for Life: An Invitation to Personal, Ecclesial, and Social Transformation.* Maryknoll: Orbis, 1999.

Korsmeyer, Carolyn. *Making Sense of Taste. Food and Philosophy.* Ithaca and London: Cornell University Press, 1999.

Kristeva, Julia. *Powers of Horror: An Essay on Abjection,* translated by Leon S. Roudiez. New York: Columbia University Press, 1982.

LaCugna, Catherine Mowry. *God for Us: The Trinity and Christian Life.* New York: HarperCollins Publishers, 1991.

Lamm, Nomy. 'It's a Big Fat Revolution'. Accessed 23 June 2018. http://www.tehomet.net/nomy.html

Lane, Anthony N. S. 'Lust: The Human Person as Affected by Disordered Desires', *Evangelical Quarterly* 78, no. 1 (2006): 21–35.

Lazar, Michelle, 'Recuperating Feminism, Reclaiming Femininity: Hybrid Postfeminist Identity in Consumer Advertisements'. *Gender and Language* 8, no. 2 (2014): 205–24.

Leaver, Hayley. 'Companies Growing Fat as You Slim: The Growth of the Weight Loss Market'. *Metro*, 30 January 2014. http://metro.co.uk/2014/01/30/companies-growing-fat-as-you-slim-the-growth-of-the-weight-loss-market-4282903/

LeBesco, Kathleen. 'Neoliberalism, Public Health, and the Moral Perils of Fatness'. *Critical Public Health* 21, no. 2 (2011): 153–64.

LeBesco, Kathleen. *Revolting Bodies? The Struggle to Redefine Fat Identity*. Amherst and Boston: University of Massachusetts Press, 2004.

LeBesco, Kathleen and Braziel, Janna Evans. 'Editor's Introduction'. In *Bodies out of Bounds: Fatness and Transgression*, edited by J. E. Braziel and K. LeBesco, 1–17. Berkeley, Los Angeles and London: University of California Press, 2001.

Lee, Sing, Chan, Y. Y. Lydia and Hsu, L. K. George. 'The Intermediate-Term Outcome of Chinese Patients with Anorexia Nervosa in Hong Kong'. *The American Journal of Psychiatry* 160, no. 5 (2003): 967–72.

Leit, Richard A., Gray, James J. and Pope, Harrison G. 'The Media Representation of the Ideal Male'. *International Journal of Eating Disorders* 31, no. 3 (2002): 334–8.

Lelwica, Michelle. *Starving for Salvation: The Spiritual Dimensions of Eating Problems among American Girls and Women*. New York and Oxford: Oxford University Press, 1999.

Lelwica, Michelle. *The Religion of Thinness: Satisfying the Spiritual Hungers behind Women's Obsession with Food and Weight*. Carlsbad: Gürze Books, 2010.

Lelwica, Michelle, Hoglund, E. and McNallie, J. 'Spreading the Religion of Thinness from California to Calcutta'. *Journal of Feminist Studies in Religion* 25, no. 1 (2009): 19–41.

Levy-Navarro, Elena. 'Fattening Queer History'. In *The Fat Studies Reader*, edited by Esther Rothblum and Sondra Solovay, 15–24. New York and London: New York University Press, 2009.

Levy-Navarro, Elena. 'I'm the New Me: Compelled Confession Diet Discourse'. *The Journal of Popular Culture* 45, no. 2 (2012): 340–56.

LighterLife. 'About Us'. Accessed 27 August 2017. http://www.lighterlife.com/about-us/

Liljeström, Marianne and Paasonen, Susanna. 'Introduction: Feeling Differences – Affect and Feminist Reading'. In *Working with Affect in Feminist Readings: Disturbing Differences*, edited by Marianne Liljeström and Susanna Paasonen, 1–7. London and New York: Routledge, 2010.

Llewellyn, Dawn and Sharma, Sonya. 'Introduction'. In *Religion, Equalities, and Inequalities*, edited by Dawn Llewellyn and Sonya Sharma, xvii–xxvii. London and New York: Routledge, 2016.

Lodge, Bethany. 'No Sins Cafe Forced to Change Its Name After Slimming World Threatens Legal Action'. *Gasette Live*, 7 July 2016. Accessed 10 May 2018. https://www.gazettelive.co.uk/news/teesside-news/no-sins-cafe-for ced-change-11580726

Longhurst, Robyn. 'Becoming Smaller: Autobiographical Spaces of Weight Loss'. *Antipode* 44, no. 3 (2012): 871–88.

Lorde, Audre. *Sister Outsider: Essays and Speeches by Audre Lorde*, New Foreword by Cheryl Clarke. Berkeley: Crossing Press [1984] 2007.

Lowe, Mary Elise. 'Theology Update: Woman Oriented Hamartiologies: A Survey of the Shift from Powerlessness to Right Relationship'. *Dialog: A Journal of Theology* 39, no. 2 (2000): 119–39.

Lowe, Michael R., Kral, Tanja V. E. and Miller-Kovach, Karen. 'Weight-loss Maintenance 1, 2 and 5 Years after Successful Completion of a Weight-loss Programme'. *The British Journal of Nutrition* 99, no. 4 (2008): 925–30.

Luckman, Thomas. *The Invisible Religion: The Problem of Religion in Modern Society*. London: Macmillan, 1967.

Lupton, Deborah. *Fat*. London and New York: Routledge, 2013.

Lupton, Deborah. *Food, the Body and the Self*. London and New Delhi: Sage, 1996.

Luther, Martin. *Galatians*, The Crossway Classic Commentaries, edited by Alister McGrath and J. I. Packer. Wheaton: Crossway Books, 1998.

Lyons, Pat. 'Fitness, Feminism and the Health of Fat Women'. In *Overcoming Fear of Fat*, edited by Laura S. Brown and Esther D. Rothblum, 65–78. London and New York: Routledge, 1989.

Lyons, Pat. 'Prescription for Harm'. In *The Fat Studies Reader*, edited by Esther Rothblum and Sondra Solovay, 75–87. New York and London: New York University Press, 2009.

Macek, Petr. 'The Doctrine of Creation in the Messianic Theology of Jürgen Moltmann'. *Communio viatorum* 49 (2007): 150–84.

Mann, Patricia. *Micro-Politics: Agency in a Post-Feminist Era*. Minneapolis: University of Minnesota Press, 1994.

Marketdata Enterprises Inc. 'The U.S. Weight Loss Market: 2014 Status Report & Forecast'. Accessed 23 April 2014. http://www.marketresearch.com/ Marketdata-Enterprises-Inc-v416/Weight-Loss-Status-Forecast-8016030/

Marketdata Enterprises Inc. 'The U.S. Weight Loss Market: 2015 Status Report'. Accessed 3 November 2016. http://www.marketresearch.com/Marketdata -Enterprises-Inc-v416/Weight-Loss-Status-8745878/

Marsh, Sarah. 'All That Striving for Healthiness is Making Millennials More Anxious than Ever'. *The Guardian* (11 March 2016). Accessed 30 August 2017. https://www.theguardian.com/commentisfree/2016/mar/11/strivi ng-for-healthiness-makes-us-unhappy-millennials

Martin, Daniel D. 'Organizational Approaches to Shame: Avowal, Management, and Contestation'. *The Sociological Quarterly* 41, no. 1 (2000): 137–40.

Martinez Beck, Amanda. 'All Bodies Are Good Bodies', *Facebook Group*. Accessed 15 June 2018. https://www.facebook.com/groups/allbodiesaregoodbodies/

Martinez Beck, Amanda. 'Fat, Catholic, and Loved', *Facebook Group*. Accessed 15 June 2018. https://www.facebook.com/fatcatholicandloved/

Massumi, Brian. *Parables of the Virtual: Movement, Affect, Sensation*. Durham and London: Duke University Press, 2002.

McAllister, Heather. 'Embodying Fat Liberation'. In *The Fat Studies Reader*, edited by Esther Rothblum and Sondra Solovay, 305–11. New York and London: New York University Press, 2009.

McFadyen, Alisair. *Bound to Sin: Abuse, Holocaust and the Christian Doctrine of Sin*. Cambridge, New York: Cambridge University Press, 2000.

McFague, Sallie. *Models of God: Theology for an Ecological, Nuclear Age*. Philadelphia: Fortress Press, 1987.

McFague, Sallie. *The Body of God: An Ecological Theology*. Minneapolis: Fortress, 1993.

McKinley, Nita Mary. 'Ideal Weight/Ideal Women: Society Constructs the Female'. In *Weight Issues: Fatness and Thinness as Social Problems*, edited by Jeffrey Sobal and Donna Maurer, 97–116. New York: Aldine de Gruyter, 1999.

McRobbie, Angela. 'Post-feminist and Popular Culture'. *Feminist Media Studies* 4, no. 3 (2004): 255–64.

Mead, Rebecca. 'Slim for Him: God Is Watching What You're Eating'. Accessed 15 April 2014. http://www.spiritwatch.org/rebeccamead.htm

Méndez Montoya, Angel F. *The Theology of Food: Eating and the Eucharist*. Chichester: Wiley-Blackwell, 2009.

Miles, Margaret R. *Fullness of Life: Historical Foundations for a New Asceticism*. Eugene: Wipf & Stock Publishers, 1981.

Miles, Margaret R. *The Image and Practice of Holiness: A Critique of the Classic Manuals of Devotion*. London: SCM, 1988.

Miller-McLemore, Bonnie J. 'Revisiting the Living Human Web: Theological Education and the Role of Clinical Pastoral Education'. *The Journal of Pastoral Care & Counseling* 62, no. 1–2 (2008): 3–18.

Miller-McLemore, Bonnie J. 'The Human Web: Reflections on the State of Pastoral Theology'. *Christian Century* 110, no. 11 (1993): 36–69.

Miller-McLemore, Bonnie J. 'The Living Human Web: Pastoral Theology at the Turn of the Century'. In *Through the Eyes of Women: Insights for Pastoral Care*, edited by Jeanne Stevenson Moessner, 9–26. Philadelphia: Westminster John Knox Press, 1996.

MiniMins.com. 'Syns'. Accessed 8 December 2016. https://www.minimins.com/threads/syns.139980/

Moltmann, Jürgen. *God in Creation: An Ecological Doctrine of Creation*. London: SCM, 1985.

Moltmann, Jürgen. 'Liberating and Anticipating the Future'. In *Liberating Eschatology: Essays in Honor of Letty M. Russell*, edited by Margaret A.

Farley and Serene Jones, 189–208. Louisville: Westminster John Knox Press, 1999.

Moltmann, Jürgen. 'Sabbath: Finishing and Beginning'. *The Living Pulpit* 7, no. 2 (1998): 4–5.

Moltmann, Jürgen. 'The Sabbath – The Feast of Creation'. *Family Ministry* 14, no. 4 (2000): 38–43.

Moltmann, Jürgen. *The Trinity and the Kingdom of God: The Doctrine of God*. Munich: SMC, 1981.

Moltmann-Wendel, Elisabeth. *I am my Body: New Ways of Embodiment*. London: SCM, 1994.

Monaghan, Lee F. *Men and the War on Obesity: A Sociological Study*. London and New York: Routledge, 2008.

Montoya, Angel F. *The Theology of Food: Eating and the Eucharist*. Chichester: Wiley-Blackwell, 2009.

Moore, Stephen D. *God's Gym: Divine Male Bodies of the Bible*. New York and London: Routledge, 1996.

Morgan, Nicole J. *Nicole J. Morgan blog*. Accessed 15 June 2018. https://jnicolemorgan.com/

Morris, Wayne. 'Christian Salvations in a Multi-Faith World: Challenging the Cult of Normalcy'. In *Alternative Salvations: Engaging the Sacred and the Secular*, edited by Hannah Bacon, Wendy Dossett and Steve Knowles, 121–31. London: Bloomsbury Academic, 2015.

Morris, Wayne. *Salvation as Praxis: A Practical Theology of Salvation for a Multi-Faith World*. London and New York: Bloomsbury T & T Clark.

Morton, Nelle. *The Journey is Home*. Boston: Beacon Press, 1985.

Moss, Candida R. 'Heavenly Healing: Eschatological Cleansing and the Resurrection of the Dead in the Early Church'. *Journal of the American Academy of Religion* 79, no. 4 (2011): 991–1017.

Mostert, Christiaan. 'Salvation's Setting: Election, Justification and the Church'. In *God of Salvation: Soteriology in Theological Perspective*, edited by Ivor J. Davidson and Murray A. Rae, 137–54. Farnham: Ashgate, 2011.

Muers, Rachel and Grummet, David. *Theology on the Menu: Asceticism, Meat and Christian Diet*. London and New York: Routledge, 2010.

Mulder, Anne-Claire, *Divine Flesh, Embodied Word: 'Incarnation' as a Hermeneutical Key to a Feminist Theologian's Reading of Irigaray's Work'*. Amsterdam: Amsterdam University Press, 2006.

Murray, Samantha. *The 'Fat' Female Body*. Basingstoke and New York: Palgrave Macmillan, 2008.

Murray, Samantha. '(Un/Be)Coming Out? Rethinking Fat Politics'. *Social Semiotics* 15, no. 2 (2005): 153–63.

Murray, Samantha. 'Women Under/In Control? Embodying Eating after Gastric Banding'. In *Whose Weight is it Anyway?: Essays on Ethics and Eating*, edited by Sofie Vandamme, Suzanne van de Vathorst and Inez de Beaufort, 43–54. Leauven: Acco Academic, 2010.

Murray-West, Rosie. 'Slimming Clubs Weigh into Trademark War over Who has the Right to "Sin"'. *The Telegraph*, 14 February 2006. Accessed 4 December 2014. http://www.telegraph.co.uk/news/uknews/1510451/Sli mming-clubs-weigh-into-trademark-war-over-whohas-the-right-to-sin.html

NAAFA. 'Education'. Accessed 1 May 2017. https://naafaonline.com/dev2/t he_issues/education.html

Nasser, Mervant. *Culture and Weight Consciousness*. London and New York: Routledge, 1997.

National Collaborating Centre for Mental Health. 'Eating Disorders: Core Interventions in the Treatment and Management of Anorexia Nervosa, Bulimia Nervosa and Related Eating Disorders'. Accessed 3 November 2016. https://www.nice.org.uk/guidance/cg9/evidence/full-guideline-243824221

National Eating Disorders Association. 'Race, Ethnicity and Culture'. Accessed 11 November 2016. http://www.nationaleatingdisorders.org/race-ethnicity-and-culture

National Education Association. 'Report on Size Discrimination'. Accessed 1 May 2017. http://www.lectlaw.com/files/con28.htm

NEDA. 'Research on Males and Eating Disorders'. Accessed 6 August 2017. https://www.nationaleatingdisorders.org/research-males-and-eating-disorders

Nelson, Derek. *What's Wrong with Sin: Sin in Individual and Social Perspective from Schleiermacher to Theologies of Liberation*. London and New York: T & T Clark, 2009.

NHS Choices. 'Helping Put You in Charge of Your Healthcare'. Accessed 10 November 2016. http://www.nhs.uk/aboutNHSChoices/Pages/NHSCh oicesintroduction.aspx

NHS Choices. 'How Your GP can Help You Lose Weight'. Accessed 16 November 2016. http://www.nhs.uk/Livewell/loseweight/Pages/WhataG Pcando.aspx

Nichter, Mimi. *Fat Talk: What Girls and their Parents Say about Dieting*. Cambridge and London: Harvard University Press, 2000.

Njoroge, Nyambura J. 'Let's Celebrate the Power of Naming'. In *African Women, Religion and Health: Essays in Honor of Mercy Amba Ewudziwa Oduyoye* (Women from the Margins), edited by Isabel Apawo Phiri and Sarojini Nadar, 59–76. New York: Orbis, 2006.

Northup, Lesley A. *Ritualising Women: Patterns of Spirituality*. Cleveland: The Pilgrim Press, 1997.

Oakley, Anne. 'Interviewing Women: A Contradiction in Terms'. In *Doing Feminist Research*, edited by H. Roberts, 30–61. London: Routledge, 1982.

O'Collins, Gerald. *Jesus Our Redeemer: A Christian Approach to Salvation*. New York and Oxford: Oxford University Press, 2007.

Ogden, Cynthia L., Carroll, Margaret D., Kit, Brian K. and Flegal, Katherine M. 'Prevalence of Obesity among Adults: United States, 2011-2012'. *NCHS*

Data Brief, no. 131 (2013). Accessed 3 November 2016. http://www.cdc.gov/nchs/data/databriefs/db131.pdf

Oliver, J. Eric. *Fat Politics: The Real Story behind America's Obesity Epidemic*. Oxford and New York: Oxford University Press, 2006.

Orbach, Susie. *Fat is a Feminist Issue*. London: Arrow Books, 1978.

Osborn, Eric. 'Tertullian'. In *The First Christian Theologians: An Introduction to Theology in the Early Church*, edited by G. R. Evans. Malden, Oxford, Carlton and Victoria: Blackwell Publishers Ltd., 2004.

Osmer, Richard. *Practical Theology: An Introduction*. Cambridge: William B. Eerdmans Publishing Company, 2008.

Papaconstantinou, Arietta. 'Introduction'. In *Conversion in Late Antiquity: Christianity, Islam, and Beyond: Papers from the Andrew W. Mellon Foundation Sawyer Seminar, University of Oxford 2009-2010*, edited by Arietta Papaconstantinou, Neil McLynn and Daniel L. Schwartz, xv–xxxvii. London and New York: Routledge, 2015.

Parker, Fiona. 'Asda Pulls Diet Ready Meals from Shelves after Slimming World Dispute'. *The Telegraph*, 19 March 2017. Accessed 10 May 2018. https://www.telegraph.co.uk/news/2017/03/19/asda-pulls-diet-ready-meals-shelves-slimming-world-dispute/

Pattison, Stephen. *Shame: Theory, Therapy, Theology*. Cambridge: Cambridge University Press, 2000.

Pennington, Emily. *Feminist Eschatology: Embodied Futures*. Abingdon and New York: Routledge, 2017.

Petrey, Taylor G. *Resurrecting Parts: Early Christians on Desire, Reproduction and Sexual Difference*. London and New York: Routledge, 2016.

Phillips, Elizabeth. 'Charting the "Ethnographic Turn"'. In *Perspectives on Ecclesiology and Ethnography*, edited by Pete Ward, 95–106. Grand Rapids and Cambridge: William B. Eerdmans Publishing Company, 2012.

Pieper, Josef. *The Concept of Sin*. South Bend: St. Augustine Press, 2001.

Plaskow, Judith. 'Finding a God I Can Believe In'. In *Goddess and God in the World: Conversations in Embodied Theology*, edited by Carol P. Christ and Judith Plaskow, 107–30. Minneapolis: Fortress Press, 2016.

Plaskow, Judith. *Goddess and God in the World: Conversations in Embodied Theology*, edited by Carol P. Christ and Judith Plaskow, 107–30. Minneapolis: Fortress Press, 2016.

Plaskow, Judith. *Sex, Sin and Grace: Women's Experience and the Theologies of Reinhold Niebuhr and Paul Tillich*. Lanham and London: University Press of America, 1980.

Pohl, Christine D. 'Hospitality and the Mental Health of Children and Families'. *American Journal of Orthopsychiatry* 81, no. 4 (2011): 482–8.

Pohl, Christine D. *Making Room: Recovering Hospitality as a Christian Tradition*. Grand Rapids and Cambridge: William B. Eerdmans Publishing Company, 1999.

Pope, Harrison G. Jr, Gruber, Amanda J., Mangweth, Barbara, Bureau, Benjamin, deCol, Christine, Jouvent, Roland and Hudson, James I. 'Body

Image Perception among Men in Three Countries'. *American Journal of Psychiatry* 157, no. 8 (2000): 1297–301.

Popenoe, Rebecca. 'Ideal'. In *Fat: The Anthropology of an Obsession*, edited by Don Kulick and Anne Meneley, 9–28. London: Penguin, 2005.

Prentice, Andrew M. and Jebb, Susan A. 'Obesity in Britain: Gluttony or Sloth?'. *British Medical Journal* 311 (1995): 437–9.

Probyn, Elspeth. 'Silences behind the Mantra: Critiquing Feminist Fat'. *Feminism & Psychology* 18, no. 3 (2008): 401–4.

Procter-Smith, Marjorie. 'Feminist Ritual Strategies'. In *Toward a New Heaven and a New Earth: Essays in Honour of Elisabeth Schüssler Fiorenza*, edited by Fernando F. Segovia, 498–515. Maryknoll: Orbis, 2003.

Procter-Smith, Marjorie. *In Her Own Rite: Constructing Feminist Liturgical Tradition*. CreateSpace Independent Publishing Platform, 2013.

Procter-Smith, Marjorie. 'Reconciliation: Hope and Risk', *Liturgy* 23, no. 4 (2008): 1–2.

PRWeb. 'Number of American Dieters Soars to 108 Million'. Accessed 23 April 2014. http://www.prweb.com/releases/2012/1/prweb9084688.htm

Public Health England. 'Health Inequalities'. Accessed 11 November 2016. http://www.noo.org.uk/NOO_about_obesity/inequalities

Quinn, Diane M. and Crocker, Jennifer. 'When Ideology Hurts: Effects of Belief in the Protestant Ethic and Feeling Overweight on the Psychological Well-Being of Women'. *Journal of Personality and Social Psychology* 77, no. 2 (1999): 402–14.

Raphael, Melissa, *Theology and Embodiment: The Post-Patriarchal Reconstruction of Female Sacrality*. Sheffield: Sheffield Academic Press, 1996.

Reid, Barbara. 'Sabbath: Recreation and Liberation'. *The Living Pulpit* 7, no. 2 (1998): 42.

Reynolds, M. 'In the Matter of Application No. 2389949 in the Name of A Different Limited and in the Matter of Opposition thereto under No. 93939 by Miles-Bramwell Executive Services Limited'. Accessed 4 December 2014. http://www.ipo.gov.uk/t-challenge-decision-results/o36607.pdf

Reynolds, Thomas E. *Vulnerable Communion: A Theology of Disability and Hospitality*. Grand Rapids: Brazos Press, 2008.

Rigby, Cynthia L. 'Scandalous Presence: Incarnation and Trinity'. In *Feminist and Womanist Essays in Reformed Dogmatics*, edited by Amy Plantinga Pauw and Serene Jones, 58–74. Louisville, London: Westminster John Knox Press, 2006.

Robinson, Eric, Hunger, Jeffrey and Daly, Michael. 'Perceived Weight Status and Risk of Weight Gain across Life in US and UK Adults', *International Journal of Obesity* 39, no. 12 (2015): 1721–6.

Rondini, Ashley C. 'The Internet and Medicalization: Reshaping the Global Body and Illness'. In *Bodies and the Sociology of Health*, edited by Elizabeth Ettorre, 107–20. London and New York: Routledge, 2010.

Ross, Susan A. *Extravagant Affections: A Feminist Sacramental Theology*. New York: Continuum, 1998.
Rossignol, Rina. 'Fat Liberation (?) Assumptions of a Thin World'. *Journal of Progressive Human Services* 14, no. 1 (2003): 5–14.
Roth, Geneen. *Women, Food and God. An Unexpected Path to Almost Everything*. London, New York, Sydney and Toronto: Simon & Schuster, 2010.
Rothblum, Ester, and Soloway, Sondra, eds. *The Fat Studies Reader*. New York and London: New York University Press 2009.
Ruether, Rosemary Radford. 'Augustine: Sexuality, Gender and Women'. In *Feminist Interpretations of Augustine*, edited by Judith Chelius Stark, 47–68. Pennsylvania: The Pennsylvania State University, 2007.
Ruether, Rosemary Radford. 'Dualism and the Nature of Evil in Feminist Theology'. *Studies in Christian Ethics* 5, no. 1 (1992): 26–39.
Ruether, Rosemary Radford. *Gaia and God: An Ecofeminist Theology of Earth Healing*. New York: HarperCollins, 1992.
Ruether, Rosemary Radford. 'Gender and Redemption in Christian Theological History'. *Feminist Theology* 7, no. 21 (1999): 98–108.
Ruether, Rosemary Radford. *Introducing Redemption in Christian Feminism*. Sheffield: Sheffield Academic Press, 1998.
Ruether, Rosemary Radford. *Sexism and God-Talk: Towards a Feminist Theology*. Boston: Beacon Press, 1983.
Ruether, Rosemary Radford. *Women and Redemption: A Theological History*, 2nd edition. Minneapolis: Fortress, 2012.
Ruether, Rosemary Radford. 'Women and Sin: Response to Mary Elise Lowe'. *Dialog: A Journal of Theology* 39, no. 3 (2000): 233–5.
Russell, Letty M. *Human Liberation in a Feminist Perspective – A Theology*. Philadelphia: The Westminster Press, 1974.
Saguy, Abigail. *What's Wrong with Fat?*. New York: Oxford University Press, 2014.
Saguy, Abigail C. and Ward, Anna. 'Coming Out as Fat: Rethinking Stigma'. *Social Psychology Quarterly* 74, no. 1 (2011): 53–75.
Saiving, Valerie. 'The Human Situation: A Feminine View'. *The Journal of Religion* 40, no. 2 (1960): 100–12.
Sands, Kathleen. 'Uses of the Thea(o)logian: Sex and Theodicy in Religious Feminism'. *Journal of Feminist Studies in Religion* 8, no. 1 (1992): 7–33.
Sands, Kathleen M. *Escape From Paradise: Evil and Tragedy in Feminist Theology*. Minneapolis: Fortress Press, 1994.
Sawyer, Deborah. 'Hidden Subjects: Rereading Eve and Mary'. *Theology and Sexuality* 14, no. 3 (2008): 305–20.
Schleiermacher, Friedrich. *The Christian Faith*, translated and edited by H. R. Mackintosh and J. S. Stewart, 2nd edition. Edinburgh: T & T Clark, 1999.
Schwartz, Hillel. *Never Satisfied: A Cultural History of Diets, Fantasies and Fat*. New York: The Free Press, 1986.

Schweitzer, Don. 'Food as Gift, Necessity and Possibility'. *Religious Studies and Theology* 20, no. 2 (2001): 1–19.

Scott, Joan W. 'The Evidence of Experience'. *Critical Inquiry* 17, no. 4 (1991): 773–97.

Scrutton, Anastasia Philippa. *Thinking Through Feeling: God, Emotion and Passibility*. London and New York: Bloomsbury, 2011.

Seid, Roberta Pollack. *Never Too Thin: Why Women Are At War with their Bodies*. New York: Prentice Hall Press, 1989.

Shamblin, Gwen. *Rise Above: God Can Set you Free from Your Weight Problem Forever*. Nashville: Thomas Nelson Publishers, 2000.

Shamblin, Gwen. 'The Pioneer of Faith-Based Weight Loss'. Accessed 2 August 2017. http://www.gwenshamblin.com/my-biography/

Shamblin, Gwen. 'The Remnant of the Kingdom of God'. Accessed 8 May 2018. http://www.remnantfellowship.org/About-Our-Church/Our-History

Shamblin, Gwen. *The Weigh Down Diet: Inspirational Way to Lose Weight, Stay Slim, and Find a New You*. New York: Galilee Doubleday, 2002.

Sharma, Sonya. *Good Girls, Good Sex: Women Talk about Church and Sexuality*. Halifax: Fernwood Publishing, 2012.

Shildrick, Margrit. *Leaky Bodies and Boundaries: Feminism, Postmodernism and (Bio) ethics*. London and New York: Routledge, 1997.

Showalter, Carol. *Your Whole Life: The 3D Plan for Eating Right, Living Well, and Loving God*. Brewster: Paraclete Press, 2007.

Simic, Zora. 'Fat as a Feminist Issue: A History'. In *Fat Sex: New Directions in Theory and Activism*, edited by Helen Hester and Caroline Walters, 15–36. Farnham and Burlington: Ashgate, 2015.

Slater, Nigel. *A Year of Good Eating: The Kitchen Diaries III*. London: Fourth Estate, 2015.

Slee, Nicola. 'Into the Woods – and Out Again: Reflecting on Sabbath and Sabbatical Time' (unpublished).

Slee, Nicola. *Praying Like a Woman*. London: Society for Promoting Christian Knowledge, 2004.

Slee, Nicola. *Women's Faith Development: Patterns and Processes*. Farnham: Ashgate, 2004.

Slee, Nicola, Porter, Fran and Phillips, Anne. *The Faith Lives of Women and Girls: Qualitative Research Perspectives*. Farnham: Ashgate, 2013.

Smith, Gordon T. *Transforming Conversion: Rethinking the Language and Contours of Christian Initiation*. Grand Rapids: Baker Academic, 2010.

Snider, Stefanie. 'Fatness and Visual Culture: A Brief Look at Some Contemporary Projects'. *Fat Studies* 1, no. 1 (2012): 13–31.

Sobal, Jeffrey. 'The Size Acceptance Movement and the Social Construction of Body Weight'. In *Weighty Issues: Fatness and Thinness as Social Problems*, edited by Jeffrey Sobal and Donna Maurer, 231–50. New York: Aldine de Gruyter, 1999.

Sobal, Jeffery, Bove, Caron and Rauschenbach, Barbara. 'Weight and Weddings: The Social Construction of Beautiful Brides'. In *Interpreting*

Weight: *The Social Management of Fatness and Thinness*, edited by Jeffery Sobal and Donna Maurer, 113–38. New York: Aldine de Gruyter, 1999.

Sog, Nerissa L., Touyz, Stephen W. and Surgenor, Lois J. 'Eating and Body Image Disturbances Across Cultures: A Review', *European Eating Disorders Review* 14, no. 1 (2006): 54–65.

Solenn, Carof. 'Eating with the Fear of Weight Gain: The Relationship with Food for Overweight Women in France'. *Menu: Journal of Food and Hospitality Research* 1, no. 1 (2012): 67–76.

Soloman, Robert, eds. *Wicked Pleasures: Meditations on the Seven Deadly Sins.* Maryland: Rowman and Littlefield Publishers, 1999.

South Carolina Department of Mental Health. 'Eating Disorder Statistics'. Accessed 3 November 2016. http://www.state.sc.us/dmh/anorexia/statistics.htm

Spitzack, Carole. *Confessing Excess: Women and the Politics of Body Reduction.* Albany: State University of New York Press, 1990.

Stearns, Peter N. *Fat History: Bodies and Beauty in the Modern West.* New York and London: New York University Press.

Steele, Jayne. 'Chocolate and Bread: Gendering Sacred and Profane Foods in Contemporary Cultural Representations'. *Theology and Sexuality* 14, no. 3 (2008): 321–34.

Stinson, Kandi M. *Women and Dieting Culture: Inside a Commercial Weight Loss Group.* New Brunswick and London: Rutgers University Press, 2001.

Stone, Kenneth. *Practicing Safer Texts: Food, Sex and Bible In Queer Perspective.* London and New York: T & T Clark International, 2005.

Stuart, Elizabeth. 'Disruptive Bodies: Disability, Embodiment and Sexuality'. In *The Good News of the Body. Sexual Theology and Feminism*, edited by Lisa Isherwood, 166–84. New York: New York University Press, 2000.

Suchocki, Marjorie. *Fall to Violence: Original Sin in Relational Theology.* New York: Continuum, 1994.

Suchocki, Marjorie. 'God, Sexism and Transformation'. In *Reconstructing Christian Theology*, edited by Rebecca S. Chopp and Mark Lewis Taylor, 25–48. Minneapolis: Fortress, 1994.

Sullender, Scott. 'The Seven Deadly Sins as a Pastoral Diagnostic System'. *Pastoral Psychology* 64, no. 2 (2015): 217–27.

Sung, Jung Mo. *Desire, Market and Religion: Reclaiming Liberation Theology.* London: SCM, 2007.

Swinton, John and Mowat, Harriet. *Practical Theology and Qualitative Research.* London: SCM, 2006.

Tavard, George H. *The Church, Community of Salvation: An Ecumenical Ecclesiology.* Collegeville: The Liturgical Press, 1992.

Taylor, Chloë. *The Culture of Confession from Augustine to Foucault: A Genealogy of the 'Confessing Animal'.* Oxon and New York: Routledge, 2008.

Tertullian. 'On the Apparel of Women'. In *Ante-Nicene Fathers*, vol. 4, edited by Rev. Alexander Roberts and James Donaldson. Peabody: Hendrickson Publishers Inc., 1995.

Tertullian. 'On Fasting'. In *Ante-Nicene Fathers*, vol. 4, edited by Rev. Alexander Roberts and James Donaldson. Peabody: Hendrickson Publishers Inc., 1995.

Therrien, Alex. 'Rise in Cancers "Caused By Weight"', *BBC News*. Accessed 4 May 2018. http://www.bbc.co.uk/news/health-43502144

Thistlethwaite, Susan Brooks. *Sex, Race, and God: Christian Feminism in Black and White*. Eugene: Wipf & Stock, 1989.

Throsby, Kate and Gimlin, Debra. 'Critiquing Thinness and Wanting To Be Thin'. In *Secrecy and Silence in the Research Process: Feminist Reflections*, edited by Róisín Ryan-Flood and Rosalind Gill, 105–16. London and New York: Routledge, 2013.

TOS Obesity as a Disease Writing Group. 'Obesity as a Disease: A White Paper on Evidence and Arguments Commissioned by the Council of The Obesity Society'. *Obesity* 16 (2008): 1161–77.

Towler, Robert. *Homo Religiosus: Sociological Problems in the Study of Religion*. London: Constable, 1974.

Townes, Emilie M. *In a Blaze of Glory: Womanist Spirituality as Social Witness*. Nashville: Abingdon Press, 1995.

Tran, Jonathan. *Foucault and Theology*. London and New York: T & T Clark, 2011.

Trust for America's Health and Robert Wood Johnson Foundation. 'Race and Ethnic Disparities in Obesity'. Accessed 11 November 2016. http://stateofobesity.org/disparities/

Tsakiridis, George. *Evagrius Ponticus and Cognitive Science: A Look at Moral Evil and the Thoughts*. Eugene: Pickwick, 2010.

United States Census Bureau. 'US and World Population Clock'. Accessed 3 November 2016. http://www.census.gov/popclock/

Walton, Janet R. *Feminist Liturgy: A Matter of Justice*. Collegeville: The Liturgical Press, 2000.

Wann, Marilyn. 'Fat & Choice: A Personal Essay'. *MP: An Online Feminist Journal*. Accessed 5 May 2018. http://academinist.org/wp-content/uploads/2005/09/010308Wann_Fat.pdf

Wann, Marilyn. *FAT! SO? Because You Don't Have to Apologize For Your Size*. Berkeley: Ten Speed Press, 1998.

Wann, Marilyn. 'Foreword: Fat Studies: An Invitation to Revolution'. In *The Fat Studies Reader*, edited by Esther Rothblum and Sondra Solovay, xi–xxvi. New York and London: New York University Press, 2009.

Ward, Peter. *Perspectives on Ecclesiology and Ethnography*. Grand Rapids and Cambridge: William B. Eerdmans Publishing Company, 2012.

Waschenfelder, J. 'Rethinking God for the Sake of a Planet in Peril: Reflections on the Socially Transformative Power of Sallie McFague's Progressive Theology'. *Feminist Theology* 19, no. 1 (2010): 86–106.

Weber, Max. *The Protestant Ethic and the Spirit of Capitalism*. London and New York: Routledge, 1992.

West, Angela. *Deadly Innocence: Feminist Theology and the Mythology of Sin*. London: Cassell, 1995.
Whelehan, Imelda. *The Feminist Bestseller: From Sex and the Single Girl to Sex and the City*. Basingstoke: Palgrave Macmillan, 2005.
Wiley, Tatha. *Original Sin. Origins, Developments, Contemporary Meanings*. New York and Mahwah: Paulist Press, 2002.
Williams, Rowan. 'The Theology of Health and Healing - Hildegard Lecture, Thirsk' (7th February 2003). Accessed 21 February 2017. http://rowanwilliams.archbishopofcanterbury.org/articles.php/2111/the-theology-of-health-and-healing-hildegard-lecture-thirsk
Wirzba, Norman. *Food & Faith: A Theology of Eating*. New York: Cambridge University Press, 2011.
Wirzba, Norman. *Living the Sabbath: Discovering the Rhythms of Rest and Delight*. Grand Rapids: Brazos Press, 2006.
Wittig, Monique. 'The Straight Mind', *Feminist Issues* 1, no. 1 (1980): 103–12.
Wolf, Naomi. *The Beauty Myth: How Images of Beauty are Used Against Women*. New York and London: Doubleday, 1991.
Woodhead, Linda. '"Because I'm Worth It!" Religion and Women's Changing Lives in the West'. In *Women and Religion in the West: Challenging Secularization*, edited by Kristin Aune, Sonya Sharma and Giselle Vincett. Aldershot: Ashgate, 2008.
Woodley, Randy. 'An Indigenous Theological Perspective on Sabbath'. *Vision: A Journal for Church and Theology* 16, no. 1 (2015): 63–71.
Yancey, Antronette K., Leslie, Joanne and Abel, Emily K. 'Obesity at the Crossroads: Feminist and Public Health Perspective'. *Signs* 31, no. 2 (2006): 425–33.
Yong, Amos. *Theology and Down Syndrome: Reimaging Disability in Late Modernity*. Texas: Baylor University Press, 2007.
Yoshino, Kenji. *Covering: The Hidden Assault on American Civil Rights*. New York: Random House Publishing Group, 2006.
Young, Iris Marion. *Justice and the Politics of Difference*. Princeton: Princeton University Press, 1990.
Young, Pamela Dickey. *Feminist Theology/Christian Theology: In Search of Method*. Eugene: Wipf and Stock, 1990.

INDEX

7/7 15
9/11 15–16

Abel, Emily 298
abjection 108, 160
activism 280, 286
   Christian 288
   fat (*see* fat activism)
   micro- 280, 294, 297, 305
ACT-Up 293
aliveness 6, 20, 46, 124, 126, 187, 191, 218, 221, 224, 241, 259, 261, 271, 206, 308–9
Althaus-Reid, Marcella 216–17, 227
Ambrose 64, 92
anorexia nervosa 11, 33–4, 43, 127
Anselm 64
Anthony the Great 110, 112, 124, 127, 130
anti-obesity discourse 81, 298, 301
Aquinas, Thomas 61, 64–5, 176–7, 239
Aristotle 90
asceticism 217
   Christian 87, 123–7, 130, 138–9, 259
   women's 128
ascetic(s) 11, 239
   Christian 110, 123
   food practices 123
   practices 100, 124–5, 127, 129, 131, 149, 239
   women 171
Athanasius 110
atonement 155, 191
Augustine 60–8, 70–2, 76, 80–1, 83, 87, 90, 92–3, 106, 111–12, 124, 127, 145, 158, 166–7, 173, 176, 184–6, 196, 200–1, 209, 217, 255

baptism 145, 154, 158–9
Barth, Karl 9
Bartky, Sandra 120
Basil of Caesarea 60–1, 71
beauty myth 10, 40, 140
Bell, Kristen 35–7, 39
Berry, Jan 283
Berry, Wendell 267
Bieler, Andrea 233
Biltekoff, Charlotte 15–16
Blevins, Kent 270
bodies
   dissatisfaction 33, 37, 42, 190
   female 3, 10–11, 36, 41, 52, 92, 115, 130, 166, 170–1, 274–5
   sensual 242, 244, 250
   size 44–5, 67, 284, 301
   of women 20, 216, 246, 294, 308
   women's 7, 10–11, 16, 20–1, 31, 38–9, 41, 43, 46, 52, 69, 88–9, 92, 95, 97, 99, 117, 139, 142, 164–5, 171, 177, 189, 192–3, 207, 216, 218, 238, 241, 282, 288, 283, 294
Body Mass Index (BMI) 44, 67, 300
bodyself/selves 47, 191, 217–21, 227, 247, 272, 273, 278–9, 282, 304–5, 309
Bordo, Susan 23, 24, 75, 104–5, 120
Bourdieu, Pierre 3
Bovey, Shelley 10, 140
Boyce, James 64, 147
Braziel, Jana Evans 38
Bringle, Mary 8–9, 141, 174
Brock, Rita Nakashima 178–9, 200

Brueggemann, Walter   263
bulimia   11, 33–4, 105, 109, *see also* eating, disorders
   political economy of   105, 109
Burgard, Deb   300
Butler, Judith   229, 294
Bynum, Caroline Walker   128–9

Cairus, Kate   100, 102
Calvin, John   64, 80, 146
capitalism   84, 87, 106, 186, 214–15, 217–18, 227, 234, 263, 308
Cassian, John   123, 126, 153, 295
Catherine of Siena   128–9
Centers for Disease Control and Prevention (CDC)   14
Chen, Eva   76, 102
Chernin, Kim   10, 39, 171
Christ, Carol   149
Christian
   asceticism   87, 123–7, 130, 138–9, 259
   eschatology   179, 227
   practices   4, 88
   thought   16, 27, 56, 91–2, 94, 106, 139, 144–6, 149, 156, 167, 189, 217, 246, 308
   weight loss
      industry   3–4
      organizations   1, 3
         First Place   1, 3
         Weigh Down Ministries (*see* Shamblin, Gwen)
         Weigh Down Workshop   1
Christianity
   evangelical   4
   neo-orthodox   146
   Protestant   3, 38, 49
   Western   56, 142, 144, 146, 178, 277
Chrysostom, John   72–3
Church Fathers   68, 152
Cixous, Hélène   113, 245

Clement of Alexandria   61, 68, 70, 72, 126
Clough, Patricia   254
Colbert, Don   1
Colls, R.   45
community   8, 21, 23, 80, 83, 96, 110, 145, 163, 179, 180, 183–6, 198–200, 225, 231, 242, 249, 258–9, 269, 280, 282, 284–6, 291, 306, 308
Cooper, Charlotte   24, 205, 276, 280, 286, 293
crucifixion   154, 191, 225–6
cultural
   capital   3, 120, 162, 183
   norms   117, 122, 125
   plastic   75, 78, 152
   war on fat (*see* fat)
culture
   consumer   104
   Euro-American   13, 131, 207
   weight loss   3, 5, 11, 68, 174, 189, 278, 310
   Western   5, 42, 92, 147, 219, 309
   women's   5, 102

Daly, Mary   94, 130, 190, 217, 257, 301
Dark, Kimberly   276, 290
Davis, Sally   81
Department of Health   14–15
desert fathers   61, 110, 130
desire for food, *see* food
detachment   75, 126, 142, 152, 218, 239, 277, 309
discipline   1, 3, 12, 26, 38, 61, 78, 88, 92, 99, 104, 108, 110, 118, 121, 132–3, 137, 177, 268, 308, 310
distorted relationality   192, 202, 216
Donne, John   73
Douglas, Mary   7
DuPuis, Melanie   17

eating
  disorders (*see* anorexia; bulimia)
  sensible   47, 69, 212, 223–4,
    238–43, 247, 251–60, 289,
    309
Eden   50, 60, 62–3, 93, 173, 233, 244
Edwards, Katie   94
Eglon   79
Ellmann, Maud   109
Enlightenment   64, 67, 190
Eucharist   128, 184–5, 233–4, 244,
    259
Evagrius Ponticus   61, 295
evangelical
  Christian culture   3
  weight loss culture (*see* weight
    loss, culture)
Evans, Bethan   51, 67
Eve   60–62, 91–5, 244–7, 291

fall   58, 61, 63–4, 81, 92–3, 194
fat
  activism (*see* fat activism)
  bodies   13, 16, 19, 51, 84, 172,
    209, 273, 276–7, 287–8,
    290, 294, 297, 302
  burning   47, 150–1, 153, 306,
    308–10
  as discredited identity   88, 277
  as disease   13, 298
  as feminine   139
  fighting   1, 278
  and genetics   50, 301
  -liberation (*see* fat liberation)
  as moral impediment   298
  people   2, 4, 6, 13, 18, 122, 140,
    159–60, 204–5, 207–8,
    274, 276, 285–6, 288, 290,
    292–4, 300–1, 303, 309
  as headless (*see* 'headless
    fatty')
  as perception   45, 294
  -phobia   17, 35, 137–8, 184, 202,
    204, 207, 210, 274, 276,
    279, 281–2, 285, 291, 305

politics   10, 275–8, 287, 310
positivity (*see* fat pride)
pride (*see* fat pride; sin)
  as risk   13, 16–17
  as sexually attractive   274
  stigmatization of   205
  studies   26, 33, 38, 310
  war on   4, 15–16, 285, 310
fat acceptance   209, 274, 277, 288,
    292–4, 302
fat activism   274, 277, 286–9, 297
  as Christian activism   288
  and 'micro-activism'   290, 294,
    297, 305
  and 'micro-salvation'   226, 160
fat liberation   274, 287, 292, *see
    also* fat acceptance; fat
    pride
fat pride   47, 261, 292–5, 297–8,
    302–6, 309
  and 'coming out' as fat   290,
    293, 297, 306
  as coming out from the closet of
    fat shame   282, 284, 291,
    297, 305–6
  and fat acceptance and
    fat liberation
    movement   209, 274,
    277, 287–8, 292–4,
    302
  and fat positivity   274
  and LGBTQI politics   293
  as a Sabbath sensibility   261,
    263, 268–70, 276–8,
    281, 286, 292–3, 302–3,
    305–6
Fat Underground   287
female
  body (*see* bodies)
  embodiment   38, 128
feminine
  fat as (*see* fat)
  Mystique   40, 119
femininity   39, 41, 78, 91, 170,
    182–3, 207

feminism
  post- 135–6, 183
  second wave 39, 136
Fiorenza, Elizabeth Schüssler 5, 284–5
  ekklēsia gynaikon 284
Fisk, Anna 214–15
food
  desire for 2, 60, 72, 88, 251
  feminist theology of 251, 253
  as a gift from God 233–4, 259
  joy of 212, 241, 257
  love of 203, 307
  nourishing gift of 224
  pleasure 8, 241
  practices 10, 101, 120, 123, 125, 129, 221, 230, 232, 249, 261
  rationalization of 224
  as shaping intentional attitudes and behaviours 309
  victimization of 46–7, 189, 191, 203, 211–16, 219, 224, 229–30, 236, 243, 259, 309
Foucault, Michel 86–7, 118, 123, 132–5, 137, 201
Friedan, Betty 40
Friedman, Jeffrey 301
Fulkerson, Mary McClintock 26, 203, 310

Gebara, Ivone 94, 224–6, 229, 258
gender 36, 38–40, 43, 88–9, 96, 118–20, 131, 139, 207, 229–30, 253, 256–7, 259, 284, 296
Gerber, Lynne 3, 49
Gill, Rosalind 135–6
Gilman, Sander 36
Gimlin, Debra 24
gluttony 50–1, 60–2, 67, 71, 93, 124, 126, 131, 295
God
  Creator 199, 249–50
  image of 68, 198–9, 249, 265, 290
  Son of 93, 153 (*see also* Jesus)

Spirit Sustainer 199
  as Trinity/Trinitarian 2, 198–201, 220–1, 249, 290
Goffman, Erving 88
Granberg, Ellen 157, 161
Greene-McCreight, Kathryn 189
Gregory of Nyssa 166, 173
Gregory the Great 295
Griffith, R. Marie 3, 23, 87
Gross, Glenda 22
Grosz, Elizabeth 84
Guthman, Judith 17, 105, 109

Hampson, Daphne 153, 189
Harrison, Beverly 252–3, 257
'headless fatty' 276
health
  and anti-obesity discourse 81, 298, 301
  and fat (*see* fat)
  individual 14
  mental 34, 122
  physical 17
  as social construct 256
Hebrew Bible 9, 79, 143, 146, 156, 220, 223, 230, 232, 261–2
Hesse-Biber, Sharlene Nagy 10
heteronormative 2, 177, 275–6
heteropatriarchal 3, 41, 207, 274
heterosexuality 32, 204, 229
Heyes, Cressida 23, 134–5
Heyward, Carter 248–9, 253
Hill, Susan 79, 150–1, 233
House of Commons 50–1
hubris 56, 101, 295
Hull, John 257

ideology 75, 89, 211
  capitalist 76
  consumer 162
  neoliberal 101
  sexist 198
Ignatius of Antioch 68
imago Dei 6, 20, 193, 197, 200
incarnation 7–8, 109, 153, 249

Irenaeus 68, 124, 168–9
Irigaray, Luce 91, 250
Isasi-Díaz, Ada María 227, 307
Isherwood, Lisa 7–8, 216–17, 230–1, 241

Jaggar, Alison 256
Jantzen, Grace 142, 145, 171–2
Jebb, Susan 50
Jerome 61, 72–3
Jesus 1, 27, 109, 140, 143, 153–4, 156–8, 162–4, 167–9, 171, 185, 190, 197, 223–4, 226, 238, 246–50, 270, 288, *see also* God, Son of
  blood of 186
  body of 129
  the bread of life 7, 109, 223, 233–4
  fat 8
Jesus's ministry of food 230–4, 244, 259
Johnson, Elizabeth 6, 220
Johnston, Josée 100, 102
Jones, Serene 191

Kent, Le'a 153
Kingdom of God 145, 176
Korsmeyer, Carolyn 243
Kristeva, Julia 108, 113

Lady Fest 287
Lamm, Nomy 274
language 7, 12, 21, 25, 51, 97, 154, 219, 281, 288
  about fat 209, 291, 293
  Christian 50
  embodied 247
  of gluttony 51
  of 'good' and 'bad' 74
  male 290
  moral 50
  religious 96
  of sin 50, 96–7, 190, 219
  of war 145

Last Supper 223, 232
Lazar, Michelle 136
LeBesco, Kathleen 38, 274–5
Lelwica, Michelle 11, 41, 78, 141–2, 174–5, 179, 181
Leslie, Joanne 298
Levy-Navarro, Elena 86, 159
LGBTQI 293
  politics and links with fat pride (*see* fat pride)
liberation theology, *see* theology
liturgy 280–1, 283, 286, 288, 291
logismoi 61, 295
Longhurst, Robyn 162
Lorde, Audre 239–40, 242, 252–3
Lowe, Mary Elise 198
Lupton, Deborah 120, 212
Luther, Martin 64, 146

McAllister, Heather 276
McFadyen, Alistair 198
McFague, Sallie 192, 200, 205
McKinley, Nita 88
McNaughton, Darlene 35–7, 39
male gaze 32, 275
Margaret of Cortona 129
Martin, Daniel 85, 87
Martyr, Justin 168
martyrdom 123, 172
masculinity 36–7, 195
Massumi, Brian 254
Méndez Montoya, Angel F. 244
Miles, Margaret 124
Moltmann, Jürgen 199, 201, 264–5, 273
Moore, Stephen 154
Morris, Wayne 163
Mo Sung, Jung 237
Murray, Samantha 84, 274–5, 277–9, 293, 303–4

National Eating Disorders Association (NEDA) 35, 43
National Health Service (NHS) 17–19

neoliberal
    discourse   106, 136
    governmentality   102, 105, 111
    political anatomy   139
    rationality   76
neoliberalism   76, 102, 115, 135–6, 160, 186
Nichter, Mimi   217

obesity 'epidemic'   14, 16, 216
Oliver, Jamie   206
    Ministry of Food   208
oral pleasure   240, 245, 259
Orbach, Susie   39
Origen   68, 124
original sin, *see* sin

Papaconstantinou, Arietta   158
Parker, Rebecca   155, 178–9
patriarchal norms   99, 139
patriarchy   36, 38–9, 170, 206
Pattison, Stephen   82, 289
Paul   63–5, 68, 70, 79–80, 143–4, 154, 156–9, 217, 255, 296
Pelagius   64
Pennington, Emily   247
Pharaoh   263
Pieper, Josef   96
Plato   90
Pohl, Christine   233
Prentice, Andrew   50
Procter-Smith, Marjorie   280, 285
prohibition   99, 106, 151, 245–6
Promised Land   2, 140, 176
Protestant work ethic   78

Qohelet   234–6, 238
Queer   160, 229, 293
    nation   293

Raphael, Melissa   150
reconciliation   142, 191, 221, 227, 259, 266, 280, 307, 309
Reformation   146
righteousness   2, 79, 111, 158–9

Riot Grrrl   287
Roth, Geneen   180
Ruether, Rosemary Radford   46, 130–1, 144, 178, 191–8, 200–4, 206–7, 210, 215, 219, 229, 247, 309
Russell, Letty   228

Sabbath
    as breathing space   269, 278
    as call to suspend 'obvious' truths about fat   282, 286
    as challenge to modern capitalism   263
    as challenge to sizeism   273
    command   261, 266, 270, 295
    as corporate duty and communal practice   265, 280, 309
    and delight   264–7, 269, 272, 274, 276–7, 279, 281, 284, 286, 297, 305–6, 309
    and facing fat in the mirror   276–7
    and fat acceptance   274, 277, 294
    and fat pride   47, 261, 292–3, 295, 297, 303–6, 309
    as the 'feast of redemption'   265
    as the finishing of creation   265, 268
    as the hope of creation   266
    as interval   268, 273, 282
    and liberation of the oppressed   262
    as 'meaningful work'   228, 265–7
    and *měnûhâ*   264–5
    and 'mini-salvation'   225, 265, 280
    as observance of 'No Diet Day'   271
    as performance of agency   306
    as performance of salvation   261
    as refraining from 'fat-talk' and 'diet talk'   271

as resistance to coercion and
domination   263–5, 273,
305
as respite from fat
shaming   279, 305
as rest for the earth and its
inhabitants   262
as rest from anxious
productivity   264–6, 281
as rest from dieting and
patrolling weight   271
as rest from ordinary work   266,
270, 286, 305–6
and self-care   270
sensibility   261, 263, 268–70,
276–8, 281, 286, 292–3,
302–3, 305–6
signs   277
and slimming   268–70
space   265–6, 269, 272–3, 277,
279–82, 285, 289–91, 304–5
as welcome and refreshing   279
and women's liturgical
groups   279–92
and the year of jubilee   262
sacrifice   12, 101, 141–2, 147, 149,
150, 154, 175, 186–7, 224,
226–7, 239, 260, 270
salvation
and fat pride (*see* fat pride)
futurizing of   178
as 'getting rid'   139, 141–2, 147,
153, 155, 169, 171–2, 179
as living the Sabbath   261, 292
as meaningful work   228, 231,
259, 265–7, 286, 297, 309
micro-   226, 260
mini-   225, 265, 280
as a queer performance   229
and reconciliation   142, 191,
221, 227, 259, 309
and Sabbath   265–9, 279–81,
285–6, 292, 302–6
as 'sensible eating'   223–4, 238,
260

weigh loss and (*see* weight loss)
Sands, Kathleen   202, 253
Schleiermacher, Friedrich   146
Schottroff, Luise   233
Schwartz, Hillel   36
Scott, Joan   26
Seid, Roberta   140–1
self
-acceptance   162, 217, 293
agonistic   104, 217–18
-assertion   123, 134
-authorization   242, 258, 306
-awareness   117, 134, 138
-care   46, 106, 120, 123–7, 132,
135–9, 149, 238, 240, 258,
270, 281, 283, 288, 294,
297, 302, 304
-determinism   99, 135, 306
-denial   126, 139, 153, 239, 242,
251, 260
divided   46–7, 106, 189, 191,
203, 216–19, 309
-division   217–19, 220, 230, 307
-esteem   142, 162, 164, 187,
287, 302, 306
-governance   102, 105, 132, 159
-harm   46, 123, 126–8
-loathing   130, 204
-negation   123, 149, 239, 256,
296–7
-permission   184, 245, 308
-possession   113, 117–18, 134,
138
-sacrifice   154, 260
-starvation   126–9, 131, 139
-surveillance   46, 99, 106,
120–1, 123, 127, 133,
139
-worth   182, 184
selfhood   153, 182–3, 198, 296
sensual   2, 234, 239–42, 244, 248,
250, 253, 259, 274
sensuality   47, 92, 233, 239, 241,
252–3, 255, 258, 309
seven deadly sins   52, 62

Index

sexism 9, 46, 137, 195–6, 202–6, 276
sexuality 11, 32, 36, 38–9, 43, 62, 126, 131, 204, 220, 229–30, 234, 240–1, 253, 256, 292
Shamblin, Gwen 1–3
Showalter, Carol 1
sin, *see also* Syn
   and the 'deadly sins' 50, 62, 295
   and the divided self 46–7, 106, 189, 191, 203, 216–19, 309
   as exploitative patterns of relationship 194, 219
   ideological–cultural dimension of 194, 197, 204, 211, 218–19
   as life-diminishing 221, 309
   original 62, 64–6, 76, 80–1, 92, 190, 195–6, 220
   personal–interpersonal dimension of 194, 204–5, 212, 218–19
   and the politics of domination 247, 266, 309
   and pride 295–7
   as a relational tear 200, 201, 309
   and salvation 4–5, 16, 21, 27–8, 46–7, 189–92, 309
   sizeism as 203–4
   social–historical dimension of 194, 196, 204, 207, 214, 218–19
   as the victimization of food 46–7, 189, 191, 203, 211–16, 219, 224, 229–30, 236, 243, 259, 309
size-acceptance 310, *see also* fat liberation; fat pride
sizeism
   as sin (*see* sin)
   sins of 47, 220, 230, 309
Slater, Nigel 211–12
Slee, Nicola 268–9, 272, 291
slimming
   community 258–9, 282
   and sacrifice 12, 101, 142, 147, 149, 175, 186–7, 224, 227, 270
   and self-permission 308 (*see also* self, -permission)
   and social bonds 142, 182, 259, 282, 306, 308
   techniques 99–100, 103, 106, 121, 123, 125, 128, 135, 139, 271 (*see also* Syn-, watching
Stinson, Kandi 12, 51, 66, 103, 108, 120, 148
Stone, Ken 59, 235–6
Streams, Peter 36
Suchocki, Marjorie 219
Syn 21, 39, 45–7, 49, 51–8, 64–5, 67, 69, 73–6, 79–84, 86–9, 92, 95–7, 99–109, 111–15, 117–21, 123–5, 135–40, 151–2, 155, 168, 180, 186, 189, 191, 212, 215, 223–4, 238, 243–4, 269, 271, 277, 281, 309
   -talk 51, 56, 58, 74, 82, 89, 97, 99, 139, 187, 191
   -watching 99, 106–7, 111, 115, 117–21, 123, 125, 128, 131, 134–9, 201, 270

taste 69–70, 212–13, 215, 224, 227, 237, 239–46, 253, 256–9, 289
Tertullian 60, 68, 93
theology
   classical 189, 240
   dualistic 8
   feminist theology of food (*see* food)
   liberation 5
   of sin 62, 93, 191, 219

thinness
    compulsory 204, 230, 290
    God of 8, 290
    pursuit of 5, 11, 21, 39–40, 141,
        174, 181, 208, 294, 308
    religion of 11, 141, 179
thin privilege 135, 180, 182, 184,
    275, 309
Throsby, Kate 24
touch 47, 160, 224, 242–3, 246–51,
    256–7, 259, 265, 289, 306–7
tradition 26
    ascetic 88
    Augustinian–Lutheran 74
    Augustinian–Pauline 203, 207,
        216
    Christian 4, 8, 233, 261, 275
    classical 94, 96
    Protestant 148
    theological 5–6, 21, 46–7, 89,
        139, 141, 171, 189, 224,
        295, 309
        discourse 46, 56, 99
        Western 62
Trinitarian
    community 199
    God 200, 220–1
    image of God 198–9, 249
    model of God 201
    principle 249
    self-sharing and embrace 2
    understanding of God 199

Wann, Marilyn 206, 209, 293–4,
    303
war
    Afghanistan–Iraq 16
    against appetite 258
    against fat 299
    against flesh 129
    holy 285
    language of 145
    self at 216
    on terror 15–16
Weber, Max 78
weight cycling 175, 300
weight loss
    book 29, 307
    culture (*see* culture)
    industry 10, 121, 227
        Christian 3–4
    narratives 5, 47, 51, 65, 309
Weight Watchers 85, 134, 179
Wiley, Tatha 62
Wirzba, Norman 213, 232,
    271–2
Wittig, Monique 204
Wolf, Naomi 10, 39–40, 140, 181
women-church 284–6, 290, 305,
    see also Fiorenza
women's liturgical groups, *see*
    Sabbath
Woodhead, Linda 182–3

Yancey, Antronette K. 237, 298